Nerad

Everydog

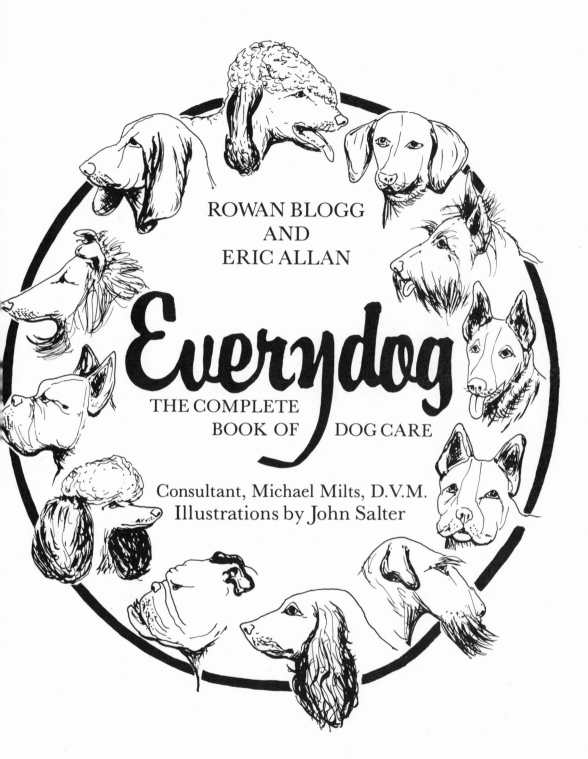

ROWAN BLOGG
AND
ERIC ALLAN

Everydog

THE COMPLETE
BOOK OF DOG CARE

Consultant, Michael Milts, D.V.M.
Illustrations by John Salter

William Morrow and Company, Inc.
NEW YORK

To our wives: Sue, Barbara and Eve

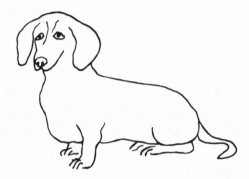

Contents

Acknowledgements

Our sincere thanks for the generous and freely given help we received from Uncle Ben's of Australia, Pfizer (Australia), the staff of Malvern Veterinary Hospital and in particular to Dr John Stirling, Dr Sonya Bettenay, Dr Murray Clarke, Dr Roger Lavelle, Dr Jack Arundel, the late Dr Geoff Rosenblum, David Weston, Angelo Zamagni and especially to Maynie Gibbins for her patience and suffering in typing the manuscript.

Introduction

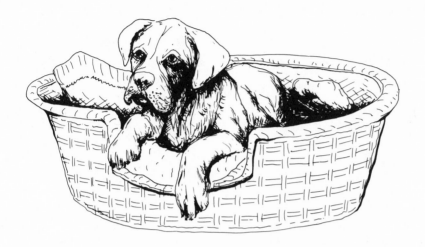

Every vet wishes he had the time to sit down and talk with dog owners. Not only about the crises and the more serious illnesses when the dog must come to the surgery, but also about the best ways to identify and cope with the common problems and conditions that can respond to home treatment.

This is not just a book on pet first aid. *Everydog* encompasses the dog in health as well as sickness. The subject matter has been suggested piecemeal by thousands of clients over the years: it is what *they* wanted to know, and covers what the vet would like to tell every owner—if only he had the time.

It is written in plain English. Jargon and unnecessary technical terms have been avoided, and instead numerous diagrams and cartoons have been used to ensure that accuracy does not suffer at the expense of clarity.

Some chapters are included mainly for interest, such as *The senses.* Others are designed for use when an urgent situation arises, such as a prolonged whelping, a poisoning or a car accident. All chapters are written according to the principle that you, the owner, have a much better chance of successfully bringing up a dog or properly caring for him during times of trauma, if you understand clearly what's gone wrong and why.

The aim of this book is to allow you and your dog to enjoy each other more. With its help you should have fewer anxieties about his health. You can find out more about matters you are uncertain of as well as ones that are completely novel to you. Although dogs depend on us entirely to look after their feeding, well-being and health, in return they give unstinting loyalty and a great deal of happiness.

Perhaps Lord Byron (1788-1824) expressed it best:

Near this spot are deposited the remains of one who possessed Beauty without Vanity, Strength without Insolence, Courage without Ferocity, and all the Virtues of Man, without his vices. This praise, which would be unmeaning Flattery if inscribed over human ashes is but a just tribute to the memory of Boatswain, a Dog.

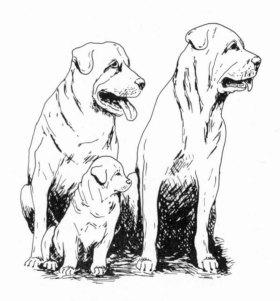

Everydog

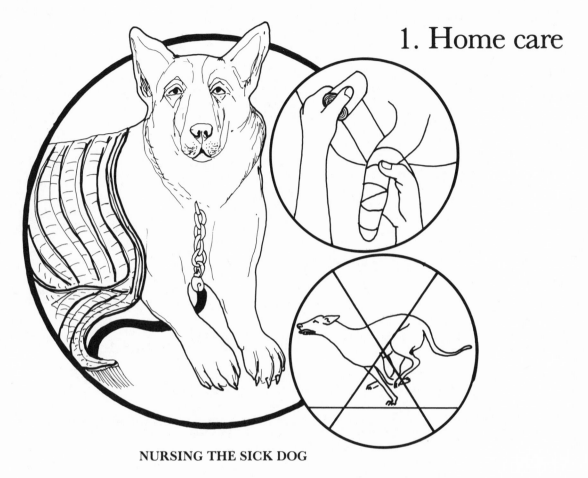

1. Home care

NURSING THE SICK DOG

No exercise should be allowed. Do not take your dog for a run to "brighten him up." Keep the patient dry and warm and free from draughts. Let the dog outside two to three times a day for bowel movements or to urinate. There should be no games or forced exercise.

Tempt the dog with food he likes and which are nutritious and easily digested, such as:

- Meat broths
- Cooked hamburger or chicken
- Baby foods
- Mashed liver
- Cottage cheese or cooked egg

Force feeding may be necessary. With solids, select small pieces of cheese, meat, etc. Gently open the dog's mouth, tilt his head back, and push the food well to the back of his mouth. With liquids, one person holds the dog, another person lifts his chin up, pulls the corner of the mouth aside to form a pocket or pouch and pours the liquid *gently* in from a bottle or syringe.

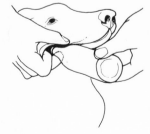

Caution: make sure the dog can swallow or the liquid could go to the lungs.

*, **, *** indicate increasing likelihood of a particular trait or problem occurring.

9

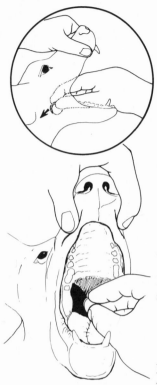

Tablets and capsules

Any of the following ways may be used to administer medicine:
- Open the mouth very wide and push the tablet well over the back of the tongue (Fig. 1:3).
- Hide the tablet in a piece of meat (see opposite).
- Conceal a crushed tablet in flavored milk and pour in to the pocket formed by pulling the check out.
- Coat the tablet with honey or butter to make it more appealing and easier to swallow.

Fluid must be given if the patient is not eating or drinking. Give water plus glucose (*not* white table sugar). Do not give milk if the dog has a bowel upset. Essential daily fluid intake is at least 30 ml (¼ cup) per 5 kg (10 lbs) body weight. This is the total daily amount and should be halved and given twice daily. Also give vitamin drops such as 5-10 drops of Pentavite or Abdec daily.

Vomiting and diarrhea

Fluids and body salt loss from persistent vomiting and diarrhea can be serious, especially in puppies; early treatment is imperative.

PROTECTION FROM SELF MUTILATION

Dogs with skin and eye irritations and those recovering from surgery often attempt to rub, bite or scratch the affected area. To prevent this:
- Cut the base out of a suitable sized plastic bucket.
- Punch holes in the lower edge of the bucket (which will be placed over the dog's head) by use of a small screwdriver.
- Place the bucket over the patient's head, base first.
- Tie the bucket in position to the collar with pipe cleaners or strong string.
- Or cut an Elizabethan collar from hard plastic or cardboard using the design in Fig. 1.4.

1.3 The tablet must be placed as far back as possible over the base of the tongue

1.4 Cut the Elizabethan collar from a flat sheet of cardboard of firm plastic. When fitted around the dog's neck it will assume a cone-like shape. The protective Elizabeth collar should fit snugly around the neck; if it is too loose the dog will be able to remove it

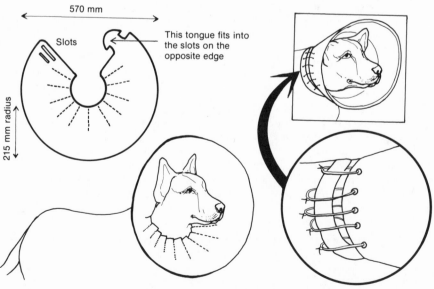

570 mm

Slots

215 mm radius

This tongue fits into the slots on the opposite edge

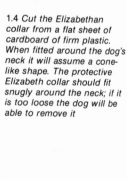

ADMINISTERING

Tablets, capsules or pills

Make the dog sit. Grasp the upper jaw just behind the long canine teeth and push his lips over his upper teeth. This should make his mouth open slightly. Pull the head back and up—the bottom jaw should drop open. If the mouth does not open, pull it open with your other hand, keeping your fingers at the front of the mouth over the incisor teeth. Be gentle.

Drop the pill right down the back of the mouth—you will notice a distinct "hump" on the tongue. Push the pill over the hump as far back as you can using two fingers.

Close the mouth and gently massage the throat to encourage the dog to swallow.

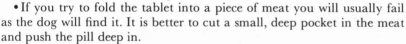

Tricks to make pill-giving easier
Disguising the tablet:

• Remember the dog has an acute sense of smell. When trying to hide the medicine in food choose something he likes which also has a strong taste or smell, such as cheese.

• If you try to fold the tablet into a piece of meat you will usually fail as the dog will find it. It is better to cut a small, deep pocket in the meat and push the pill deep in.

• Melt some chocolate and turn the tablets into chocolate drops. First give the dog a couple of "blank" chocolate drops. He may be suspicious and investigate them. After this taste, further chocolate drops (some containing the tablet) are readily eaten. It is wise to give the disguised pills as a "reward" after the dog has done something good. This allays the dog's suspicion of the gift.

• Some tablets can be powdered and mixed with the food (but not many, so ask your vet first).
Caution is needed: Many pills are "sugar coated." This is often because the inside is bitter tasting. If you crush these tablets the dog will almost always refuse food containing them.

• Some tablets have a coating to prevent them being digested too quickly. If you crush this coating it allows digestion to occur more quickly and reduces the effect of the drug.

HOME CARE OF THE SICK EYE

Proper home care, which in some cases may be over a period of many months, is essential for serious diseases of the eye.

Position of the patient for eye treatment

Treating the eye is much easier if the patient is positioned properly. Ask a neighbor to help if you live alone. Do *not* chase the patient about trying to treat the eye. Teach your dog to sit *still* while the eyes are being treated.

11

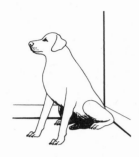

1.6 *Put larger dogs into a corner so that they cannot back away*

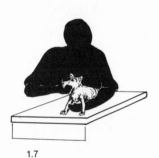

1.7

Lack of discipline leads to poorer chances of good care and therefore recovery. Firmly place the patient in a special treatment area. Place a large dog in a corner of a room so that he cannot back away, then lift the nose with one hand under the chin (Fig. 1:6). A smaller dog is placed on a table in a sitting position. Get somebody to place their hands on the dog's rear end to stop the dog backing away. Your dog may struggle initially, especially if the eye is sore, but you must be firm. The medication *must* be applied.

A small dog may be held in the arms or between your knees when seated (Fig. 1:7) with the nose and legs facing uppermost—as though you were cuddling a baby. Try to approach with the eye ointment from behind where it is not readily seen.

A dog that struggles vigorously should be made to lie on a table with your forearms on the neck and the body. Note that the left hand holds the lower front legs stretched upwards and the right hand holds the lower hind legs stretched upward. An assistant holds the head still on the table and applies the eye medication.

What is the most important part of home care?

Make sure the medication reaches the affected area. Your vet will show you how. Make sure you take home *written instructions* for each drug.

How to apply eye drops

Do not allow the tube or dropper bottle to touch the eye. When applying ointment or drops to the eye, make a bridge by placing your hands firmly on the forehead or side of the face. This avoids the eye being touched if the patient suddenly moves. Always approach from behind the eye.

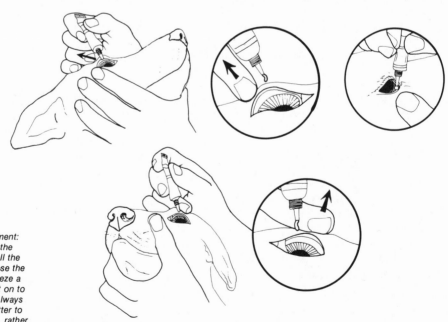

1.8 *Applying eye ointment: rest the right hand on the dog's forehead and pull the upper lid back to expose the white of the eye. Squeeze a small drop of ointment on to the white of the eye. Always remember that it is better to approach from behind, rather than in front of the eye*

After applying eye drops, apply pressure to the corner of the eye near the nose to prevent drainage down the tear duct. Alternatively, raise the nose of small animals for 3 minutes. Hold the eyelids open for a minute or two so that forceful blinking does not squeeze out medication.

How to apply eye ointment

You will need to warm some ointments before use for easier application. Cold ointments are less likely to reach deep conjunctival surfaces and if the animal moves during application, the ointment may not reach the eye at all. Remove the cap of the tube. Warm the naked end of the tube in warm water (Fig. 1:9). Running water may be used or sit the tube upside down in a shallow glass of warm water.

Eyelids stuck together

When copious pus is present the upper and lower lids may stick together. Pus which is trapped inside closed eyelids can cause serious eyeball infection. A gentle pull may be needed to open the lids. If sticky discharge is present apply antibiotic ointment liberally to prevent the lids sticking together again. For this reason it is a good idea to apply liberal amounts of ointment last thing at night.

My dog rubs his eyes after I treat them with prescribed eye drops. What should I do?

Check the label, are you using the right drug? When you have confirmed the treatment as correct, place the drops in and after you have held the eye up for minutes, take your dog for a short walk to distract his attention. If the eye drops continue to irritate, check with your vet.

Warm water

Egg cup

1.9 *Eye ointments that are thick can be warmed gently to make them flow more easily out of the tube*

CLEANING THE EYE

Cleaning the eye may be necessary in the following situations:
  • Foreign matter like sand needs washing out (especially for greyhounds after racing).
  • The eye has been burnt.
  • There is copious pus present in the eye (note that antibiotics and veterinary supervision will also be needed).
  • The eyeball is dislocated. (Note that this is an emergency situation and veterinary assistance must be sought immediately. The washing of the eye merely keeps the eyeball wet and is for temporary relief only.)
  • When severely injured eyelids cannot cover the eyeball.
  • When marked swelling stops the eyelids from covering the eyeball.

How to clean the eye

Use a syringe to squirt warm sterile saline onto the eyeball or drop on artificial tears such as Adapettes. Sometimes discharge will tend to stick to the eyeball and moving the upper and lower eyelids over the eyeball with the fingers can help to clean the eye. Your vet will tell you when this is necessary. When foreign material sticks to the eyeball never wipe the eyeball itself, but try to wash the foreign body off the eyeball with saline. Note that a healthy eye never needs to be cleaned.

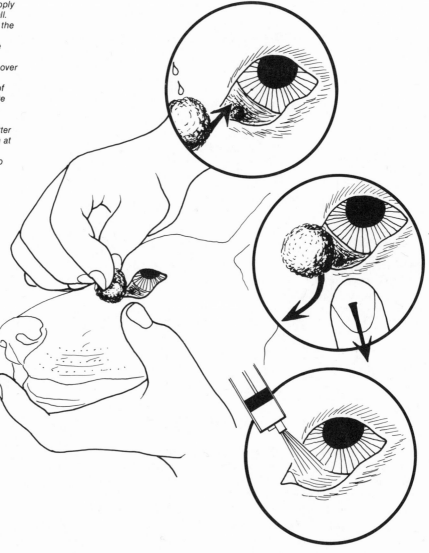

1.10 *Cleaning the eye: apply sterile water to the eyeball. Sweep the lower lid over the eyeball to move debris towards the corner of the eye near the nose.*

The upper lid is swept over the eyeball moving the debris toward the corner of the eye near the nose. Note that the eyeball is never touched.

Debris and foreign matter is then wiped off the skin at the corner of the eye. Foreign matter sticking to the eyeball requires immediate veterinary attention

2. First aid

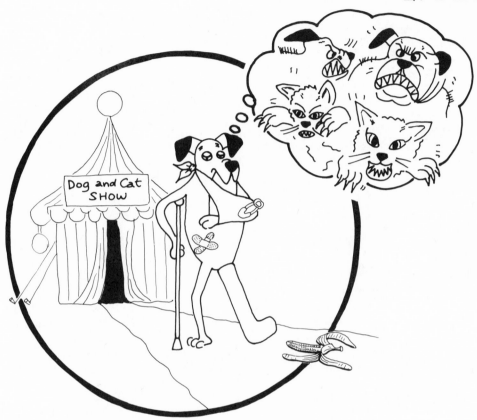

Pain

—can often be relieved with aspirin. The dose is one 300mg tablet per 30kg (66lbs). Repeat in 12 hours if necessary. If pain persists or there is no response, see a vet.

ROAD ACCIDENT INJURY

First aid

> Place a muzzle on an injured dog before you move him or touch a badly injured part—he may bite from pain.

If the dog cannot walk, slide a blanket or piece of board to act as a stretcher under the dog (Fig. 2:3). Bear in mind that internal damage can be severe with no external signs obvious to you.

If the dog can walk, carefully assist the dog into the car with support under his chest or hindquarters.

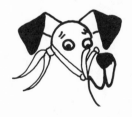

2.2 *Beware of the injured dog as he may be sore and terrified and may bite. Be cautious: muzzle an injured dog before attempting to move or treat him*

*, **, *** indicate increasing likelihood of a particular trait or problem occurring.

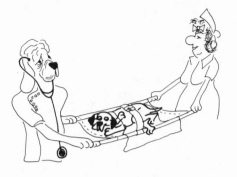
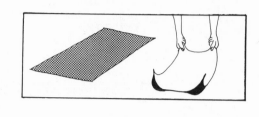

2.3 *In an emergency a piece of hardboard can be used as a stretcher. For small dogs, a blanket may suffice, but beware of bending the dog's spine*

If the dog can stand, carry him carefully to a safe place where first aid can be given. Support the chest area and also under the hindquarters and let a hurt leg dangle free, away from your body.

BLEEDING

First aid

First remember to muzzle a dog in pain. Place fingers firmly on the area which is bleeding. If the leg is bleeding, apply pressure to the groin. If the paw is bleeding, apply pressure above the paw (Fig.2:4a). Bleeding skin wounds are treated by applying a pack (made from wet cotton wool, gauze, or a clean handkerchief) to the bleeding area. A bleeding part may be controlled by pinching (Fig. 2:4b).

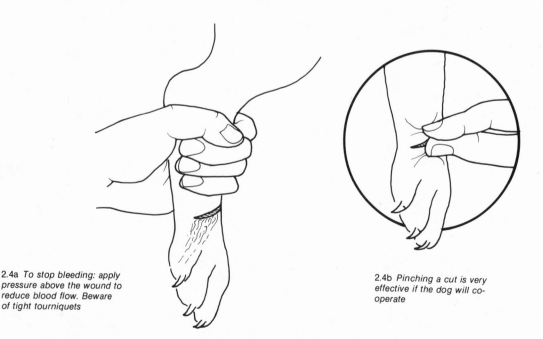

2.4a *To stop bleeding: apply pressure above the wound to reduce blood flow. Beware of tight tourniquets*

2.4b *Pinching a cut is very effective if the dog will co-operate*

> Most bleeding can be controlled by firm continuous finger
> pressure applied until the bleeding stops.

If blood soaks into the first pad applied, place a new clean pad on top and press firmly. Do not remove the bottom pad.

Tourniquets may be used for very severe hemorrhaging. Remember that they cause pain and are not well tolerated by dogs. Tourniquets should be released every 10 minutes to prevent damage to the limb due to lack of blood.

Nose bleed

Examine the nose in good light to see if you can find the cause of bleeding. If you see a cut on the nose, apply pressure with your fingers. If you cannot see the cause of bleeding keep your dog still and if possible apply cold compresses or ice cubes to the bridge of the nose. Do not try to pack the nostrils as the lining of the nose is very sensitive and easily injured.

SHOCK

Shock does not mean a "fright" but describes several physiological changes in the body after injury. Most dogs that die from road accidents die from shock.

Some causes of shock:

- Severe blood loss.
- Severe diarrhea, vomiting.
- Severe bruising.
- Blood poisoning, e.g., from womb infection.
- Bloat (twisted stomach).
- Severe heart disease.

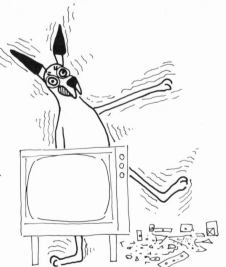

Signs of shock

- Pale and cold gums (lift the lips back to check gums).
- Rapid shallow breathing.
- Pulse is weak and rapid.
- Often dog will lie down and may be unable to stand.
- Low body temperature.
- Cold extremities, i.e., ears, paws.
- Dry and shrivelled tongue.

First aid

Time is of the utmost importance. The dog in shock needs intensive, *immediate* treatment. Reassure the dog—try to calm him and keep him warm. Do *not* attempt to give the animal any food or drinks. Seek vet's attention as soon as possible.

HEAT STRESS

If a dog becomes overheated he will be extremely uncomfortable and the condition can progress to the point where the dog collapses and may die.

What causes heat stress?

Dogs lose heat by panting. Panting has the same cooling effect that humans achieve through sweating. (Dogs cannot sweat except through their foot pads.) If the build up of heat is faster than the rate at which the dog can cool himself by panting, then his body temperature rises and heat stress begins. Breeding dogs with short noses such as the English Bulldog***, Pekingese**, and Pug** has seriously interfered with their ability to pant (Fig. 2:6). A short-nosed breed is more likely to die if kept in a car in the hot summer sun. Old and very young dogs are especially susceptible to heat stress.

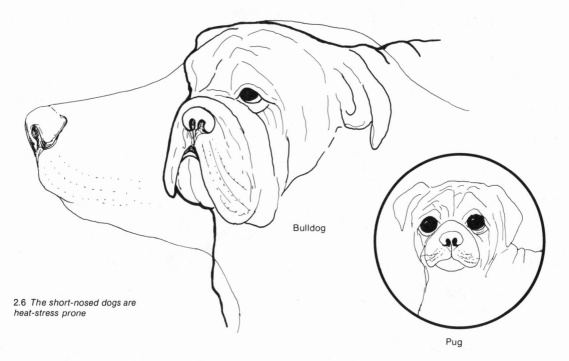

Bulldog

2.6 *The short-nosed dogs are heat-stress prone*

Pug

Signs of heat stress

At first—panting. This panting becomes very rapid and the dog will appear to be in a stupor. The heart rate (or pulse) will become very rapid and the gums will turn bright red. The legs and head become hot to the touch and there may be watery or blood-stained diarrhea. Eventually the dog collapses and may lose consciousness. Death may follow.

First aid

- First get the dog into fresh cooler air.
- Cool the dog by submerging him in a cold bath, or by playing a cold

stream of water over his head and body for a few minutes. If needed, repeat.

• Get the dog to a vet for treatment to stop swelling of the brain (cerebral edema).

How you can prevent heat stress

• Avoid confinement in a hot place, such as a car. A dog left in a closed car on a hot day is in great danger of developing heat stress. It is not enough to leave the window open a little—the dog simply must *not* be left for more than a short time in a hot, closed car.

• See that inside ventilation is good especially on days of high humidity.

• Always breed for normal length of mouth and face as dogs with flat faces are more prone to heat stress.

2.7 *First aid for heat stress: cool the patient and apply moisture internally and externally*

COLD INJURY: FROSTBITE, FREEZING, HYPOTHERMIA

Healthy, long-haired acclimatized dogs can survive temperatures as low as –50°C if they are well fed. Frostbite is rarely seen.

Dogs can be affected by the cold if they are sick, old, wet and unable to move. The tips of ears, the scrotum, the tip of the tail and sometimes the lower parts of their legs may be affected.

If a dog is, for example, accidentally locked in a freezer or caught in the snow, early veterinary attention is essential.

Neglected newborn pups are very sensitive to cold.

Treatment

Warm the dog with a warm water bath, or warm water bottles and electric blankets in a warm room. Warm the animal slowly and to a moderate heat only.

CUTS/LACERATIONS

First aid

• Control the bleeding (see p. 16-17). If the cut has perforated the chest squeeze the wound together holding a moist pad (a clean handkerchief in an emergency) firmly over the area to try and prevent air being sucked in.

• Remove any hair, glass or gravel from a superficial cut. (Leave the cleaning of deep wounds to the vet.) Pieces of cotton wool soaked in *mild* antiseptic solution or clean water may be used to stroke dirt from inside the wound to the edges of the cut (Fig. 2:8). Use a clean swab for each cleaning stroke.

• If a deep cut exposes abdominal contents (guts) which have become dirty, wash off the debris with running water and hold a broad bandage over the guts and attempt to pack them back into the abdomen. Go immediately to a vet.

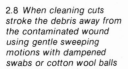

2.8 *When cleaning cuts stroke the debris away from the contaminated wound using gentle sweeping motions with dampened swabs or cotton wool balls*

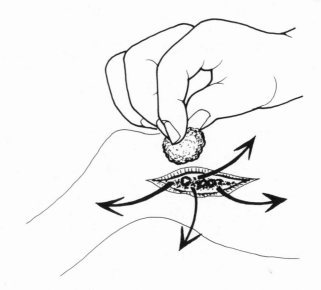

ABRASIONS

(when outer skin layers are removed but the skin is not cut through).

First aid

Clean the wound (see above) and flush liberally with clean water if necessary. The dog will usually clean the wound by licking and saliva is mildly antiseptic. A mild drying, antiseptic paint such as Mercurochrome, acriflavine or gentian violet, may speed healing.

BITES AND PUNCTURE WOUNDS

First aid

Infection is a hazard. If bleeding is profuse, apply a clean pad (such as a handkerchief) over the area and apply firm pressure until bleeding is controlled.

• Veterinary treatment may include antitetanus as well as antibiotics.

Seek early treatment for fight wounds as infection can lead to blood poisoning.

BRUISES

Usually no particular form of treatment is necessary for a bruise. Do *not* apply liniments or any other medicines designed for human use. Bruising *can* be associated with hidden, severe internal damage or broken bones. Confine your dog and if he does not move about easily, seek professional advice.

SCALDS/BURNS

Immediately immerse the burnt area (the whole dog if necessary) in cool water—a bath, swimming pool or dam can be used. Rush to the vet. A small dog can be continually immersed in a baby's bath in the car. Ice may be applied if only small areas are affected.

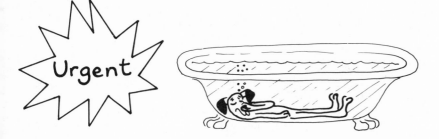

2.9 *For severe scalds and burns, try to immerse the patient in clean, cool water to minimize the shock and fluid loss*

BEE STINGS AND WASP AND INSECT BITES

Bee stings produce sudden pain and swelling, usually on the paws or the mouth. If the patient is bitten inside the mouth, swelling of the throat can make breathing difficult. Some dogs are extremely sensitive *(anaphylaxis)* and can show severe signs which include swellings under the skin and all over the body; vomiting; diarrhea; swollen head; and swollen throat.

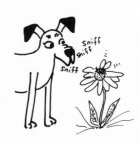

First aid

Minor swellings go down on their own. An ice pack used on a swollen part will give some relief.

Call the vet if you suspect multiple bee stings, or a severe reaction to one sting, or if the dog is bitten inside the mouth.

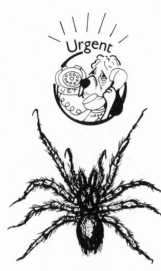

2.11 *Spider bites: some species — such as this funnelweb — are dangerous and urgent treatment gives your dog the best chance for survival*

SPIDER BITES

Spiders rarely bite dogs as their mouth parts cannot penetrate the coat and skin of dogs except where it is thin. (Between the toes of young pups or inside the mouth.)

In man, spider bites cause a spreading pain at the site of the bite, plus nausea, sweating and muscle cramps. Dogs react similarly and will hold a bitten paw up and shake it frantically.

Treatment

An antivenene is available for funnelweb spiders, but may be hard to obtain.

First aid

- Apply cold compresses over the bite area.
- Apply a pressure bandage to reduce spread of venom.
- Take the animal to the vet as soon as possible.

SNAKE BITE

Many more animals than humans are bitten by snakes.

These are the signs to look for if you suspect snake bite:

- Trembling; sweating; dilated pupils; the animal becomes excited; saliva drools from the mouth; vomiting; sudden collapse a few minutes after being bitten. Death may occur from a paralysis of breathing.
- Venomous snakes usually leave two puncture marks at the site of the bite wound. Non-venomous snakes leave a *row* of small teeth marks. There is little swelling at the bite site in most species of venomous snakes.
- Red urine may be passed later on.

2.12 *The bite of a venomous snake usually produces two puncture marks. These may not be obvious, especially in a long-haired dog. Non-venomous snakes leave a row of teeth marks.*

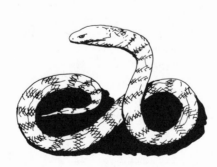

Tiger snake

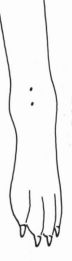

Bite of a venomous snake

What to do if you know your dog has been bitten

• Assume it is poisonous if the type of snake is not identified.
• Minimize the dog's movement. Too much movement will make the poison speed more quickly through the animal's body.
• If a leg is bitten, bandage the leg. Tourniquets are not as effective as firm bandages in minimising speed of poison spread.
• Wash the wound liberally with cold water to remove any surface venom.
• *Do not* attempt to suck the venom out.
• *Do not* cut into the wound.

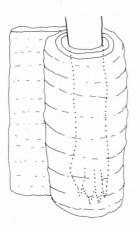 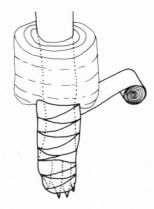

2.13 *The Robert Jones dressing: first apply a large amount of cotton wool. Layer it on in sheets.*
An elastic adhesive bandage is then firmly applied over the cotton wool. Start at the bottom of the foot and work up. The Robert Jones dressing can also be used as a temporary splint in fracture cases — even in large dogs or horses

What can the vet do?

Veterinary surgeons in most areas carry antivenen. If given promptly, antiserum and cortisone can be life saving.

Should the dog owner carry antivenen, just in case?

No. It is not legally available to the public and can be dangerous if given incorrectly.

TICKS

Some ticks are capable of causing paralysis and death. These ticks include the Scrub and Bush tick *(Ixodes)* found in warm coastal areas such as in Australia and Southern California.

Signs

Paralysis starts with the hind legs weakening and progresses to an inability to stand and eventually death from paralysis of breathing muscles. A single tick takes 3 or 4 days to cause paralysis so a thorough daily check will prevent problems.

2.14 *Ticks are elusive: You must check all possible hiding places. When you find one keep looking for more*

Top

Underneath

Between toes

Ears

Under lips

Under tail

2.15 *Tick removal*

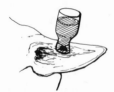

An inverted bottle
of methylated spirits
or acetone
(nail polish remover)

Treatment

Remove the tick (by placing an inverted bottle of alcohol or methylated spirits over it). Do not squeeze the tick or you risk injecting more poison into the dog.

If paralysis has started, see the vet immediately as antiserum will usually save the dog.

Prevention

Suitable anti-tick rinses and powders are available from your vet.

JELLYFISH STINGS

If your dog shows signs of extreme pain after swimming in the sea then treat it for jellyfish sting. Look for tentacles of jellyfish clinging to the dog's skin. Be careful when you remove these as they can still sting you. Give the dog one or two tablets of aspirin (dose, 1 tablet per 30 kg) and apply dilute ammonia 1:10 water to the areas of the sting. Keep your dog warm and if the symptoms do not disappear go *at once* to your vet. If your dog stops breathing then give it mouth-to-nose respiration. When removing tentacles, avoid rubbing. Pull cleanly and rapidly in one direction.

ARTIFICIAL RESPIRATION

Artificial respiration moves air in and out of the lungs and must be given as soon as the animal stops breathing. Three minutes after breathing has stopped the dog is beyond recovery. This means you have no time to lose.

Technique

• Lie the animal on its right side, open the animal's mouth, check that there are no obstructions inside the mouth.
• Pull out any sand and gravel with your finger and make sure that the tongue is lolling out clear of the back of the throat.
• Hold the dog's mouth closed and cup your hand around the nose. Blow into the nostrils until the chest rises. Wait for 10 seconds and repeat.

HEART MASSAGE

Lie the dog on its right side, place your thumb on one side of the breast bone and your fingers on the other just behind the elbow. Compress the chest rapidly and firmly six times, wait 5 seconds to let the chest expand, and repeat. Heart massage is a vigorous exercise—if the heart stops "get tough with it." Continue massaging until the heart beats on its own or until no heart beat is felt for 10 minutes. For larger dogs place the heel of your hand on the ribcage just behind the elbow and over the heart. Compress the chest firmly six times as above.

DROWNING AND SUFFOCATION

Suffocation occurs when oxygen is prevented from getting into the lungs. Drowning, inhalation of smoke, gasoline, refrigerant fluid, carbon monoxide poisoning, and being locked up in a small air-tight space are among the causes of suffocation. The tongue and inside the mouth turn blue. The dog gasps for breath and may lose consciousness. If drowning is the cause, hold the dog upside down by its hind legs to let the water run out of the windpipe and lungs, then give mouth-to-nose respiration and heart massage.

How to induce vomiting

Any one of the following ways may be used to induce vomiting:
• Give 1-3 teaspoonfuls of hydrogen peroxide. Repeat in 10 minutes if unsuccessful.
• Place ½-1 teaspoonful of table salt on the back of the tongue.
• Give syrup of ipecac: 1 teaspoonful per 5 kg (10 lbs) bodyweight.
Note that vomiting should *not* be induced if the dog is:
• Severely depressed or comatose (semi conscious).
• If an acid, alkali, solvent or corrosive substance is swallowed.
• If the animal is struggling for breath.

FISH HOOKS

Take your dog to the vet as soon as possible if a fish hook is caught in the dog's mouth or elsewhere in the body. You may be able to snip the barb off a hook by use of pliers (Fig 2:16). Do not attempt to pull the barb back through the skin.

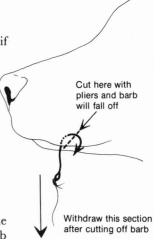

Cut here with pliers and barb will fall off

Withdraw this section after cutting off barb

2.16 *Removal of fish hooks*

FITS

The best you can do when your dog is having a fit is to prevent it from hurting itself. Do not try to calm your dog by petting or stroking it—you may get bitten. Put blankets or pillows into a small room or corner of the room and remove any furniture. Very carefully put the dog into this padded area. Move the dog by pulling it along by the back legs approaching the dog from behind. Once the patient is in a safe place, leave it alone. If recovery does not occur within 5 minutes, call your vet. If you have not previously consulted your vet about fits do so immediately.

CHOKING

Choking occurs when a foreign body blocks the back of the throat or windpipe. If the dog has passed out from lack of oxygen, open the mouth, pull the tongue out and look for a blockage in the windpipe. If you locate a foreign body, hook it out with your finger. Hold the mouth open with a block of wood and attempt to remove any foreign matter with a pair of pliers or similar long-nosed instrument. Once the throat is clear give mouth-to-nose respiration and perhaps heart massage. Do not attempt home treatment if you are able to seek immediate veterinary attention.

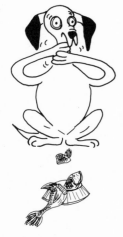

2.17 Small, sharp bones should never be fed to dogs

PENIS WILL NOT GO BACK INTO THE SHEATH

If the penis protrudes from the sheath and will not slide back into place, apply warm olive oil to the shaft of the penis and around the opening of the sheath. Pull the sheath over the penis. With smaller dogs place the dog into a cold bath. The penis should automatically go back as the cold water reduces the swelling.

EYE INJURIES

• All injuries to the eye need immediate veterinary attention and treatment given shortly after injury determines whether or not vision is saved. If you suspect injury call your vet at once, sometimes the full "storm of inflammation" may take hours to develop. Read the section on eye inflammation (see p. 161-4).

• If you cannot see your vet *within the hour,* phone for first aid advice. Treatment is vital *before* the eye looks bad.

How do I know the eye is injured?

• Compare one eye with the other. The only external signs may be closed or half-closed eyelids and a watery eye.

• When the eye is inflamed, the white of the eye is red and the pupil may be small. Do remember, however, that many injuries are hidden from casual view. An eye suffering from serious disease can appear very similar to an eye mildly diseased.

• Head injuries commonly harm the eye—a blow to the head can damage delicate eye tissue.

> If your dog comes home with one eye half closed, presume
> a serious injury is present until it is proven otherwise.

The eyelids are swollen and bruised, is this dangerous?

Yes, if the eyelids cannot sweep across the eyeball it will be dry and *the eye can be destroyed overnight.* Always keep the eyeball wet in this situation. Also the inside of the eyeball might be seriously sick.

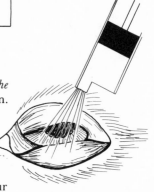

2.18 *Keep a swollen eye constantly wet*

My dog has been hit on the head. Will this hurt the eyes?

Yes. A blow to the head "shakes up" the eyes and can cause blindness. Your dog needs immediate treatment for eye inflammation following a severe head injury (even if eye injury is not obvious to you).

Why the vet needs to see the eye injury early

• It is extremely important to have a cortisone injection "before the storm" of eye inflammation destroys the eye.
• Cortisone antibiotic eye drops administered six or more times a day may be prescribed. Ask your vet if there is a cortisone derivative in the ointment you plan to use. Cortisone is *not* used on the eyeball if an ulcer develops.
• The vet may wish to dispense atropine 1 per cent eye drops. (*Caution:* Keep atropine away from children—a dropper bottle of atropine can kill several children.)

How to reduce eye injuries

• Keep a new puppy away from the family cat.
• Have the eyelid openings on pop-eyed dogs like Pekingeses surgically made smaller when they are young.
• Always check your dog's eyes after hunting or racing or if it's been involved in a road accident or a dog fight.

Eyeball dislocated out of its socket

If the eye is displaced out of the socket (e.g. Pekingese dogs) make sure the eye is *kept wet. Rush* to your vet and in the meantime constantly drip clean water onto the eye. Sometimes it is possible to put the eye back yourself if the eye is only slightly displaced (see p. 174).

Bruised or torn eyelids

Keep the eyeball continually wet with clean water. The eyeball may also be damaged internally. Get to your vet without delay.

Lime or cement burns

Burns to the eye are best treated by immediately washing the eyeball with copious amounts of saline (use clean tap water in an emergency). General anesthesia is often necessary to remove all foreign matter.

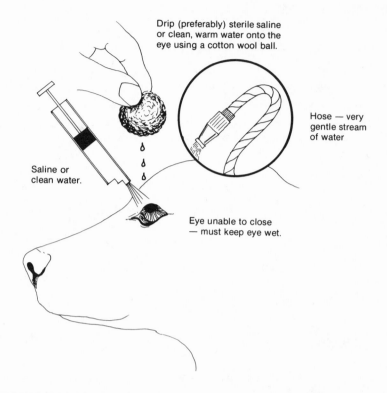

2.19 *Keeping an injured eye wet: the injured eye must be kept wet, especially when the eyelid is damaged or if it is unable to close. Seek veterinary attention immediately*

Drip (preferably) sterile saline or clean, warm water onto the eye using a cotton wool ball.

Hose — very gentle stream of water

Saline or clean water.

Eye unable to close — must keep eye wet.

> When the eye is injured make sure the lids can cover the eye.
> If the lids cannot blink over the eye keep the cornea continually
> wet with saline or water. Call the vet.

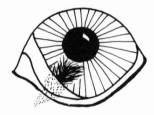

2.20 *Grass seeds, awns or other foreign bodies can lodge under the lids, especially under the third eyelid, causing severe eye irritation. Some seeds may be fairly obvious, as in the diagram, but many are almost completely hidden under the lid.*

Roll the lids back, and look carefully in a good light. A pen torch is useful. You may see a few strands of the grass seed's tail, or only pus issuing from under the third eyelid

Foreign matter in the eye

Grass seeds

If grass seeds cannot be washed out with a syringe (Fig. 2:19) go to your vet at once for removal with anesthetic drops. Grass seeds can burrow into the eye socket and destroy the eye.

Note that dogs can have a dark line of pigment on the whole of the eye under the upper lid which can be mistaken for a splinter.

Sand on the eyeball

Wash foreign matter off using copious saline in a syringe. Sweeping the upper lid over the eyeball may help to clean the eye.

Caution: Matter on the eyeball can be the result of a dry eye (see p. 176). See your vet if continuous eye discharge is present.

Gunshot in the eye

Surprisingly, shotgun pellets in the eye are often overlooked. Gunshot through the eyeball causes severe eye damage with signs which may not be noticed by the owner. A weeping red eye in a hunting dog may be due to his owner's poor marksmanship.

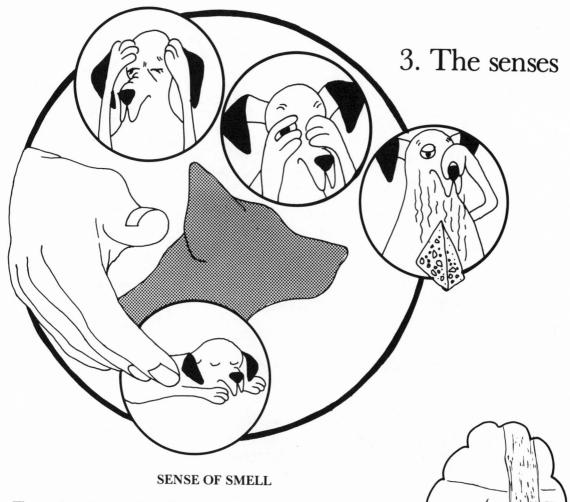

3. The senses

SENSE OF SMELL

The newborn's sense of smell

Smell is the newborn pup's most important sense. Newborn puppies start off life deaf and blind but respond to smell.

Around the time of birth the bitch emit scents (called pheromones) especially from her mammary glands. These scents cause the pup to seek the nipple and so learn that this smell means warm milk. As the sense of smell develops, pups react to new stimuli. Right at the time that meat becomes a part of their diet (at 3 or 4 weeks) pups are stimulated by the smell of meat.

As with all senses, the sense of smell depends to some degree on training and practice. Foxhounds are specially trained to find foxes, Bassets to find hares, Pointers to find game birds, and Bloodhounds to find people.

The adult dog's sense of smell

The dog's sense of smell is possibly 100 times greater than man's and is used more than short-range vision is for moving about a dog's world. A

*, **, *** indicate increasing likelihood of a particular trait or problem occurring.

3.2 Scents give dogs a lot more information than humans

large nose indicates the significant role this highly developed sense of smell plays in the dog's life (p. 30). The dog's nose is unlike the simple nose of man. Inside the dog's nose are many rolls of cartilage lined by sensitive nerve endings. These give the dog an extremely subtle sense of smell and enable him to perform such feats as finding hidden heroin and lost people. Dogs bred for short noses may be largely deprived of this acute sense of smell. The dog also has an additional scent organ buried behind the canine teeth on the roof of the mouth. This is called the vomeronasal organ and does not exist in man. Brain development also reflects the importance of smell to the dog. The part of the dog's brain responsible for sense of smell is far larger than in the human brain.

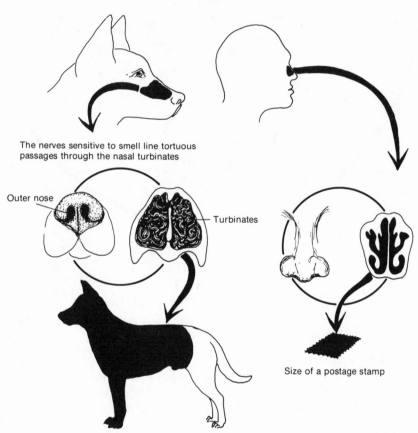

The nerves sensitive to smell line tortuous passages through the nasal turbinates

Outer nose

Turbinates

Size of a postage stamp

3.3 The sense of smell. Dog and man compared: the nerve cells sensitive to smell line scrolls of bone and cartilage in the dog's nose. These are arranged so that they present a huge surface area to air samples sniffed in. This area is approximately equal to 2.3 of the dog's skin surface area. Compare this to the relatively tiny area in man's nose responsible for smell detection which is about the size of a large postage stamp.

The significance of smell to some hunting dogs is shown when a fox, running before the hounds, doubles back through a Foxhound pack. The dogs fail to recognize the fox by sight but continue their chase, running on and then doubling back in the same loop taken by the fox.

When adult dogs first meet, sniffing is an important ritual which identifies the newcomer—including the smell of the anal glands with which the dog marks his territory at each bowel motion (see p. 114). Sniffing trees

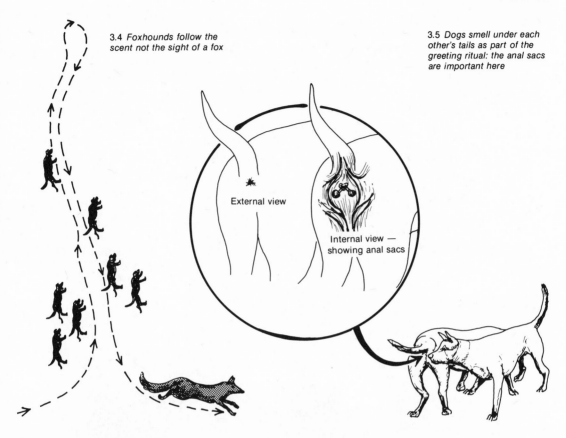

3.4 *Foxhounds follow the scent not the sight of a fox*

3.5 *Dogs smell under each other's tails as part of the greeting ritual: the anal sacs are important here*

External view

Internal view — showing anal sacs

or posts tells the dog which dogs have urinated there before—again a method of marking out territory in the wild. When a bitch is in season and urinates she is telling the canine world she is ready to mate. Males come from all over in reaction to this strong odor. If you allow your bitch to pass urine in your front garden when she is in season, it is little wonder that your garden is suddenly filled with enthusiastic canine visitors.

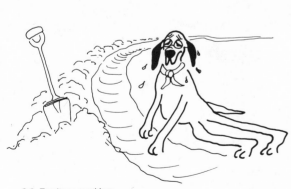

3.6 *Territory marking: digging or scraping in a new territory serves to mark out the dog's "claim."*

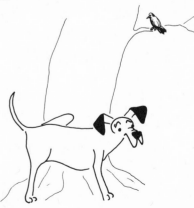

3.7 *Territory-marking signs: urinating over a previously 'marked' tree, the dog covers the previous scent with his own*

Senses of dog and man compared

	Dog	Man
Smell	Excellent. Used instead of close vision	Comparatively poor.
Hearing	Greater range of sounds detected. e.g. can detect impending thunderstorm before man.	Less than the dog.
Color vision	Very poor.	Good.
Vision in dim light.	Good.	Poor.
Main function of vision	To pick up moving prey, even at night.	For fine, close work, tool making, handcraft.

3.8 *Senses of dog and man compared*

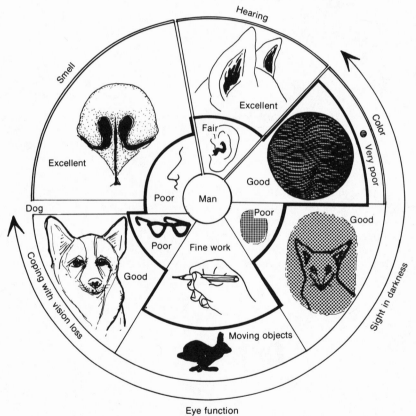

Eye function

HEARING

The newborn's sense of hearing

All newborn pups are deaf—they have flattened ears and closed ear canals. The pup will react to sound when it is 10 days old, but it will be 6 weeks before the brain is adult-like in form, size, weight and volume and it is the brain which is taught to hear or which contains inherited ability regarding hearing. No senses can be fully developed until this time.

The adult dog's sense of hearing

The dog hears sounds which are not only too faint for the human ear, but also too high-pitched and outside our hearing range. This is the basis of the "silent" dog whistle.

The dog appears to be able to tell the footsteps of his owner from those of someone else. He can also detect the direction of the sound. You will notice he cocks his head to one side to locate where the sound is coming from. Dogs can also tell that the family car is arriving home long before we, at home, are sure of this ourselves.

There is a breed difference in the ability to hear very well. Dogs with erect ears such as German Shepherds and Foxhounds are better equipped to collect sound waves than dogs with long floppy ears which have hair falling over the ear canal.

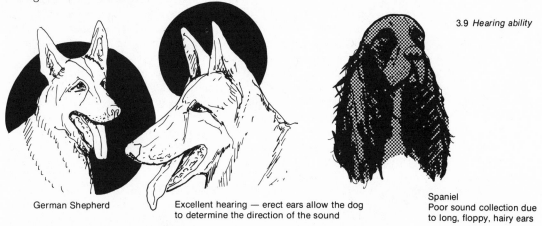

3.9 *Hearing ability*

German Shepherd

Excellent hearing — erect ears allow the dog to determine the direction of the sound

Spaniel
Poor sound collection due to long, floppy, hairy ears

Can dogs understand many words?

Your dog can, with training, pick up key words such as "sit," "stay," "heel," "here," and his name. Most of our vocabulary, however, is lost on our canine friends. The exact meaning is not understood, but the dog can pick up what our mood is by the tone of our voice, our body language and our scent.

Although we say, 'He understands every word I say', we really mean he reads our manner, mood and body language well—and what being is as dedicated to every move we make as man's best friend?

VISION

Vision in the puppy

The puppy is born blind. Not only are his eyelids closed but the eye and brain are poorly developed. At 10-14 days the eyes open and the eye—still not well developed—begins to receive light. There is great variation from breed to breed in the time the eyes open, for example: 9 days for the Cocker Spaniel or Maltese, 11-13 days for the Wirehaired Terrier and 16 days for Airedale pups.

Until the puppy is 3 weeks of age vision plays very little part in his life. He has other senses—mainly smell and warmth—to keep him close to his mother.

By about 6 weeks the pup has some useful vision as the retina is mature.

Generally speaking, vision is slow to develop in dogs. Other senses such as smell, warmth and hearing guide the pups in a protected world by their mother's side. It is some months before vision develops fully. Good vision does not occur until perhaps 4 months of age.

Vision in the adult dog

The factors which determine how well a dog sees are not only the design of the eye (see p. 162), but also where the dog was brought up, inheritance and education.

How does the dog's vision compare with ours?

The answer to this question is that a dog sees only what he must in order to survive—just as ancient man had to be equipped with the eyesight needed for survival. If we look at the dog's life in the wild, and at human life, we have the basis of a comparison of sight in the two species. Man is omnivorous (we eat everything) and we need near vision and color vision to pick ripe fruit and vegetables. We rely on sight as our sense of smell helps us little when compared with the dog.

Man and dog are both hunters—but our vision needs are different. Man hunts with weapons—and for weapon-making we need close vision. The dog is a different sort of hunter. The dog is no craftsman or weapon-maker—his weapons are his teeth. The dog needs to locate his prey. The dog's eyes are designed not only to find a meal but also to avoid becoming one.

Nature has given the dog more vision out of the corners of the eye than we have. His long vision is good and his night vision is much better than ours. A dog's close vision is not nearly as good as man's. When close to his prey the nose takes over. The dog looks for his prey at night and has limited color vision. Why does a dog not see much color? Because he doesn't need to.

Vision is a learning or taught process and is a function of the brain as well as the eye. The eye does not actually see, but only receives the light and the brain then interprets the information.

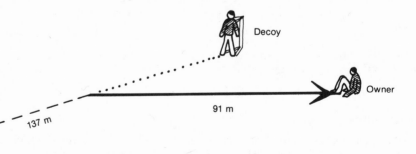

3.10 *At over 100 metres, most dogs can be fooled by a cardboard replica of their master — but within 100 metres the sense of smell takes over and the real owner can be detected*

Decoy

Owner

91 m

137 m

Dog

What colors can the dog see?

The dog has limited color vision but appears to be able to distinguish red, green and yellow from grey. Red and pink are most probably seen as different shades of grey. With training, we could expect a dog to pick out more colors—although to him he may be choosing between different greys.

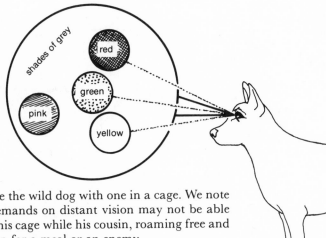

3.11 *Dogs have very poor colour vision*

Wild dog vs. dog in captivity

It is interesting for us to compare the wild dog with one in a cage. We note that a caged animal with no demands on distant vision may not be able to see much beyond the bars of his cage while his cousin, roaming free and taught to hunt, scans the horizon for a meal or an enemy.

Breed difference in vision

Some breeds use their eyes more than others. The "gaze" hounds: Greyhounds, Afghans, Borzois, Deerhounds, Italian Greyhounds, Whippets and Irish Wolfhounds are dogs that hunt by sight. They will pick up moving prey much more readily than a dog that relies more on smell, such as a Bloodhound or Foxhound. If a rabbit crouches still in the grass, a Greyhound may run straight past as dogs which hunt by sight need movement to stimulate the corners of the eye (peripheral vision). Contrast this with "the sniffers":—a Foxhound would be delighted if his prey sat still— and would smell his way right up to the tasty meal.

Sheepdogs, similarly, have good vision and are trained to react to hand signals more than a kilometer away. Sheepdogs also use their eyes to control the sheep in much the same way as we hold people in our gaze. If one eye becomes cloudy or absent the sheepfarmer will say his sheepdog is no longer able to 'hold' the sheep with his eyes.

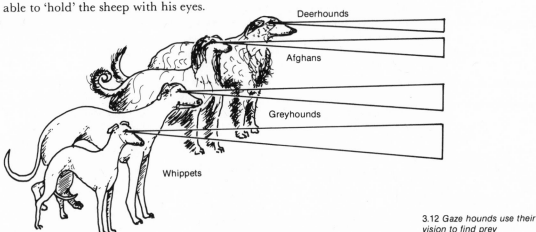

3.12 *Gaze hounds use their vision to find prey*

Other dogs in the field, such as the Labrador Retriever, are able to see shot birds falling from the sky, locate the bird and bring back the game to their master. If the Retriever does not see the movement of the falling prey, however, retrieval by nose alone is more difficult.

35

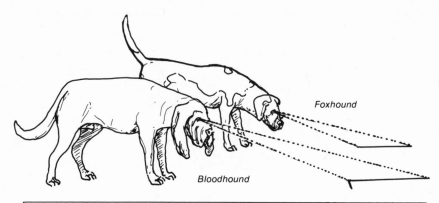

3.13 *'The sniffers' use their sense of smell rather than vision to find prey*

Foxhound

Bloodhound

> Compared with man, dogs are more aware of movement out of the corner of the eye and focus less on objects in front.

Does age cause vision loss in dogs?

One of the penalties of age in man is that we are less able to focus in our middle to later years. The dog—without our refinements of sight—does not suffer our loss of near vision. *Provided no disease occurs,* the old dog sees as well as the young.

> Inherited diseases—not old age—are the greatest threat to vision in the dog.

MENTAL TELEPATHY AND EXTRA-SENSORY PERCEPTION

Many stories exist of man communicating with his dog which suggest mental telepathy exists between man and his dog. So many people ask: How did my dog know I was on that train? How did he know I was going to take him for a walk? (He ran to the door before I had even moved from my chair.) The canine powers of telepathy or extra-sensory perception we can only continue to observe and document. When we know more about ESP we will better understand the deep bond between man and dog.

PAIN

As a general rule dogs tolerate pain well—in fact better than most people. Dogs may react to pain by being depressed, quiet and lethargic. They may also lick, rub or scratch at an irritated part.

Do we always know when our dog is in pain?

Although we believe they *feel* pain much as we do, dogs may *show* no sign at all when experiencing pain. Some dogs will even allow you to manipulate a broken leg without uttering a sound.

Some diseases, such as glaucoma and blockage of the bladder, may be associated with very little outward signs. One of the authors vividly remembers a sheepdog working the sheep at full speed with a completely blocked bladder. Nothing in the dog's behavior changed, even when the bladder became so swollen it occupied the whole abdomen.

4. Inherited Diseases— Before you buy

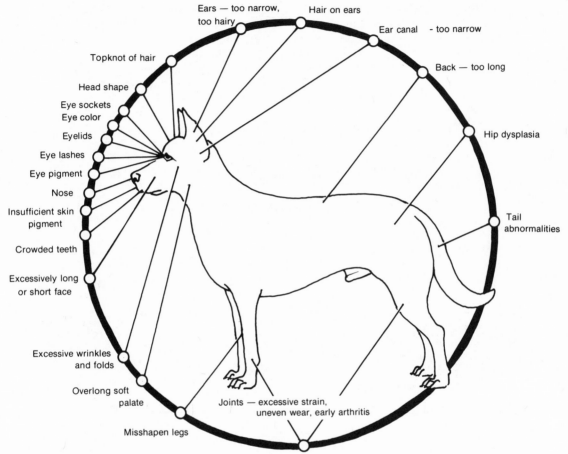

Ears — too narrow, too hairy

Hair on ears

Ear canal - too narrow

Back — too long

Topknot of hair

Head shape

Eye sockets
Eye color

Eyelids

Eye lashes

Eye pigment

Nose

Insufficient skin pigment

Crowded teeth

Excessively long or short face

Excessive wrinkles and folds

Overlong soft palate

Misshapen legs

Joints — excessive strain, uneven wear, early arthritis

Hip dysplasia

Tail abnormalities

4.1 *Areas where breed faults can occur*

FASHION AND DISEASE

This section is a breed-by-breed list of some diseases with an inherited basis or presumed inherited basis. These diseases either have spread in some families or threaten to become widespread if breeding controls are not established. This list will vary considerably from time to time and place to place. Consult your local veterinarian or the relevant breed society to establish the prevalence of these inherited diseases in a particular breed. Some of these conditions are restricted to certain geographical areas, and dog breeders should be aware of these before importing new bloodlines. In Britain in 1974, for example, the Kennel Council showed 116 breeds and of these, 43 breeds showed patella luxation and 40 showed hip dysplasia[1].

[1]**Harmar H.,** *Dogs and how to breed them,* John Gifford Ltd., London, 1974

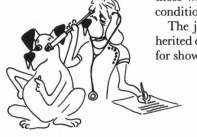

4.2 *All show dogs should pass a thorough physical examination by independent experts before being awarded champion status. This could clear many inherited conditions and lead to a more realistic approach to breeding and judging*

The incidence of an inherited disease is increased in a breed when a championship is awarded to a dog either with an inherited disease, or prone to develop inherited disease later. Even though he appears to be normal, the dog may be carrying a gene for an inherited disease.

While widespread use of an affected stud animal can rapidly increase the incidence of inherited disease, disease control schemes, on the other hand, can eliminate diseases listed here. On occasions, zealous breeder co-operation has been shown to reduce inherited diseases such as hereditary cataract and progressive retinal atrophy (PRA).

Note that breeds with long lists of defects are not necessarily inferior to those with short lists of inherited disease. The frequency with which the condition occurs is also important.

The judge in the show ring has a vital role to play in eliminating inherited diseases. Comments on showing and inherited defects with a routine for show judge's examination are given at the end of the chapter.

INHERITED DISEASES*

Afghan Hound

Blood
　　Blood group incompatibility.
Eyes
　　Juvenile cataract.
　　Corneal degeneration (dystrophy).
　　Third eyelid turned out (everted).
　　Oversized eyelid opening.
　　Primary glaucoma (abnormal drainage angle).
　　PPM (persistent pupillary membrane).
Bones
　　Elbow joint malformation.
Behavior
　　Behavioral abnormalities.
Testicles
　　Testicles do not 'drop' (cryptorchidism).

Airedale Terrier

Brain/nervous system
　　Trembling of the hindquarters.
　　Cerebellar hypoplasia.
Abdomen
　　Umbilical hernia.
Eye
　　Corneal degeneration (dystrophy).
　　Extra eyelashes.
 • Long eyelid hair.
　　Entropion.

Akita

Eye
　　Corneal degeneration (dystrophy).

Alaskan Malamute

Blood and bone disease
　　Anemia with chondrodysplasia.
Kidney
　　Renal cortical hypoplasia.
Eye
　　Corneal degeneration (dystrophy).
　　Day blindness.
Behavior
　　Aggressiveness.

American Cocker Spaniel *(See Cocker Spaniel)*

American Foxhound

Eye
　　Small eye (microphthalmia).
Ear
　　Deafness.

*Look in the glossary for an explanation of technical terms.　• High incidence in each breed

"Australian" (Californian) Shepherd

Eye

PPM (persistent pupillary membrane).
Retinal dysplasia (detachment).
• Malformed eye tunic (scleral ectasia).

Australian Terriers

Bones
• Dislocated patellas.
Dislocated shoulders.

Eye
Cataracts.
PRA (progressive retinal atrophy).

Basenji

Eye
• PPM (persistent pupillary membrane).
Pits (colobomas) of the optic disc.

Abdomen
Umbilical hernia.
Inguinal hernia.
Gut infection (coliform enteritis).

Kidney
Renal tubular dysfunction.

Basset Hound

Eye
• Droopy lower lids (ectropion).
• Redundant forehead skin.
• Oversized eyelid opening.
Extra eyelashes.
PPM (persistent pupillary membrane).
• Glaucoma (abnormal drainage angle).
Glaucoma due to dislocated lens.

Bones
• Deformed legs.
Abnormal neck vertebra.

Blood
Platelet disorder.

Abdomen
Inguinal hernia.

Beagle

Eye
Cataract.
Droopy lower lids (ectropion).
Glaucoma.
Underdeveloped optic nerve (hypoplasia
of the optic nerve).
PPM (persistent pupillary membrane).

PRA (progressive retinal atrophy).
Cherry eye.
Deformed eye tunic (ectasia syndrome).

Nervous system
Epilepsy.

Mouth
Clefts of lip and palate.

Spine
• Intervertebral disc disease.

Skin
Atopic (allergic) dermatitis.

Bedlington Terrier

Eye
Absent tear duct drainage.
Extra eyelashes.
Retinal detachment (dysplasia).

Kidney
Renal cortical hypoplasia.

Bernese Mountain Dog

Mouth
Clefts of lip and palate.

Bichon

Eye
Corneal degeneration (dystrophy).

Black and Tan Coonhound

Blood
Hemophilia.

Bloodhound

Defective immunity:
Susceptibility to disease, e.g., distemper.

Eye
• Droopy lower lids (ectropion).
• Entropion.
• Redundant forehead skin.

Border Collie

Eye
CRA (central retinal atrophy).
Pinkish "lumps" on the eyeball (proliferative
keratoconjunctivitis).

Border Terrier

Womb
Failure to expel pups at term (uterine inertia).

Borzoi

Eye
> Retinal dysplasia.

Boston Terrier

Eye
> Corneal degeneration (dystrophy).
> Extra lashes (distichiasis).
> • Entropion (medial entropion).
> Corneal ulcer.
> Juvenile cataract.
> Cherry eye.
> "Turned" eyeball or squint.

Bones
> Deformity of the jaw (craniomandibular
> osteopathy).
> Hemivertebra.
> Slipping kneecap (patella luxation).

Cancer
> Mastocytoma.
> Pituitary tumor.
> Mast cell tumors.

Boxer

Eye
> Extra eyelashes.
> • Boxer ulcer (corneal epithelial erosion).

Heart and blood vessels
> Aortic stenosis.
> Pulmonic stenosis.
> Atrial septal defects.

Mouth
> Gingival hyperplasia (epulis).
> • Abnormal dentition (extra incisor teeth).

Skin
> Dermoid sinus.
> Dermoid cysts.

Tumours
> Mast cell tumors.
> Histiocytoma.

Kidneys
> Cystine crystals in urine.

Briard

Eye
> Extra eyelashes.
> CRA (central retinal atrophy).
> Oversized eyelid opening.

Bones
> Hip dysplasia.

Brittany Spaniel

Eye
> Retinal detachment (dysplasia).

Brussells Griffon

Eye
> Extra lashes.

Bulldog

(See English Bulldog)

Bull Mastiff

Eye
> Entropion.
> Folded out third eyelid.
> Diamond eye (greatly oversized eyelid
> opening).

Teeth
> Abnormal dentition (extra incisor).

Bull Terrier

Ear
> • Deafness.

Abdomen
> • Umbilical hernia.
> Inguinal and midline hernias.

Cairn Terrier

Kidney
> Cystine crystals in urine.

Blood
> Hemophilia.

Abdomen
> Inguinal hernia.

Eye
> Extra lashes.
> PRA (progressive retinal atrophy).
> Glaucoma (due to lens dislocation).

Brain and eye
> Globoid cell leukodystrophy
> (Krabbe's disease).

Bone/jaw
> Craniomandibular osteopathy.

• High incidence in each breed

Chesapeake Bay Retriever

Eye

Entropion.
Folded-out third eyelid.
Juvenile cataract.
PRA (progressive retinal atrophy).
CRA (central retinal atrophy).

Chihuahua

Eye

Corneal degeneration (dystrophy).
Thin iris (iris atrophy).
Dry eye (KCS keratoconjunctivitis sicca).
Glaucoma (due to dislocation of lens).
Deviated eyelashes (trichiasis).

Brain

• Hemophilia.

Blood

Haemophilia.

Heart

Pulmonic stenosis.
Mitral valve defects.

Windpipe

Collapsed trachea.

Bones

• Patella luxation.
Dislocation of the shoulder.

Chow Chow

Eye

Displaced tear duct openings
(lacrimal puncta).
Entropion (eyelids rolled in at the outer
angle of the eyelids or lateral canthus).
• Narrow eyelid opening.
Oversized eyelid opening.
PPM (persistent pupillary membrane).
• Redundant forehead skin.

Clumber Spaniel

Eye

Diamond eye (greatly oversized
eyelid opening).

Cocker Spaniel (American and English)

Eye

Absent tear drainage.
• Droopy lower lids (ectropion).
• Entropion.
Upper lid entropion.

• Redundant skin of the forehead.
Extra lashes.
• Oversized eyelid opening.
• Oversized upper eyelashes.
Cherry eye.
Corneal degeneration (dystrophy).
Juvenile cataract.
Glaucoma (abnormal drainage angle).
Glaucoma (due to lens dislocation).
PPM (persistent pupillary membrane).
PRA (progressive retinal atrophy).
Retinal detachment (dysplasia).
Underdeveloped optic nerve.

Brain

Hydrocephalus.

Kidney

Renal cortical hypoplasia.

Heart

Patent ductus arteriosus.

Mouth

Clefts of lip and palate.
Overshot and undershot jaw.

Bones

• Hip dysplasia.
Intervertebral disc disease.

Abdomen

Umbilical hernia.

Behavior

• Behavioral abnormalities.

Collie (Rough or Scotch)

Eye

• Extra eyelashes.
Entropion (related to enlarged eye socket
or orbit).
Corneal degeneration (dystrophy).
Pinkish "lumps" on the eyeball (proliferative
keratoconjunctivitis).
PPM (persistent pupillary membrane).
Small eye (microphthalmia).
• Collie eye anomaly (ectasia syndrome).
• PRA (progressive retinal atrophy).
CRA (central retinal atrophy).
Retinal detachment (dysplasia).
Underdeveloped optic nerve.

Ear

Deafness.

Brain

Epilepsy.

*Look in the glossary for an explanation of technical terms.

Blood
> Haemophilia.

Abdomen
> Umbilical hernia.
> Inguinal hernia.

Nose
> • Nasal solar dermatitis.

Curly Coated Retriever

Eye
> Entropion.

Dachshund

Eye
> Hairy growth (conjunctival dermoid).
> Extra lashes.
> Corneal ulcer.
> Glaucoma (inherited defect in the
>   drainage angle).
> Inflamed cornea (chronic superficial
>   keratitis).
> Dry eye (keratoconjunctivitis sicca).
> PPM (persistent pupillary membrane).
> PRA (progressive retinal atrophy).
> Underdeveloped optic nerve.

Ear
> Deafness.

Abdomen
> Diabetes mellitus.

Mouth
> Clefts of lip and palate.
> Overshot and undershot jaw
>   (Longhaired Dachshund).

Spine
> • Intervertebral disc disease.

Kidney
> Renal cortical hypoplasia.
> Cystine crystals in urine.

Dachshund (Miniature)

Eyes
> Inflamed cornea (chronic superficial
>   keratitis).
> PRA (progressive retinal atrophy).
> Extra lashes.

Dalmatian

Ear
> • Deafness.

Brain and eye
> Globoid cell leukodystrophy
>   (Krabbe's disease).

Kidney
> • Excess uric acid excretion.

Skin
> • Atopic (allergic) dermatitis.

Eye
> Hairy growth (conjunctival dermoid).

Dandie Dinmont Terrier

Eye
> Subluxated lens.

Doberman Pinscher

Kidney
> Renal cortical hypoplasia.

Eye
> • Deepset eyes due to oversized eye socket
>   (enlarged orbit).
> Folded-out third eyelid.
> PPM (persistent pupillary membrane).

English Bulldog

Brain
> Water on the brain (hydrocephalus).

Pelvis
> • Small birth canal, therefore difficult birth.

Heart
> Pulmonic stenosis.
> Mitral valve defects.

Windpipe
> Underdeveloped windpipe.

Mouth
> Clefts of lip and palate.
> • Abnormal dentition (extra incisor tooth).

Spine
> Hemivertebra.

Eye
> • Redundant forehead skin.
> • Oversized lid opening.
> • Entropion (lower lid, medial entropion,
>   lateral entropion).
> • Droopy lower lids (ectropion).
> • Extra lashes.
> PPM (persistent pupillary membrane).

Head
> • Excessive facial folds.
> • Overlong soft palate

---

*Look in the glossary for an explanation of technical terms.   • High incidence in each breed

English Setter

Blood
Haemophilia
Eye
Cataract.
• Droopy lower lids (ectropion).
Entropion.
Brain and eye
Storage diseases due to enzyme deficiency.

Foxhound

Spine
Osteochondrosis of the spine.
Ear
Deafness.

Fox Terrier (smooth and wire-haired)

Eye
Extra lashes.
Deviated eyelashes (seen in Toy Fox Terrier).
Corneal degeneration (dystrophy—seen in Wire-haired Terriers).
Corneal ulcer (seen in Wire-haired Terriers).
Juvenile cataract.
• Glaucoma (due to lens dislocation).
Ear
Deafness.
Brain
Ataxia.
Heart
Pulmonic stenosis.
Bones
Dislocation of the shoulder.
Throat
Oesophageal achalasia (seen in Wire-haired Terriers).
Goitre.
Skin
• Atopic dermatitis (seen in Wire-haired Terriers).

French Bulldog
Spine
Hemivertebra.

German Shepherd Dog

Eye
Hairy growth on eye (dermoid).
Folded out third eyelid (eversion of the third eyelid).
Inflammation of the third eyelid.
• Red mass on the cornea (chronic superficial keratitis, degenerative pannus).

Senile cataract.
Brain
Epilepsy.
Kidney
Renal cortical hypoplasia.
Cystine crystals in urine.
Blood
Hemophilia.
Heart
Persistent right aortic arch.
Mouth
Clefts of lip and palate.
Gullet
Esophageal achalasia.
Behavior
Behavioral abnormalities.
Bones
Hip dysplasia.
Skin
Anal furunculosis.

German Shorthaired Pointer

Eye
Extra lashes.
Corneal degeneration (dystrophy).
Entropion.
Folded-out third eyelid.
Turned eyeball (strabismus).
Lymph system
Lymphoedema
Blood vessel
Subaortic stenosis.
Brain and eye
Storage disease due to enzmye deficiency.

Giant breeds

Bones
Osteogenic sarcoma.
Elbow dysplasia.
Hip dysplasia.

Golden Retriever

Eye
• Cataract.
PRA (progressive retinal atrophy).
CRA (central retinal atrophy).
Extra lashes.
Entropion (lower lid and lateral entropion).
Bones
Hip dysplasia.

Gordon Setter

Eye
- Entropion.
  Droopy lower lids (ectropion).
- PRA (progressive retinal atrophy).

Great Dane

Eye
  Extra lashes.
- Droopy lower lids (ectropion) due to
    oversized eyelid opening.
- Entropion (includes entropion related to
    oversized eye socket [enlarged orbit] and
    entropion unrelated to orbit size).
- Third eyelid turned in and turned out.
  Primary glaucoma (abnormal
    drainage angle).
  Retinal displacement (dysplasia) in
    the Harlequin Dane.

Ear
  Deafness.
Kidney
  Cystine crystals in urine.
Heart
  Mitral valve defects.

Greyhound

Eye
- Inflamed cornea (chronic
    superficial keratitis).
  PPM (persistent pupillary membrane).
  GRD (retinal degeneration).
Pelvis
  Predisposition to difficult whelping.
Blood
  Hemophilia.

Griffon, Brussels

Bones
  Dislocation of the shoulder.

Irish Setter

Eye
  Corneal degeneration (dystrophy).
  Extra lashes.
- Deepset eyes due to enlarged eye socket
    (orbit).
  PPM (persistent
    pupillary membrane).

rod-cone dysplasia).
- PRA (progressive retinal atrophy,
Paralysis and blindness
  Quadriplegia with amblyopia.
Blood
  Haemophilia.
Chest
  Persistent right aortic arch.
Muscles
  Generalized muscle disease (myopathy).

Irish Terrier

Kidney
  Cystine crystals in urine.

Jack Russell Terrier

Eye
- Lens dislocation leading to glaucoma.
Movement
  Lack of balance (ataxia).

Keeshond

Brain
  Epilepsy.
Heart
  Tetralogy of Fallot.
  Mitral valve defects.
Eye
  Extra lashes.

Kerry Blue Terrier

Eye
  Extra lashes.
  Entropion.
- Narrow eyelid opening.
  Deviated eyelashes of upper lid.
  Dry eye (keratoconjunctivitis sicca).

King Charles Spaniel

Abdomen
  Diabetes mellitus.
Eye
  Extra lashes.
- Medial entropion.

King Charles Spaniel, Cavalier

Eye
- Extra lashes.
  Oversized eyelid opening.

Labrador Retriever

Eye
  CRA (central retinal atrophy).
  Cloudy cornea (corneal opacity).
  Extra lashes.
  Entropion.
  Juvenile cataract.
  Retinal detachment (dysplasia).
Kidney
  Cystine crystals in urine.
Blood
  Hemophilia.
Bone
  Deformity of the jaw
    (craniomandibular osteopathy).
  Dislocation above the front paw
    (carpal subluxation).
  • Hip dysplasia.

Lakeland Terrier

Eye
  Extra lashes.
  Dislocated lens leading to glaucoma.

Lhasa Apso

Kidney
  Renal cortical hypoplasia.
Abdomen
  Inguinal hernia.
Eye
  Extra lashes.
  • Entropion (medial entropion).
  • Long eyelid hair.
  • Dry eye (keratoconjunctivitis sicca).
  • Poorly developed eye socket

Manchester Terrier

Eye
  Glaucoma due to dislocation of the lens.

Mastiff

Eye
  Droopy lower lids (ectropion).
  Entropion.
  PPM (persistent pupillary membrane).

Mexican, Turkish and Chinese Breeds

Skin
  Hairlessness.

Miniature Breeds

Pelvis
  • Predisposition to difficult birth (dystocia).
Throat
  • Collapsed trachea.

Miniature Pinscher

Bones
  • Dislocation of the shoulder.
Eyes
  Entropion (medial entropion).
  Dry eye (keratoconjunctivitis sicca).
  PRA (progressive retinal atrophy).

Miniature and Toy Poodle

Eye
  Absent tear duct (atresia of lacrimal puncta
    and nasolacrimal duct).
  • Watery eye/facial staining.
  • Extra lashes.
  • Overly long hairs (on the eyelid skin) and
    overly long upper lashes.
  • Entropion (medial entropion).
  Inflamed cornea (chronic superficial
    keratitis in Miniature Poodles).
  Corneal degeneration (dystrophy).
  Thin iris (iris atrophy).
  Juvenile cataract.
  Small eye (microphthalmia).
  Glaucoma (primary narrow-angle glaucoma).
  • PRA (progressive retinal atrophy, rod-cone
    degeneration).
  Day blindness (Miniature Poodles).
  Underdeveloped optic nerve
    (Miniature Poodles).
Brain and eye
  Globoid cell leukodystrophy
    (Krabbe's disease).
Kidney
  Cystine crystals in urine.
Chest
  Patent ductus arteriosus.
Skin
  Partial hair loss (alopecia).

• High incidence in each breed

*Look in the glossary for an explanation of technical terms.

Bones
Achondroplasia.
- Patella luxation.
Dislocation of the shoulder.

Abdomen
Diabetes mellitus (Miniature).

Throat
Collapsed windpipe

Behavior
- Behavioral abnormalities.

Miniature Schnauzer

Eye
Absent tear drainage apparatus.
Corneal degeneration (dystrophy).
Extra lashes.
Juvenile cataract.
Small eye (microphthalmia).
PPM (persistent pupillary membrane).

Heart
Pulmonic stenosis.

Newfoundland

Eye
- Droopy lower lid.
- Entropion.
- Folded-out cartilage of the third eyelid.
- Oversized eye socket (orbit).
- Oversized eyelid opening.

Heart
Subaortic stenosis.

Norwegian Dunkerhund

Eye
Small eye (microphthalmia).

Ear
Deafness.

Norwegian Elkhound

Eye
Extra lashes.
Glaucoma.
- PRA (progressive retinal atrophy).

Kidney
Small kidneys (renal cortical hypoplasia).

Old English Sheepdog

Eye
- Extra lashes.
Cataract (congenital).

PRA (progressive retinal atrophy).

Pekingese

Eye
Absent tear drainage apparatus.
- Extra lashes.
- Entropion (medial entropion).
- Hairy caruncle.
- Nasal fold irritation (trichiasis).
- Pigment on cornea.
Corneal ulceration.
Deviated eyelashes.
- Oversized eyelid opening.
- Poorly developed eye socket.

Bones
- Patella dislocation.

Pointer

Eye
- Entropion.
PRA (progressive retinal atrophy).

Abdomen
Umbilical hernia.

Pomeranian

Eye
Absent tear duct.
Extra lashes.
Watery eye.
Deviated eyelashes.

Bones
- Patella luxation.
Dislocation of the shoulder.

Chest
Patent ductus arteriosus.
Windpipe (tracheal) collapse.

Pug

Eye
Extra eyelashes.
Entropion (medial entropion).
Deviated eyelashes.
Hairy caruncle.
Pigment on the cornea.
Corneal degeneration (dystrophy).

Pyrenean Mountain Dog

Eye
Droopy lower lids (ectropion).
Entropion.

PPM (persistent pupillary membrane).

Redbone Coonhound

Eye
> CRA (central retinal atrophy).

Rhodesian Ridgeback

Skin
> Dermoid sinus.

Eye
> Extra eyelashes.
> Entropion.

Rottweiler

Eye
> Entropion.
> • Oversized eyelids.
> • Oversized socket (orbit).
> Retinal displacement (dysplasia).

Abdomen
> Diabetes mellitus.

Bones
> • Hip dysplasia.
> • Tendency to osteochondritis dissecans.

St Bernard

Eye
> Hairy growth (dermoid).
> Extra lashes.
> • Droopy lids.
> • Entropion.
> Third eyelid turned in or turned out.
> • Oversized eyelid opening.
> • Oversized eye socket (orbit).
> • Redundant forehead skin.
> Redundant facial skin.

Blood
> Hemophilia.

Bones
> • Hip dysplasia.

Saluki

Eye
> Glaucoma (abnormal drainage angle).
> PPM (persistent pupillary membrane).
> PRA (progressive retinal atrophy).
> Retinal detachment.

Samoyed

Eye
> • Extra lashes.
> Glaucoma.
> PPM (persistent pupillary membrane).
> • PRA (progressive retinal atrophy).
> Retinal displacement (dysplasia).

Blood
> Hemophilia.

Heart
> Pulmonic stenosis.
> Atrial septal defects.

Abdomen
> Diabetes mellitus.

Schipperke

Eye
> Entropion.
> Narrow eyelid opening.

Schnauzer

Eye
> PHPV (persistent hyperplastic primary vitreous).

Scottish Terrier

Eye
> PPM (persistent pupillary membrane).

Ear
> Deafness.

Muscles
> "Scottie cramp" syndrome.

Kidney
> Cystine crystals in urine.

Womb
> Failure to express pups at term (uterine inertia).

Bones
> Deformity of the jaw (craniomandibular osteopathy).
> Achondroplasia.

Skin
> Atopic dermatitis.
> Cancer (melanoma).

Sealyham Terrier

Eye
> Absent tear duct.

---

*Look in the glossary for an explanation of technical terms.

• High incidence in each breed

Cataract.
Glaucoma due to lens dislocation.
Retinal detachment (dysplasia).

Shetland Sheepdog

Eye
Corneal degeneration (dystrophy).
• Extra eyelashes.
PPM (persistent pupillary membrane).
• Collie eye anomaly (ectasia syndrome).
CRA (central retinal atrophy).
Blood
Hemophilia.
Chest
Patent ductus arteriosus.
Bones
Hip dysplasia.
Nose
Nasal solar dermatitis.

Shiba Inu

Bones
Short spine.

Shih Tzu

Eye
Entropion (medial entropion).
• Poorly developed eye socket.
Kidney
Renal cortical hypoplasia.
Mouth
Clefts of lip and palate.

Short-nosed breeds

Nose
Small nose and elongated soft palate.
Pituitary gland
Pituitary cysts.

Siberian Husky

Eye
Corneal degeneration (dystrophy).
PPM (persistent pupillary membrane).

Silky Terriers, Australian

Eye
Cataracts.

Silver-grey Collie

Blood
Cyclic neutropenia.
Eye
Deformed eyeball.

Skye Terrier

Throat
Underdeveloped larynx (hypoplasia).

Springer Spaniel

Eye
Extra lashes.
Droopy lower lid (ectropion).
PPM (persistent pupillary membrane).
PRA (progressive retinal atrophy).
CRA (central retinal atrophy).
Faulty development of retina
(retinal dysplasia).
Skin
Skin weakness (hyperelasticity, fragility).

Staffordshire Bull Terrier

Eye
Juvenile cataract.

Staffordshire Terrier

Mouth
Cleft lip and palate.

Standard Poodle

Eye
Cataract.
Oversized eye socket (orbit).
• Oversized eyelid opening.

Swedish Laphund

Limbs
Neuronal abiotrophy.

Tibetan Terrier

Eye
Lens dislocation.
PPM (persistent pupillary membrane).
PRA (progressive retinal atrophy).

*Look in the glossary for an explanation of technical terms.   • High incidence in each breed

Toy Breeds

Brain
Glycogen storage disease.
Windpipe
Windpipe collapse (especially Toy Poodle).
Skin
Cancer (melanoma).

Toy Poodle *(See also Miniature and Toy Poodle)*

Toy Terrier

Eye
Lens dislocation.

Vizsla

Blood
Hemophilia.

Weimaraner

Eye
Extra lashes.
Oversized eye socket (orbit).
Entropion.
Third eyelid turned in or out.
Blood
Hemophilia.
Abdomen
Umbilical hernia.

Welsh Corgi

Eye
• Corneal ulcer.
PPM (persistent pupillary membrane).
Glaucoma due to dislocated lens.
PRA (progressive retinal atrophy).
CRA (central retinal atrophy).
Pelvis
Predisposition to difficult birth due
to narrow birth canal (dystocia).
Kidney
Cystine crystals in urine.
Behavior
• Behavioral abnormalities.

Welsh Terrier

Eye
Glaucoma due to dislocated lens.
Overlong eyelashes.

West Highland White Terrier

Brain and eye
Globoid cell leukodystrophy.
Bones
Deformity of the jaw
(craniomandibular osteopathy).
Abdomen
Inguinal hernia.
Skin
• Atopic dermatitis.

Whippet

Skin
Partial alopecia.

White dogs of various breeds

• Deafness.

Yorkshire Terrier

Eye
Extra lashes.
Dry eye (keratoconjunctivitis sicca).
Retinal displacement (dysplasia).
Bones
• Patella dislocation.

Most breeds

Testicles
• Undescended testicles (cryptorchidism).

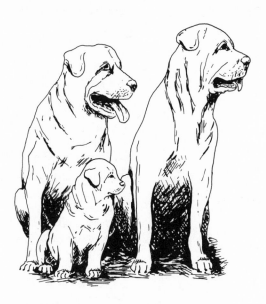

IMPORTING DOGS FREE OF INHERITED FAULTS

A veterinary certificate stating the bloodline is free of inherited diseases helps to make sure your new pup will not suffer later from the results of careless breeding.

Contact your vet to determine what inherited faults exist in the breed of your choice $\longrightarrow$ For some diseases you may be referred to a specialist

$\downarrow$ $\downarrow$

Contact overseas or interstate veterinarians to represent *your* interest *before* you buy and carry out an independent examination of breeding stock—sire, dam and progeny from which you intend to buy.

$\swarrow$ $\searrow$

Certificate issued that stud is free of inherited disease

Examination suggests inherited fault may exist

$\downarrow$ $\downarrow$

Sale continues   Cancelled sale

Veterinary advice is essential *before* you import breeding stock.

SHOWING AND INHERITED DEFECTS

The aim of showing is supposedly to improve the overall standard of the breed. Special status is given to the stud animals of future generations.

It is the dogs which prove themselves in the show ring which are used as a basis for the next generation, so it is vital that any dogs which have, or carry, inherited defects are not allowed the opportunity to gain status in the show ring, and thus become "in demand" for stud use.

Acceptance of dogs with inherited defects such as PRA and collie eye anomaly, small dogs with chronic patella luxation or larger dogs with hip dysplasia can be avoided by introducing compulsory certification of all dogs, prior to acceptance in the show ring.

Certificates for show dogs

Before acceptance in the ring, veterinary certification is needed in those breeds prone to inherited diseases (p. 38-49).

The certificate indicates:

• Freedom from the inherited defect. (Many are not obvious, such as hip dysplasia, extra lashes, PRA, collie eye anomaly.)

• Temporary certification of freedom. (This is for a dog not old enough for permanent certification. See PRA p. 184-6.)

• Freedom from the carrier state. (Complete genetic freedom from the disease, p. 37.)

An alternative method would be to require veterinary certification before a dog may be awarded a Championship title. Preferably, the family from which the show entrant comes should be certified free of inherited defects.

Can some defects be allowed in the show ring?

Yes. *Non*-inherited conditions such as scars (due to injury) which do not alter the conformation or mobility of the dog, nor greatly detract from the dog's appearance can be accepted. Some "battle" scars incurred in the life of a working dog should certainly not cost him show points. In the same way a spayed bitch may be shown if the removal of the ovaries and womb was necessary to save her life.

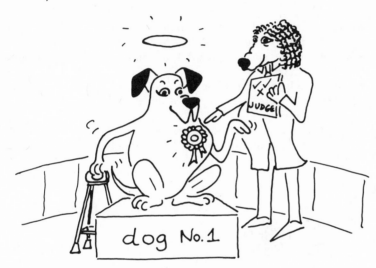

4.3 *Dogs have been shown with hidden or disfigured inherited defects, to the detriment of that breed.*

Exercise tolerance

We hardly need to emphasize that a dog must be able to run around without distress. A simple test of nose, windpipe, heart and lungs is to put the dog through vigorous exercise before acceptance. Snuffly or difficult breathing or excessive panting suggest disqualification.

Pre-show vision test

Dogs with collie eye anomaly have been presented in the show ring with one blind eye. In dogs which are prone to collie eye anomaly (Scotch Collie and Shetland Sheepdog) vision can be tested prior to acceptance.

4.4 *Blind dogs have actually won at shows. A vision test should be part of a potential champion's examination*

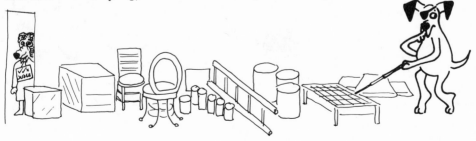

Test the dog through an obstacle (maze) course (Fig. 4:4) in light and also in the dark with one eye covered at a time (hurdles may be used as well). Use a piece of black cloth over each eye in turn.

Check points of examination by the show judge for risky conformation and possible disease.

Head

- Are there any folds where skin disease may start?
- Is the forehead skin tight when the head is lowered?
- Are there any skin folds which may allow the eyelids to fall onto the eyeball? (Fig. 4:5)

Eyes

- Are the eyelids tight on the eyeball?
- Is the eyelid opening the correct size?
- No folds in the eyelid edge? Pull the outer angle of the eye to test for the correct eyelid opening size. (Fig. 4:6)
- Are the eyelid hairs or lashes too long?
- Is the eye bloodshot? A red eye means disease.
- Is the eye watery?
- Are the pupils the same size? Are the pupils small in bright light?
- Are the eyes pigmented (dark)? They should be.
- Do the eyes move together?

4.5 *Excessive folds — especially obvious in a lowered head*

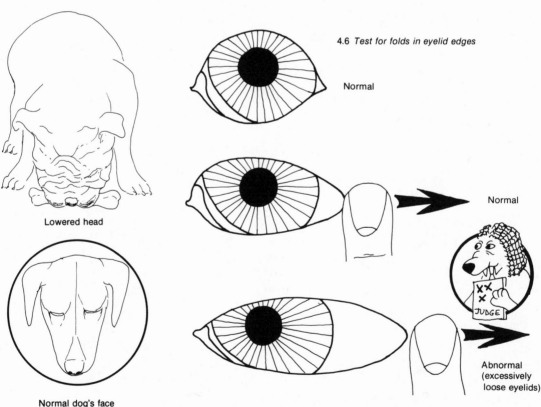

Lowered head

Normal dog's face

4.6 *Test for folds in eyelid edges*

Normal

Normal

Abnormal (excessively loose eyelids)

Teeth and mouth

- How many incisor teeth? Twelve is the correct number. (Fig. 4:7)
- Are they straight?
- Do the teeth meet exactly (or at least touch)?
- Are the gums a normal pink color? (Fig. 4:8)

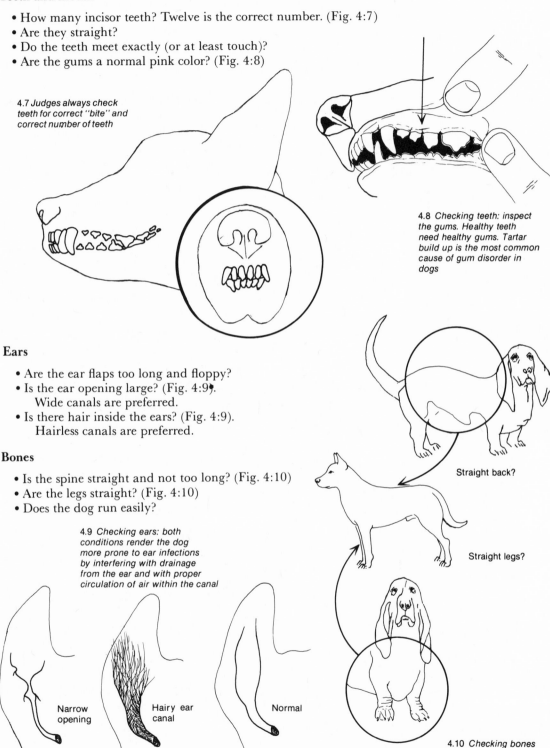

4.7 Judges always check teeth for correct "bite" and correct number of teeth

4.8 Checking teeth: inspect the gums. Healthy teeth need healthy gums. Tartar build up is the most common cause of gum disorder in dogs

Ears

- Are the ear flaps too long and floppy?
- Is the ear opening large? (Fig. 4:9). Wide canals are preferred.
- Is there hair inside the ears? (Fig. 4:9). Hairless canals are preferred.

Bones

- Is the spine straight and not too long? (Fig. 4:10)
- Are the legs straight? (Fig. 4:10)
- Does the dog run easily?

4.9 Checking ears: both conditions render the dog more prone to ear infections by interfering with drainage from the ear and with proper circulation of air within the canal

Narrow opening

Hairy ear canal

Normal

Straight back?

Straight legs?

4.10 Checking bones

53

Testicles

• Are both present? Do they feel the same?

Body

• Any excessive skin folds?
• Any skin disease?
• Is the skin correctly pigmented, especially around the eyes and nose?

Tail

• Can it move freely?

4.11 Checking testicles: two testicles of current size and consistency must be present

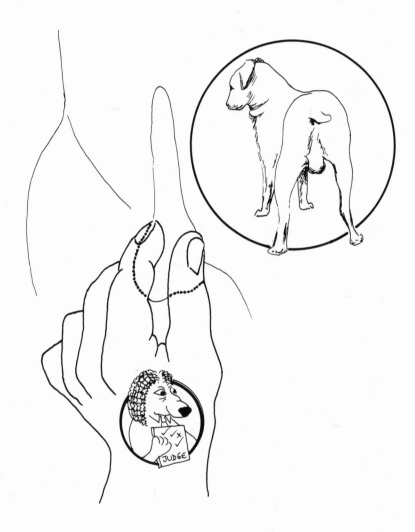

5. The young pup

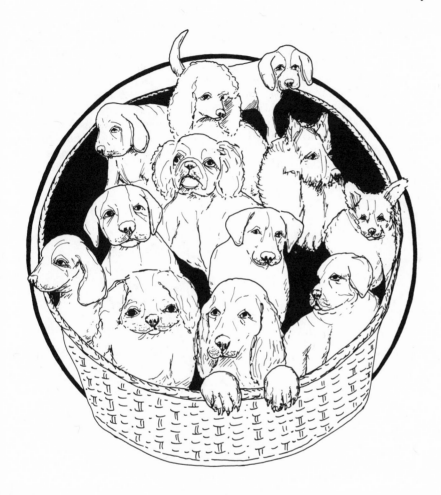

SELECTING A PUP

The age to buy a pup

The best age to bring a pup home is between 6 and 18 weeks, preferably between 6 and 12 weeks. It is at this age that the pup will form the closest attachment to you and at which you can commence to train him to eat and behave as you want. Refer to p. 241-4 for behavior in pups.

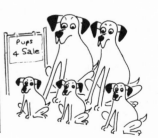

> Before you buy, look at the parents and other progeny as this is more significant than a study of the pedigree.

Which breed should I buy?

Think hard about what you want a dog for. Will you jog with your dog and always give him a daily run in the park? No? Then get a small breed. Will you groom your dog constantly? No? Then do *not* get an Afghan or a Cocker Spaniel. Will you take him to the country? Yes? Then get a short-coated, easy to wash dog. Do you want a lovable pet free of inherited disease? Make out a list of which breeds you prefer and look up a list of inherited diseases these breeds suffer from (see p. 38). Ask your vet to recommend studs free of inherited disease. At any stud you visit, it is more important to ask to see a veterinary certificate of freedom from these diseases than it is to look at the stud's show ribbons. A mongrel (cross-bred) may be ideal for you. (Cross-breds have less inherited diseases than the pure-breds.) Do you live in a flat? Yes? Your dog must be small. Do you want a watchdog for your business? Nobody gets past a Rottweiler or Australian Cattle dog (Queensland Heeler) on guard.

5.3 *Pups can be a health risk to young children and should be treated for roundworm on their arrival home*

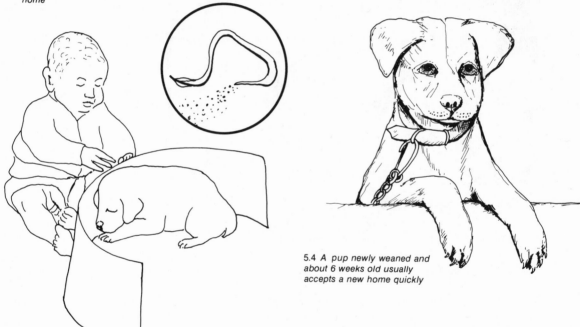

5.4 *A pup newly weaned and about 6 weeks old usually accepts a new home quickly*

Should I get a small or large dog?

In the city a small dog is usually better, cheaper to feed, requires less space and less exercise. Also a small dog passes far less feces than a large animal. This is certainly a consideration in built-up areas.

What about the choice of coat color?

Generally speaking it is better to select a dark coat color. Dogs with light color tend to have more skin trouble.

What about the shape of the ears?

Small upright short-haired ears are better than long floppy hairy ears. Floppy ears produce more ear disease.

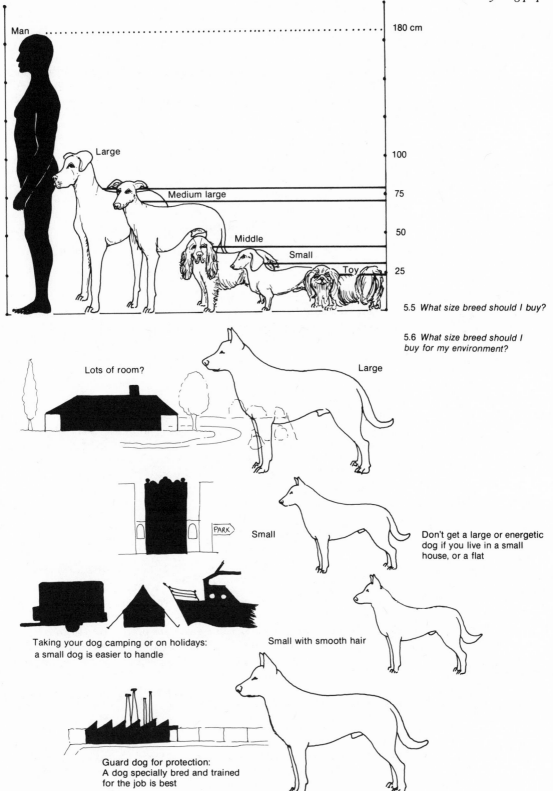

Man .... 180 cm

Large

100

Medium large

75

50

Middle

Small

25

Toy

Lots of room? Large

5.5 *What size breed should I buy?*

5.6 *What size breed should I buy for my environment?*

Don't get a large or energetic dog if you live in a small house, or a flat

PARK

Small

Taking your dog camping or on holidays: a small dog is easier to handle

Small with smooth hair

Guard dog for protection: A dog specially bred and trained for the job is best

57

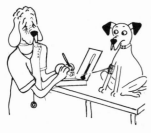

5.7 *Veterinary examination: before you buy have your prospective pet examined by an expert*

Should I have a pure-breed or a cross-breed?

A big advantage of buying a cross-breed (or a mongrel) is that the cross-breed is more likely to be free of inherited disease than many of the pure-breeds. Also, when two different pure-breeds are crossed we get what is known as hybrid vigour, that is, you often get the best of both parents in the progeny (see p. 203).

How do I know my new pup is healthy?

Before you buy, request that the sale is cancelled if your new pup does not pass the examination of your own vet. This makes it easy to return the new pup to the breeder if your vet finds fault.

How do I know how my pup will turn out?

Look at the parents of your intended purchase—are they calm and well-behaved? A good temperament is the best asset.

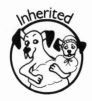

> Choose a pup from a family which is free of inherited diseases. Looking at adults from the same sire and dam will tell you more than the show ribbons of the parents.

Should I get a male or female dog?

It is a matter of individual preference, but spayed females often make the best pets. They stay at home and are usually more devoted. Male dogs, unless intended for breeding, can be castrated at 6 months and then will make a good stay-at-home pet. A roaming dog is more prone to car accidents, dog fights and periods in the dog pound. Sexy male dogs tend to ride young children and males constantly urinate to mark their territory.

> Desexed dogs are the best pets for suburbia.

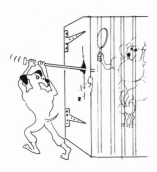

5.8 *A bitch on heat is almost irresistable to male dogs — and they are hard to keep apart. Desexed males and females make the best pets*

Should I have a dog with long or short hair?

Long-haired animals require very much more attention than short-haired dogs, and are more easily affected by heat, ticks, and grass seeds in the country. Buy a short-haired dog unless you are prepared to devote a great deal of time to the care of his coat. Long-haired dogs generally suffer from skin diseases, ear problems and are more worried by fleas and grass seeds in the coat

Owner examination when selecting the pup

• Check the dog for fleas. A pup covered with fleas tells you that the breeder is careless.

• Hold the pup in your hand and feel his weight as compared with the other pups. Do not choose the runt of the litter, even if he is the most appealing.

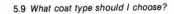

5.9 *What coat type should I choose?*

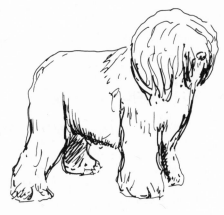

Long:
Old English Sheepdog
Afghan Hound
Collie
Chow Chow
Maltese
Samoyed
Yorkshire Terrier

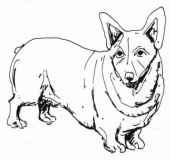

Medium length:
Corgis
Cairn Terrier
German Shepherd Dog
Labrador Retriever
Saluki
Spaniels

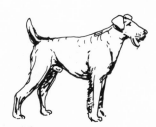

Short coat:
Whippet
Basset Hound
Beagle
Boxer
Smooth Dachshund
Greyhound
Pointer
Pug

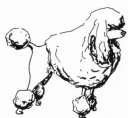

Woolly-haired:
Poodles
Wheaten Terrier
Komondor
Bichon Frise

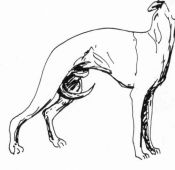

Wire-haired:
Airedale Terrier
Sealyham
Griffon
Irish Wolfhound
Schnauzer

• Check his mouth. Is the lower jaw longer or shorter than the upper?
• The eyes (inside the eyeball) should be the same color and the lids should be darkly pigmented. Eyelids should tightly fit the eyeball.
• Make sure the teeth are in line. When the mouth shuts, the upper and lower teeth should meet.
• The gums should be a healthy, pink color.
• Smell the ears. A bad smell means an infection inside the ear. If the pup is shaking his head, this suggests ear mites.
• Look at the tummy near the "belly button." Feel the abdomen for hernia, which will show as a lump in the middle part of the stomach around the navel region.
• Check that the tail is straight. Run your fingers down it to make sure it has no kinks.
• Examine all four legs and count the toes. The dog should have four toes and most breeds have one dew claw on the inside of each leg (see p. 138). Dew claws are often removed, especially if they are large as in German Shepherds.

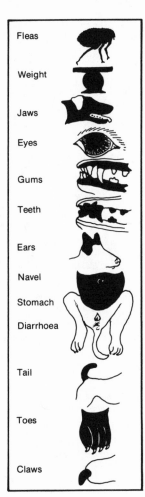

| Fleas |
| Weight |
| Jaws |
| Eyes |
| Gums |
| Teeth |
| Ears |
| Navel |
| Stomach |
| Diarrhoea |
| Tail |
| Toes |
| Claws |

5.10 *Owner's check list*

• Make sure there are no signs of diarrhea around the tail area. (Look at the other puppies to ensure that they are not suffering from diarrhea.)

CARING FOR THE NEW PUP

When your new pup arrives home, let him quietly make himself familiar with his new surroundings. Remember he is away from his mother and litter mates, probably for the first time, and after the initial excitement of a new place will feel a little forlorn and lost.

Handle him gently. When lifting him, put one hand under his rump and the other under his chest. Small puppies may be lifted by the scruff of the neck, the way the mother does.

Introduce him to his bed—somewhere warm and quiet that is free of draughts. Get him into proper routine early on and do not make the mistake of letting him sleep on your bed "just for the first night."

Pups tend to operate at one of two speeds—stop or go. They become very tired and at this time the children must leave the pup alone. The new pup needs undisturbed rest and sleep. Most pups will whimper or cry at first when left alone at night. Do not rush in too quickly to comfort him or you will often only prolong the settling-in period.

A loud ticking clock near his bed often helps the new pup to settle in more easily. Some people believe that the ticking clock substitutes for his mother's heart beat.

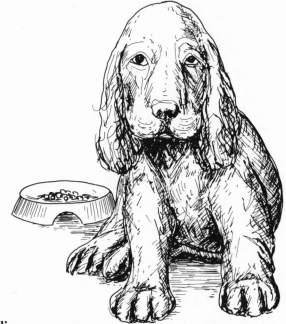

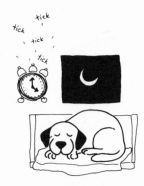

5.12 *A ticking clock soothes most pups*

Feeding

Feeding the pup is simple, as long as a few guidelines are followed.

Try to find out what the pup was fed before he came to you, and if possible start him off on a similar diet. A sudden change of diet, added to the stress of a new home, frequently results in diarrhea.

Changes in diet should be made gradually.

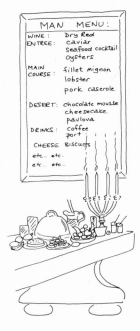

Dog food

In the United States, most vets, pet shops, breeders, and veterinary colleges recommend commercial dog food over a diet of "people food." The contents of commercial foods are regulated, and will provide a balanced diet for your pup.

Special puppy foods are marketed. They do contain a higher mixture of protein than "adult dog food," but veterinarians will tell you that regular dog food is equally good for puppies.

If you do put together a diet for your pup, remember that dogs need more than just meat. They require a balance of protein and carbohydrate and more vitamins and minerals than can be found even in the best steak. Meat, eggs, and vegetables should be cooked.

Milk

Milk is a good liquid food and most pups thrive on it. Unfortunately, it does not agree with all pups, so if your pup develops diarrhea when fed milk, you may have to water the milk down or feed him skim milk. If he still has diarrhea and milk seems to be the cause, then stop the milk altogether.

Water

Always provide plenty of fresh clean drinking water.

A commercial dog food diet is better for your pup than a diet of "people food."

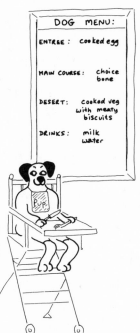

Specimen menu for a pup aged 6-12 weeks

Breakfast: Cereal, milk or puppy meal or Farex.
Lunch: Feed a selection of: minced meat, mashed table scraps, a few cooked vegetables, cooked egg, semi-moist commercial foods, dry puppy foods or canned food (chopped finely).
Tea: As for lunch, plus milk.
Bedtime: As for lunch, plus milk and cereal.

Supplements to a pup's diet

Vitamins: Although not essential if you are feeding a balanced diet, adding children's vitamin drops to the bedtime meal will overcome any deficiencies.

Vitamin supplements are very helpful in a pup that is sick or recovering from a sickness or accident. Use children's vitamin drops and give 5-15 drops daily according to size.

5.13 *Always feed your puppy a simple diet*

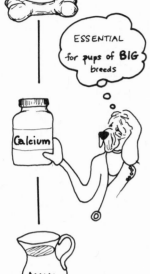

Calcium: A calcium supplement is useful in all dogs and *essential* in the breeds that mature to weighing over 60 lb (30 kg).

Use calcium carbonate powder: 1 teaspoon per ½ kg of meat fed or calcium gluconate or calcium lactate tablets. (*Dose:* 1 tablet per 5 kg bodyweight per day.)

VACCINATIONS

Temporary vaccinations may be given from 6 weeks of age onwards.

Dogs should be vaccinated against Distemper, Parvovirus and Infectious Canine Hepatitis. Rabies vaccine is needed except in Rabies-free countries such as the UK and Australia. In some areas dogs are vaccinated against Leptospirosis.

Permanent vaccinations are given at 12 weeks of age. (Although termed "permanent" the dog does need regular booster revaccinations.)

Vaccination program

This program is modified according to the areas where these diseases are a problem. In an outbreak vaccinations may be given more frequently.

Age	*Vaccine*
5-8 weeks:	Distemper Parvovirus Parainfluenza
14 weeks:	Distemper Hepatitis Leptospirosis Parainfluenza Rabies Parvovirus
15 months:	Distemper Hepatitis Leptospirosis Parainfluenza Rabies Parvovirus
Annually:	Parainfluenza Leptospirosis Parvovirus
Every 2-3 years:	Distemper Hepatitis Rabies

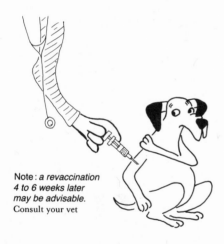

Note: *a revaccination 4 to 6 weeks later may be advisable.* Consult your vet

5.15 *Check the vaccination program given here to make sure that your pup is up to date with his injections*

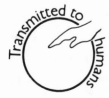

WORMING

Roundworms are a major problem in pups and all pups should be routinely treated. Pups should have had worm treatment while with the mother, but it is wise to be sure and dose the new pup yourself.

Dose with a product containing piperazine (e.g. Antoban) or as an alternative your vet may recommend pyrantel pamoate (e.g., canex). Dose at least 3 times at 21 day intervals. The dose: 100 mgm of piperazine per kg bodyweight. Tablets or syrup may be used (see p. 239).

If the pup has a lot of worms he may vomit some of them up. Otherwise, the dead worms pass out in the droppings.

Note: In some areas Roundworms are becoming resistant to drugs such as piperazine. Consult your vet for a product he recommends.

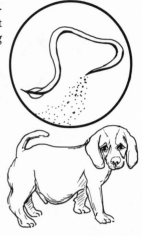

HOUSE TRAINING

See chapter on Behavior.

WASHING THE NEW PUP

Dogs do not need to be washed as often as humans. Excessive washing can leach the dog's skin of essential oils, leaving it dry and scurfy.

5.16 *Roundworms lay huge numbers of eggs daily. All pups should be routinely treated for possible roundworm infestation*

The pup's skin is very sensitive and can easily be irritated by harsh detergents, so do not use preparations designed for human use. Instead use pure soaps, without added perfumes, antiseptics or deodorants. Coconut oil shampoos or baby shampoos can also be used. Or use a product specifically designed and produced for use on pups.

In general, do not bath a pup more than once a month. Because of the pup's habit of rolling in anything with a strong smell, this rule may have to be broken, but try to minimize the number of washes you give—often a grooming with brush and comb will suffice to clean the pup.

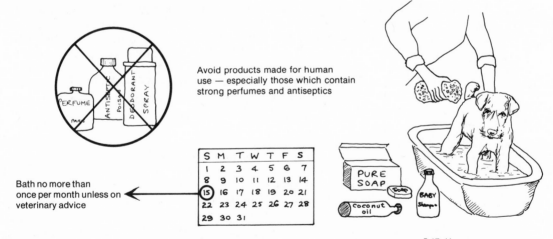

Avoid products made for human use — especially those which contain strong perfumes and antiseptics

Bath no more than once per month unless on veterinary advice

5.17 *Use pure soaps or gentle baby products*

FLEAS AND TICKS

Flea powders are the safest form of flea and tick treatment to use in the young dog. Work the powder into the coat, then take a damp cloth and wipe the surface of his coat to remove any excess that he may otherwise lick off.

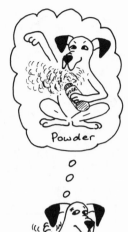

Flea rinses, flea collars and oral flea treatments should *not* be used until the pup is at least 14 weeks old and some are not used until the dog is mature. Follow the manufacturer's recommendations.

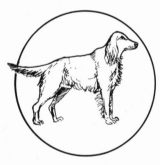

Powder

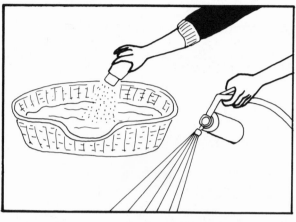

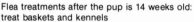

Flea treatments after the pup is 14 weeks old: treat baskets and kennels

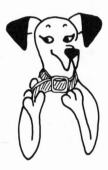

Flea collar

5.18 *Getting rid of fleas*

CAR SICKNESS (MOTION SICKNESS)

This is a common problem, especially in young dogs. Some pups (such as Irish Setter) seem especially prone to car sickness. Apprehension or fear can be a big part of the problem. Get the dog used to the car by sitting him in it while it is stationary. Most dogs gradually become accustomed to travel and the problem disappears.

Travel sickness can be controlled by giving Dramamine (25-50 mg according to size) or Acepromazine (5-10 mg for a 10 kg dog) an hour before travelling.

5.19 *Irish Setters are among the breeds most prone to car sickness*

COSMETIC SURGERY

Tail docking is unnecessary surgery to comply with demands of fashion and should not be carried out. In our opinion breed standards should be changed to state that long tails are desirable for all breeds.

Ear cropping serves no useful purpose; is a mutilation and does nothing to improve the appearance of the dog.

Plastic surgery to correct skin folds, facial folds, excess forehead skin, lip folds or incorrect eyelid position may be necessary for your dog's comfort (see p. 151-3, 168). Such animals must *not* be shown after surgery and never used for breeding.

Undescended testicles, because they represent an inherited defect, are not placed surgically in the scrotum. Do not ask your vet to rectify an undescended testicle—you are asking him to be professionally unethical.

6. Infectious diseases

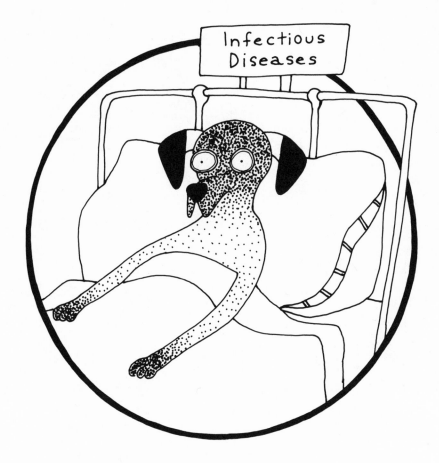

DISTEMPER (also known as "hard pad disease")

Canine distemper is a highly contagious viral infection. Dogs of any age may be affected, but young dogs are especially at risk.

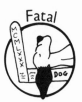

> Distemper can be a fatal disease.

Fortunately a safe and effective vaccine is available. The distemper virus also affects wild animals such as the fox, wolf, dingo, coyote, ferret, mink, skunk, badger, weasel, racoon and others.

Distemper is NOT transmissible to humans.

There are two distinct phases in the course of the disease.

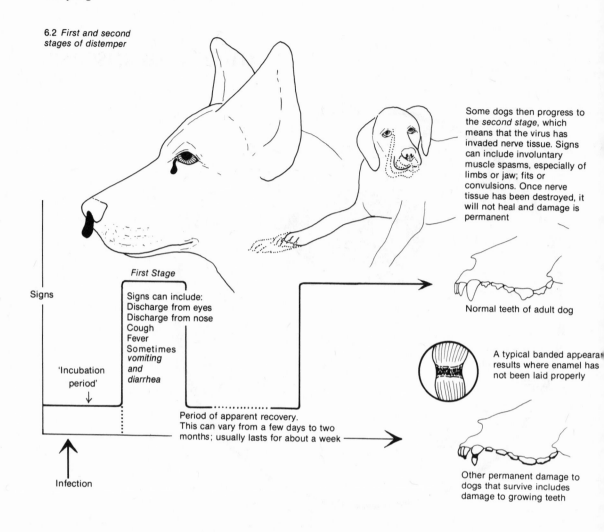

6.2 *First and second stages of distemper*

Some dogs then progress to the *second stage*, which means that the virus has invaded nerve tissue. Signs can include involuntary muscle spasms, especially of limbs or jaw; fits or convulsions. Once nerve tissue has been destroyed, it will not heal and damage is permanent

First Stage

Signs

Signs can include:
Discharge from eyes
Discharge from nose
Cough
Fever
Sometimes *vomiting and diarrhea*

'Incubation period'
↓

Infection

Period of apparent recovery. This can vary from a few days to two months; usually lasts for about a week

Normal teeth of adult dog

A typical banded appearance results where enamel has not been laid properly

Other permanent damage to dogs that survive includes damage to growing teeth

The first stage of distemper

The first signs appear about 3-5 days after the dog is infected by the virus.

Characteristically the dog will have a discharge from the eyes and nose that is at first clear but which becomes thick and yellow.

The animal will run a high fever, although this fever may last only 24-48 hours.

Other signs which *may* be seen in distemper include:

Coughing, loss of appetite, pneumonia, vomiting and diarrhea, dehydration.

Note that none of these signs are specific for distemper and can be part of other diseases.

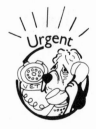

> Take no chances if your dog "has a cold"—
> early treatment is vital.

The second stage of distemper

Not all dogs suffering from distemper progress to the second stage.

Signs of the second stage usually occur about a week after the first stage, but may occur up to 2 months later.

The signs of the second stage are due to the virus invading the nervous system and destroying nerve cells. These signs vary considerably, depending on which part of the nervous system is affected:

Convulsions, fits (seizures)

Fits may be very short and infrequent at first, but often become more frequent and violent. Do not confuse these fits with rabies (see p. 72-4).

Muscle spasms and tremors

These are *rhythmic* contractions of a group of muscles. Usually a leg is involved, or the jaw muscles. The affected limb will jerk every few seconds, whether the dog is awake or asleep, and the dog cannot control this jerking motion. It continues through eating, playing or any other activity. In severe cases the dog may be unable to move properly or, if the jaw is involved, to eat or drink easily.

Other signs of stage two

Some dogs lose their sense of balance, others may be paralysed in one or more limbs. Occasionally there is stupor or a loss of awareness of surroundings.

The sequels to distemper infection

Dogs that survive may show after-effects. The most common of these in young dogs is pitted enamel of the teeth, giving a "banded" effect on the teeth. Loss vision is another occasional sequel.

The other common sequel to distemper is hardening of the pads of the feet. This used to be called "hard pad disease."

How does infection spread?

Animals suffering from distemper, or having recently recovered from it, shed the virus in enormous numbers, mainly in the air. The dog's breath contains virus particles, contained in minute droplets much the same as in human influenza. The virus is shed from the mouth (in saliva) and all other body excretions (urine, feces, tears).

How to protect your dog from contracting distemper

A very effective vaccine is available. Pups can be vaccinated at 6 weeks of age, but this is only temporary. A longer lasting vaccination can be given from 12-14 weeks of age.

All dogs should be vaccinated against distemper.

Vaccinations do *not* produce immediate immunity—protection takes about 10 days to develop.

Immunity is not life long and a *booster vaccination 12 months after the first is recommended.* Brood bitches are given booster vaccines before they are mated.

> Distemper boosters every year keep immunity high.

What treatment is available?

If the dog is showing the first signs of distemper *antibiotics* will help stop bacteria-produced complications such as pneumonia and bronchitis; and injections of antiserum—containing antibodies that neutralize the virus—may help if given *immediately.* Good nursing, good food and some loving care are very important.

Some common questions often asked about distemper

Does the pup gain any protection against distemper from the mother?

If the mother is immune she will pass on temporary protection to her pups. Part of this immunity is given before birth while the pups are still in the womb and part is given in the first milk (colostrum). The colostrum contains antibodies that protect the pup against many diseases, including distemper, in the first few weeks of life.

Can colostrum help protect pups at later stages?

No. The protecting antibodies of colostrum can only be absorbed through the pup's intestine in the first 24 hours of life. The protection is temporary only and after 6 weeks the levels of protection rapidly dwindle.

A regular source of colostrum is not available. Bitches only produce it during the last days of pregnancy and ordinary milk (without antibodies) is produced from then on.

If my dog has distemper, is he likely to die?

About 50 per cent of dogs recover without nervous signs developing. Of the other 50 per cent some die, others are so severely affected that they have to be humanely destroyed and others survive with lesser effects such as regular muscle contractions—"tics" or "chorea."

Early veterinary treatment greatly enhances a dog's chances of survival.

How long after the first signs have disappeared before I can be sure that nervous signs will not start?

Several months. After two weeks the chance of nervous signs developing decreases, but cases have been seen where the dog has started convulsing two months or more after the first stage was noted.

In most cases, if the dog is going to develop nervous signs he will do so in the first two weeks.

Is distemper dangerous to humans?

As far as we know, no.

If a dog with distemper has been in a house and garden how long before it is safe to get another dog?

We cannot be sure of the answer. It is wise to only introduce dogs that have been vaccinated at least 10 days before introducing them to the area.

Is a bite from a dog with distemper dangerous?

No more so than any other dog bite. It is the bite of a dog with rabies (see p. 72-73) that we fear, not distemper.

Once a dog has had distemper can he get it again?

It is extremely unlikely, especially in the first few years after infection, but it is possible.

INFECTIOUS CANINE HEPATITIS (ICH)
(Other names:
Canine Adenovirus Infection, CAV-1, Hepatitis.)

Infectious canine hepatitis is a highly infectious viral disease of dogs. It is contagious and can cause serious liver damage. Although infectious canine hepatitis is a disease of young dogs, dogs of any age may be affected. NB: The word "hepatitis" means inflammation of the liver. This inflammation can be due to many causes, including tumors, poisons and bacterial infection. Beware of linking the word "hepatitis" just to the viral disease. Infectious canine hepatitis is *one* form of hepatitis caused by a specific virus.

The signs of canine hepatitis

Most dogs show no signs at all. The disease in these dogs is mild and is not even apparent to the owner. However, other dogs may become severely ill. Factors such as the age of the dog, the infecting dose of virus and the resistance of the patient combine to decide whether the disease will be mild or severe.
   The signs of canine hepatitis may include:
   High fever, loss of appetite, tonsillitis, red (or inflamed) gums, pain in the abdomen, diarrhea (sometimes blood stained). An eye may turn blue during the recovery stage. Any blue eye should be examined by a vet.
 In severe cases, dogs can suddenly become ill and even collapse, have bloody diarrhea and die within a few hours.

Can canine hepatitis be prevented?

An excellent and highly effective vaccine is available. Live virus vaccine can cause blue eye, and some inflamed blue eyes go blind. Many present modified live vaccines, most of which do not cause blue eyes, are preferred. All dogs should be vaccinated and revaccinated.

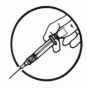

How is the virus spread?

The dog excretes virus in all body secretions—saliva, urine and feces. Other dogs pick it up by breathing in or ingesting virus loaded air, liquids or foods.

Treatment of infectious canine hepatitis

There is no specific treatment available to kill the virus once it has invaded the dog's liver. Treatment is aimed, therefore, at improving the dog's own resistance, so that his immune system can ward off the infection.

Antibiotics may be given to prevent any complicating bacterial infections. Good nursing and good food are necessary (see p. 9-14, 80-4). Vitamin supplements are essential, as the normal liver is the site of vitamin production. Fats should be avoided in the diet.

The acutely ill dog may need to be hospitalized and given intravenous fluids and drugs.

Some common questions often asked about ICH.

Is canine hepatitis dangerous to humans?

No. It is not the same hepatitis that humans suffer from.

Is repeated "booster" vaccination necessary?

Yes. Immunity conferred by vaccination is temporary and regular boosters are recommended.

Is the dog infectious after he has recovered?

Yes. The recovered dog may shed the virus in the urine for several months even after he has returned to apparent normal health.

If a dog has had infectious canine hepatitis, how long before it is safe for him to mix with other dogs?

The recovered dog can shed the infectious virus in his urine for several months after apparent recovery. Therefore, be careful not to let him mix with any *unvaccinated* dogs.

PARVOVIRUS INFECTION (contagious enteritis of dogs)

Parvovirus affects the dog in two distinct ways:
- Sudden death in pups.
- A contagious gastro-enteritis in dogs of all ages.

In 1978 a "new" disease was seen in dogs. It appeared simultaneously world wide—in Australia and America, Canada and elsewhere.

How did such a disease suddenly emerge?

Scientists believe that the widespread and well-known cat disease called "panleucopacnia" or "feline enteritis" is at the root of the mystery. This cat disease is also caused by a virus of a type termed parvovirus, and a slight alteration (or "mutation") of this virus may have allowed it to infect dogs.

The signs of parvovirus infection

The first form is a contagious gastro-enteritis (that is, a bowel infection that spreads rapidly between dogs).

The signs include vomiting, diarrhea, loss of appetite and lethargy. The bowel motions may be bloody. The condition can be fatal, especially in young pups. On recovery, diarrhea may persist for many weeks.

The second form is one of sudden death in puppies. The virus attacks the heart muscle, causing heart failure. Some pups may first stagger and show signs of difficulty breathing, others simply die suddenly.

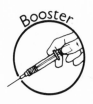

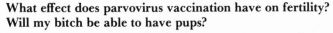

Parvovirus may cause sudden puppy death.

Treatment of parvovirus infection

Once the virus has invaded the body, treatment can only be aimed at minimizing the effect of the virus, and that may not be enough to save life—especially in the young pup. Vaccination at this stage does not help treatment, as immunity takes about 7-10 days to build up after infection.

Prevention of parvovirus

Protection prior to infection, that is, a good vaccination program, is the answer.

When to have your dog vaccinated

Pups may be vaccinated as young as 2 weeks, but the usual program is at 6 weeks and again at 14 weeks.

An annual booster may be necessary to maintain immunity. Some authorities suggest a booster shot one month after the first vaccination and boosters every 6 months.

Adult dogs may be vaccinated at any age.

Pregnant bitches: Vaccination of the pregnant bitch will result in a strong, although temporary (6 weeks) immunity being passed on to her pups.

What effect does parvovirus vaccination have on fertility?
Will my bitch be able to have pups?

Vaccinating for parvovirus does not cause reproductive disorders. The inactivated virus used in the vaccine has been studied closely and the conclusion was that it is safe to use in breeding bitches—although, as with most vaccines, vaccination during the first third of pregnancy should be avoided.

Other contagious diarrhea diseases of dogs

There are several viruses capable of causing very similar diseases to that described under "parvovirus." These include *Corona Virus* and *Rota Virus,* Consult your vet for information regarding any current outbreaks in your area. In general, it takes some years after an outbreak of a virus disease before an effective vaccine can be produced.

KENNEL COUGH

Kennel cough is an infection of the throat and sometimes of the major air passages of the lungs. It is not a specific disease and has several possible causes. A virus probably is the usual cause.

Kennel cough is more of a nuisance disease rather than a dangerous one. Very few dogs die, but the virus is highly contagious, especially in groups

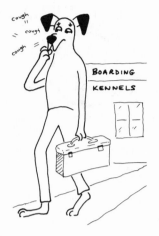

of dogs such as in kennels or a litter of pups. A high percentage of dogs exposed will contract the disease.

The signs of kennel cough

A cough: Starting as a dry cough it may become a deep hacking cough. Owners frequently telephone their vet saying that their dog has a bone in his throat, because that is often what it looks like. The dog will put his head forward, cough, gag and sometimes vomit. Once the dog starts coughing he may continue for several minutes. Kennel cough usually runs a course of about a week. Occasionally the cough may persist for much longer.

Treatment of kennel cough

Mild cases will run a course without the need of treatment similar to a cold in humans.

There is danger, however, that "secondary" infection by bacteria will turn a mild condition into a serious one. If the dog develops bronchitis and lung infection the vet may prescribe antibiotics.

Children's cough syrup may be used to reduce the severity of the cough. Consult your vet regarding a good safe product and the correct dose.

Warning: The coughing patient may not have kennel cough, but other problems such as distemper, heart problems, pneumonia or bronchitis (see p. 65, 124-31).

A persistent cough needs veterinary care.

Some common questions often asked about kennel cough:

Is kennel cough infectious to humans or other species?
No.

Once a dog has had kennel cough, can he get it again?
Yes. A temporary immunity only is produced. Also, there is more than one cause of kennel cough, so that while the dog may develop immunity to one cause he is not immune to them all.

Why is kennel cough more common in kennels?
The disease is spread by airborne droplet infection. When dogs are confined together the concentration of virus particles in the air becomes much higher and the chance of a dog breathing in air full of this virus or bacteria is far greater.

Efficient ventilation and air circulation in kennels will reduce kennel cough.

RABIES

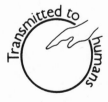

Rabies is caused by a virus. It can infect any warm-blooded animal, but is most common in carnivores (meat eaters) such as wolves, foxes, skunks and some bats. Fortunately it has been excluded from some countries by strict quarantine laws.

Rabies is the most feared disease of dogs because it is fatal and transmissible to man. (It is rare for people to survive the disease although new treatments are now available.)

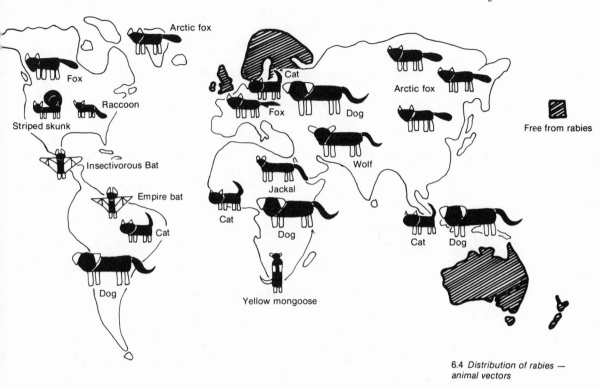

6.4 *Distribution of rabies —
animal vectors*

The saliva of an infected animal is loaded with the virus. Infection usually occurs from a bite. The virus is thus "injected" into the body where it rapidly seeks out the nervous system.

The signs of rabies

The first signs of rabies are
  • A slight fever.
  • A personality change—quiet dogs become irritable and snappy, or the opposite may happen and aggressive dogs may become fawning and affectionate.

Signs are not constant. Never take any chances at all if there is any suspicion of you or your animal having been bitten by a "rabid" animal (that is, one infected with rabies).

In countries where rabies exists a change in temperament
may be the first sign of the disease.

There are two forms rabies may take:

1. The "furious" form

The animal becomes excessively sensitive to any stimulus and bites at any moving object. Biting may be triggered by noises, lights or even vibrations.

The dog may run apparently aimlessly, biting at anything that moves.

As the disease progresses, convulsions start. These become more frequent and last longer and longer, and the dog may die during a convulsion. The final stage is paralysis and death.

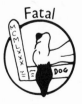

2. The "dumb" or "paralytic" form

Some infected patients do not show this furious desire to bite, but instead the virus paralyses the muscles, so that the patient has a characteristic sloppy jawed, slack tongue 'hang-dog' look. His bark may change.

The patient suffering the "dumb" form is just as infectious and dangerous as the "furious" sufferer.

What do you do if you suspect rabies?

If an animal is suspected of having rabies there is no treatment. Public health authorities *must* be informed and they will take over the case.

The dog is locked up, and if he dies his brain is examined to confirm the diagnosis. Dogs are not destroyed if they can be safely locked up.

How long after being bitten do signs appear?

Usually between 3 and 8 weeks but it can be up to 8 months. It varies with the site of the bite. Bites around the head usually kill more quickly.

Is the dog infectious before signs show?

An important question. The answer is yes. The dog (or other animal) may shed virus for up to a week before signs of the disease show.

Why is vaccination not allowed in areas where rabies is not yet present?

Vaccination can interfere with testing for the disease. If the disease gets to a free area, it is easier to control if animals have not been vaccinated.

Quarantine

Animal smugglers run a dreadful risk of introducing this horrendous disease into rabies-free countries. Strict quarantine of animals from an infected area, such as the European or North American continent, protects countries such as Australia and Great Britain from rabies.

> If it is possible that a dog has rabies and has been in contact with humans, lock the dog up and consult your vet and doctor.

BRUCELLOSIS

Brucellosis has been recognized in dogs since 1966. It is caused by a bacterium, *Brucella canis,* and causes abortion in bitches, infertility in males and is a serious transmissible venereal disease. Treatment is uncertain, expensive and prolonged. An outbreak in a breeding establishment or dog colony can be distrastrous.

> Brucellosis is a venereal disease in the dog.

In what countries does brucellosis occur?

The disease has been discovered in the USA, Germany, Japan, South America and Czechoslovakia. Undoubtedly it will spread further.

What are the signs of brucellosis?

In bitches the disease causes abortion—usually in the last third of pregnancy. Occasionally it will appear to cause infertility, but this is often due to early death of the pups.

In males brucellosis causes sterility. Two weeks after infection the testicles may be swollen. Later the testicles shrink. Both males and females may have swelling of the lymph nodes and the eyes may be inflamed.

How does it spread?

Spread is primarily through infected vaginal discharges and from aborted pups. It may also be transmitted in the bitch's milk.

Males spread the infection during mating. The bacteria is mixed with the semen, coming especially from the prostate gland (see   p. 101-2).

Diagnosis of brucellosis

Veterinary diagnosis of brucellosis includes blood tests, and examinations of discharges, and aborted material.

Treatment

Antibodies can sometimes treat the condition, but they will probably not prevent sterility. An infected animal shouldn't be bred in any case, because of the risk of infecting other dogs.

Is there any risk to humans?

There is some risk, although humans are fairly resistant to infection. The disease is not as severe in humans, and generally presents itself as fever and headache. Infertility is not a part of the human disease. (*Note:* There is another form of brucellosis that *can* be contracted from infected cows and this "undulant fever" may be severe in humans.)

What should you do if your bitch has an abortion?

Seek veterinary advice. If possible, take the aborted pups and membranes to your vet and do so with minimal delay. *Avoid handling this aborted matter—* use gloves or tongs and seal the dead pups and membranes in a plastic bag.

In the event of a brucellosis outbreak, what steps should be taken?

• Any females that have aborted or are infertile should be assumed to be infected. They should be isolated until the vet clears them.
• Any male should be isolated and considered infected until examined by a vet.
• All stock should be isolated.
• Consider euthanasia for affected animals.
• Kennels should undergo a thorough disinfection process. All people working in the kennels should be extremely careful not to transfer infection and should wear disposable gloves when handling infected animals.

LEPTOSPIROSIS

Leptospirosis is an infectious disease that can affect many species, including the dog and man. In the dog, leptospirosis can damage the liver and the kidney, and other organs may become involved.

The cause of leptospirosis is a microscopic organism called a *Spirochete* which is transmitted from infected and recovering animals to other animals, mainly via the urine. Rats are the main source of leptospirosis infection and may contaminate food and water with their infected urine.

The signs of leptospirosis

There are different types of leptospirosis, and the signs of infection vary according to the type and severity of the infection.

The kidneys and muscles are most commonly affected causing the dog to move with a painful "tucked-up" gait.

Other signs may include:
• Fever.
• Listlessness.
• Lack of appetite.
• Jaundice (a yellowing of the membranes, most easily seen in the whites of the eyes and the gums).

In cases where kidney damage is severe, the dog may develop diarrhea, vomiting and mouth ulcers and this may develop to dehydration, collapse and death.

How do dogs contract leptospirosis?

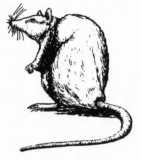

Infected animals pass the leptospira in their urine. This urine may then contaminate the food or water supplies of other animals who consequently can become infected. Rats and other rodents are the most common source of the disease, although the urine from dogs that have recovered from leptospirosis may still be infectious for up to a year after apparent recovery.

6.5 *Rats are a potent vector of Leptospirosis*

In which countries is leptospirosis common?

Leptospirosis is found in most countries, but is very common in some—notably Great Britain. In areas where the disease is common a vaccination against leptospirosis is available and routine booster vaccinations should be given. Your vet will tell you if you live in an area where vaccination is advisable.

Is leptospirosis transmissible to humans?

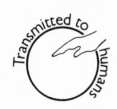

Yes, although dogs are not thought to be a great risk to man. Leptospirosis is an occupational hazard for slaughtermen and other livestock workers who may be contaminated by urine from infected animals.

To avoid infection, take care to prevent contamination by urine from an infected dog. Wear rubber gloves when clearing up any soiled bedding. Cattle are the main source of danger to man.

Treatment of leptospirosis

Treatment with antibiotics such as penicillin and streptomycin is usually effective but if there has been kidney or liver damage this may delay or prevent recovery.

FUNGAL DISEASES

Some fungi affect the skin—such as ringworm (see p. 153-4)—or the mouth area—thrush (see p. 93). Other fungi can have a more generalized effect on the body and these are called the deep mycoses or systemic fungal diseases. Systemic fungal diseases of dogs may cause illness in man, so in some cases euthanasia of the infected dog is recommended.

Many fungal diseases are acquired from soil or dust rather than an infected animal, but laboratory tests are needed to determine the type of fungus involved and the degree of risk to humans.

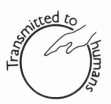

Some of the more common fungal diseases include histoplasmosis, blastomycosis, cryptococcosis, coccidioidomycosis, nocardiosis and actinomycosis.

The deep fungal diseases are limited to certain areas of the world. They are difficult to treat and you must be advised by your physician and vet whether treatment is advisable in view of the hazards to human health.

The signs of systemic fungal disease

The deep fungal diseases usually affect the lungs, liver, bowel or spleen, but some produce skin disease as well. Signs of infection are often vague and non-specific and may include a chronic cough or persistent diarrhea. Blindness occurs in some fungal diseases.

Laboratory tests are usually needed to confirm a diagnosis.

TOXOPLASMOSIS

Toxoplasmosis can affect all animals including man and dogs. It is caused by organisms called "coccidia" and the main sources of infection for man are raw meat and contamination from cats' feces.

It is estimated that in the United States about 24 per cent of all dogs have been infected and in humans the percentage of people affected rises with age.

The signs of toxoplasma infection

Most infections result in no signs and no apparent disease. When the immune system of the infected animal is inefficient, signs appear and vary from mild to severe. Toxoplasmosis can be fatal.

In dogs the main signs are:
- Lung infection (pneumonia).
- Liver infection (hepatitis).
- Brain infection (encephalitis).

How do humans become infected?

Dogs are *not* thought to be a source of infection to man. The main route of infection is by eating undercooked meat *or* from contamination from cats' excreta. When cats foul gardens or sandpits, these can remain a source of infection for up to a year. Cats' litter trays are potentially a source of infection unless they are cleaned properly *every day*.

To guard the health risk to pregnant women refer to your physician and vet.

TUBERCULOSIS

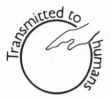

Tuberculosis affects man and all domestic animals. Dogs may infect humans and vice versa. Tuberculosis also affects cows and other livestock which in turn may infect dogs.

The signs of tuberculosis

- Low grade fever.
- Loss of weight and wasting.
- Chronic cough.
- Difficulty in breathing.

Treatment

Treatment is difficult and expensive. Euthanasia must be considered.

TETANUS

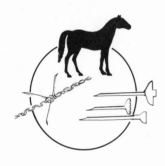

Tetanus is a disease which can affect most animals and man. Dogs have a greater natural resistance to this infection than man. Tetanus bacteria are found in soil; especially soil contaminated with horse manure and, to a lesser extent, cow manure. Any deep cut can allow entry of tetanus, but deep puncture wounds such as from nails or barbed wire are particularly dangerous.

The signs of tetanus

Signs start from one to several weeks after the initial wound, so you may not even recall the injury. The muscles are affected. The muscles of the face tighten, giving the dog a "worried" expression. As the disease progresses the legs become rigid, the lips are retracted and the eyeballs pulled back, making them appear sunken. The dog becomes acutely sensitive to any stimulus, especially to sound. Sudden or loud noises may trigger a spasm of muscles and the dog becomes rigid and may appear to be having a fit.

The chewing muscles of the face are among the first affected, so that there is difficulty in opening the mouth (hence the old name "lockjaw").

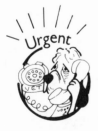

Treatment/Prevention

Temporary protection against tetanus—tetanus "antitoxin"—may be given following an injury. Protection is immediate but lasts only a few weeks.

If a dog has started to show signs, then prompt veterinary attention is essential. A very sick dog will require intensive care, but most dogs respond well if treatment is commenced early.

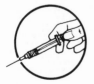

Vaccination against tetanus

Routine vaccination that would confer long-term immunity to tetanus is not usually given, as natural resistance is high in the dog. You may consider vaccinating dogs that live or work near livestock.

7. Feeding

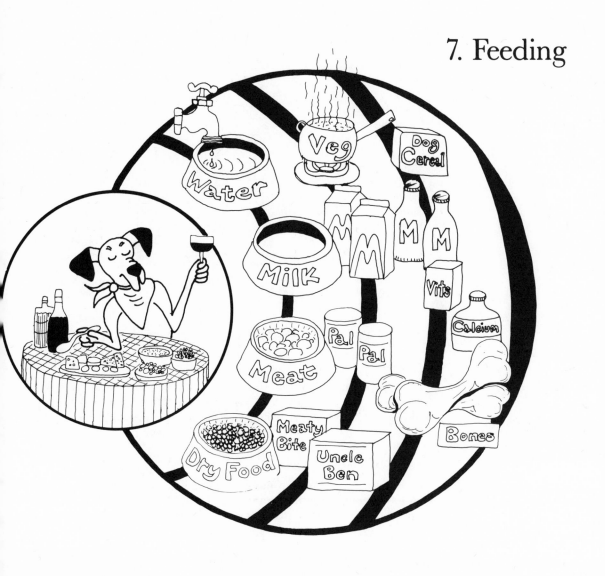

Feeding your dog is straightforward, if simple guidelines are followed. *Meat alone is not enough.*

In the wild, the dog is principally a carnivore (meat eater) but he eats the whole of his prey, not just the muscle meat, and so obtains vegetable matter from the digestive tract and calcium from the bones. Furthermore, wild dogs supplement their diet with a variety of plants, fruit and berries, especially when prey is scarce.

Remember, a pure meat diet is deficient in many things.

Nutrient	Nutrient requirement for 22 lb. dog	Raw beef supplies	Raw beef is . . .
Calories	740	740	—
Fat, g.	11	47	Too high
Calcium, mg.	2420	46	Too low
Phosphorus, mg.	1980	784	Too low
Cal./phos. ratio	1.2:1.0	1.0:17	Improper
Iron, mg.	13.2	11.5	Too low
Sodium, mg.	950	251	Too low
Copper, mg.	1.6	0.31	Too low
Magnesium, mg.	88	84.8	Too low
Iodine, mg.	0.33	0.036	Too low
Vitamin A, I.U.	1100	77.1	Too low
Vitamin D, I.U.	110	50.1	Too low
Vitamin E, I.U.	11	2.4	Too low

Adapted from "Nutrient Requirements of Dogs," National Research Council, National Academy of Sciences, USA, 1974.

TYPES OF COMMERCIAL FOOD AVAILABLE

Dry foods

These may be in the form of a meal, extruded cake or chunks. Manufacturers have now produced dry foods which are both highly palatable as well as being nutritionally balanced. Remember, always allow free access to water. Heavy feeding after exercise should be avoided.

Semi-moist food

This may be in the form of moist cubes, chunks or minces. These foods tend to be more palatable than dry food and are nutritionally complete. Remember that plenty of drinking water should always be available.

Canned food

Most veterinarians, pet shops, breeders, and veterinary colleges actually recommend commercial dog food over a diet of people food. The dog food industry is regulated by the government to ensure that its products offer a balanced diet for your dog. There are special dog foods for every stage of your dog's life, from puppy to old age. There are even special diets for dogs with cardiac conditions or kidney problems; your vet can recommend these diets for you.

If you feel that you must put together a diet for your dog, though, here are some guidelines.

ESSENTIAL COMPONENTS OF THE DOG'S DIET

Protein

Protein is well digested by the dog and is the basic building block for animal tissue. Protein utilization is variable and depends on the biological value of the protein fed. The most easily digested proteins are of animal origin, but dogs are capable of surviving very well on vegetable protein.

Eggs are a good source of protein but are best served cooked for the following reasons:
- The egg white is digested better when cooked.
- The raw white contains a substance (avidin) which can interfere with Vitamin B (biotin) metabolism.

Cheese is another good source of protein although too much may cause diarrhea. It is, however, an excellent source of calcium so a little as a "treat" will greatly benefit your dog.

Milk is an excellent food as it provides a good source of vitamins and minerals. As it also contains lactose it should not be fed to fat dogs and it should be remembered that some dogs may have difficulty in digesting it. Skim milk powder is nearly half sugar and should not be fed in large quantities.

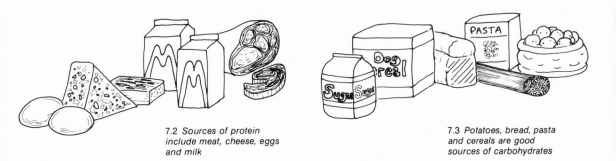

7.2 *Sources of protein include meat, cheese, eggs and milk*

7.3 *Potatoes, bread, pasta and cereals are good sources of carbohydrates*

Carbohydrates

Carbohydrates provide a ready source of energy for the dog, as they can be rapidly converted to glucose, the body's essential fuel. Cereals, bread, pasta and potatoes are all good sources of carbohydrates.

Vegetables

Vegetables should be cooked to make them more digestible—particularly the fibrous vegetables such as carrot. Grating finely is not sufficient. Mix in the cooked vegetables with the rest of the dog's food and most dogs will accept them—especially if you have got them used to vegetables during their puppy days.

Fat

A certain amount of fat should be left on the meat. Although fat is high in calories and therefore the quantity should be restricted, dogs digest fat well. The coat especially will benefit.

Vitamins and minerals

Here are two tables which show what minerals and vitamins are needed and the clinical symptoms of deficiencies or excesses:

Minerals

Mineral	Dietary sources	Main functions in body	Deficiency	Excess
Calcium	Bones, milk, cheese, bread	Bone and tooth formation, nerve function, blood clotting, muscle contraction. Requires adequate Vitamin D and Phosphorus	Poor growth, nutritional secondary hyperparathyroidism, convulsions	Lameness, joint problems
Phosphorus	Bones, milk, cheese, meat	Bone and tooth formation, many other roles in metabolism, energy utilization. Acid-base balance	Rare. Depraved appetite	Parathyroid changes, bone resorption, calcification of soft tissues.
Sulphur	Proteins containing sulphur amino acids, meats, eggs	As part of amino acids	Same deficiency as amino acids. Poor growth, poor coat	Not reported
Potassium	Meat, milk	Water balance, nerve function. Acid-base balance	Poor growth, restlessness, lesions to kidney and heart muscle	Possibly muscular weakness
Sodium and Chlorine as Salt	Salt, cereals	Acid-base balance. Gastric juices, body water balance	Fatigue, decreased water intake, poor growth, hair loss	Marked thirst, but non-toxic if water available
Magnesium	Cereals, green vegetables, bones, fish	Constituent of bones, teeth. Necessary for enzymes concerned with protein synthesis	Anorexia, muscular weakness, vomiting, convulsions	Diarrhea
Iron	Eggs, meats, bread, cereals, green vegetables	Part of hemoglobin, important in respiration and in energy metabolism	Anemia, reduced disease resistance	Anorexia, weight loss. Gastro-intestinal damage
Copper	Meats, bones	Necessary for incorporation of iron into hemoglobin	Anemia	Not reported
Zinc	Many foods, meats, cereals	Part of digestive enzymes. Probably involved in tissue repair	Growth retardation, emaciation, skin lesions	Diarrhea
Manganese	Many foods	Involved in several enzymes. Fat metabolism	Poor growth, reproductive abnormalities	Not reported. Can affect nervous system in man
Iodine	Fish, dairy products. Salt, vegetables	Part of thyroid hormone	Goitre, hairlessness in newborn pups	Probably toxic. Depression of thyroid
Cobalt	B12. Organ and muscle meats, milk	Constituent of Vitamin B12	Not demonstrated when adequate B12 present	Rare. Adverse effect on red blood cells
Selenium	Cereals, fish, meats	Associated with Vitamin E	Muscle myopathies	Diarrhea

All trace elements (shown below *Iron* in this table) are known to be toxic at very high intakes.

Vitamins

Vitamin	Dietary sources	Main functions in body	Deficiency	Excess
Vitamin A	Cod liver oil, milk, butter, cheese	Protects epithelial integrity, associated with bone growth	Keratinization of ocular tissue, thickening of skin, hardening of epithelial tissues. Susceptibility to disease. Impaired nerve function	Anorexia, pain in long bones. Remodelling and hemorrhage of cartilage.
Vitamin D	Cod liver oil, eggs, dairy produce, margarine, meats	Promotes growth and mineralization of bones. Increases absorption of calcium. Calcium transport	Rickets, bone deformities	Anorexia, bloody diarrhea. Calcification of soft tissues
Vitamin E	Green vegetables, margarine, cereals	Involved in cell membrane function probably as an antioxidant.	Possibly muscular dystrophy or anemia. Gestation failure	No harmful effects in dogs. May be toxic in other species
Vitamin K	Green vegetables, meats, cereals	Important in formation of prothrombin for blood clotting	Not demonstrated naturally. Induced deficiency leads to hemorrhage	Not observed in the dog. High doses probably cause jaundice
Thiamin (Vitamin B1)	Pig meat, organ meats, whole grains, peas, beans	Co-enzyme in various reactions involving carbohydrate metabolism	Anorexia, vomiting, peripheral nerve degeneration, heart failure	Not likely from diet
Riboflavin (Vitamin B2)	Most foods	Part of two co-enzymes involved in energy metabolism	Weight loss, anorexia, anemia, eye lesions	None known
Niacin	Liver, meats, cereal grains, legumes	Part of co-enzymes NADP and NAD, involved in many aspects of metabolism, chiefly oxidation or reduction	Black tongue or pellagra. Loss in weight, mouth ulcers, diarrhea,	Mild cutaneous flush. No adverse effect in dogs
Pyridoxine (Vitamin B6)	Meats, vegetables, cereal grains	Amino acid metabolism as co-enzyme pyridoxal phosphate	Anorexia, slow growth, possibly hair loss, convulsions	None observed in dogs
Pantothenic Acid	Most foods	Important in co-enzyme A. Central to energy utilization	Slow growth, poor reflexes, reduced appetite, hair loss, nervous degeneration, diarrhea	Not seen in dogs
Folic Acid	Legumes, green vegetables, wheat, and probably intestinal synthesis	Involved in nucleic acid and amino acid metabolism	Poor appetite, poor weight gain, watery eyes, anemia	None by oral administration
Cyanoco-bolamin (Vitamin B12)	Muscle meat, eggs, dairy produce (animal proteins)	Involved in carbon transfer like folic acid	Not described in the dog	Not reported
Biotin	Meats, legumes, vegetables	Probably amino acid metabolism.	Not described, may be linked with scaly skin	Not known
Choline	Egg yolk, liver, grains, legumes	Methyl donor mostly in fat metabolism	Fatty liver, poor blood clotting	Not reported
Vitamin C	Not required			

SOME QUESTIONS OFTEN ASKED ABOUT FEEDING

Does eating raw meat make dogs savage?

There is no evidence to suggest that raw meat makes dogs savage. What is more likely to make dogs savage are stress conditions.

What advantages are there to cooking meat?

There may not be any, although it could be agreed that it makes meat more palatable. It is, however, possible for dogs to become infected with tapeworms from uncooked meat. Raw offal should never be fed due to the danger of parasite infection and this is particularly important with sheep offal, as the dog may become infected with hydatid tapeworms, the cysts of which can infect humans. Pork is another meat which should be cooked as it may contain the parasite *trichinella* (ask your vet if it is a problem in your area). From a safety viewpoint, particularly if children play with the dog, meat should always be cooked.

> Remember, meat alone is not a balanced diet. Commercial pet foods of good quality are both nutritious and free from the dangers of parasitic infection.

If my dog eats grass is it a sign of illness?

Usually not, as many dogs may eat small amounts of grass, though if a dog eats a lot of grass he may vomit. The eating of a lot of grass may show an imbalance in the diet, so check what you are feeding. Research in America, however, has shown that the eating of grass originates from the wild dog, who will gorge its prey and then vomit in order to feed its pups. Grass is eaten to encourage the vomiting.

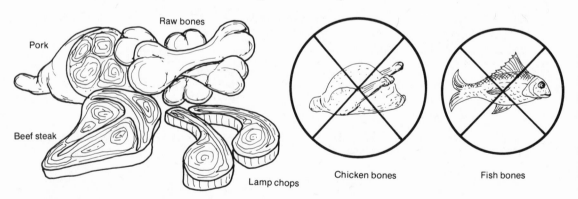

7.4 *Avoid feeding cooked bones, especially those liable to splinter, such as chop bones, or small bones, such as fish or chicken bones. Large raw bones are excellent for dental health.*

What kind of bones may be fed?

Raw bones are preferable to cooked bones which are much more likely to splinter and lodge in the dog's throat or intestine. Beef, pork and lamb bones are better than chicken bones. Raw bones are more easily digested. *Never* feed grilled chop or steak bones as these splinter easily. Bones can cause the droppings to turn a chalky white color and may cause constipation.

Should a calcium supplement be fed?

If a pup is fed a lot of meat then a calcium supplement is a good idea. Calcium carbonate is a good source. Feed one teaspoon of calcium carbonate per half kilogram of meat. Other types of calcium are calcium lactate or calcium gluconate. Calcium phosphate (e.g., D.C.P.) is *not* recommended.

Should a bitch be fed more during pregnancy?

The aim is to have a fit but not fat bitch at whelping. In order to achieve this it will be necessary to gradually increase the food during pregnancy. After the birth of the pups, the bitch does need to be fed substantially more.

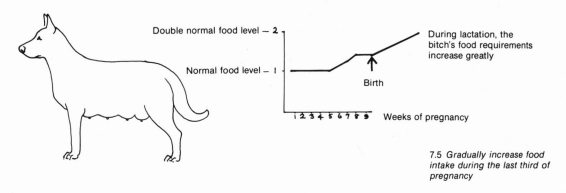

7.5 *Gradually increase food intake during the last third of pregnancy*

The normal maintenance diet for the bitch should be multiplied by the following factors during gestation.

First 5 weeks	1.0
5th week	1.1
6th week	1.2
7th–9th week	1.3

During lactation:

First week	1.5
2nd week	2.0
Peak up to	3.0
Taper off after 5 weeks	1.5

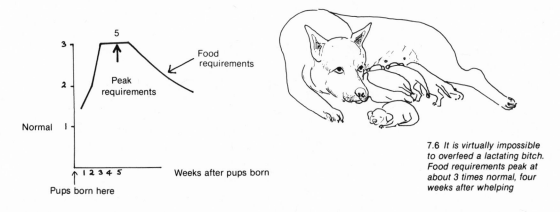

7.6 *It is virtually impossible to overfeed a lactating bitch. Food requirements peak at about 3 times normal, four weeks after whelping*

It is important that a nutritionally complete and balanced diet be given, but if a predominantly meat diet is fed, vitamin and mineral supplementation will be necessary. A note of caution is that oversupplementation is just as damaging to the dog as a deficiency. It is far easier to feed a nutritionally complete commercial food and it is virtually impossible to overfeed a lactating bitch.

Are table scraps all right for dogs?

It is claimed that most dogs fed in American kennels (fed on commercially formulated rations) are better fed than most American people. Possibly this is true. Table scraps can be a welcome addition to many a dog's diet but remember:
- No cooked bones.
- Table scraps by themselves are insufficient.

Are baby foods all right for dogs?

Baby foods are an expensive way of feeding dogs and, furthermore, babies and puppies have differing requirements due largely to different growth patterns.

Should food be fed hot or warm?

The aroma of warm food may make it more appetizing than cold food, but be careful not to feed the food too hot as this can burn the dog's mouth. Heating food, contrary to popular myth, does not really destroy food value and in some cases may actually increase it.

Does red meat make dogs itchy?

A very small number of dogs may develop an itch when fed red meats (e.g., beef). Red meat is one of the least likely causes of itching.

Obesity (overweight)

Overweight dogs are more liable to die young. In man, early death rates are 50 per cent higher for those who are 20 per cent overweight and it is thought that the rate may be similar for dogs. Overweight dogs are more likely to develop arthritis, disc disease, heart and lung disease, diabetes and liver disease. They are an increased surgical risk and may have a reduced resistance to infection.

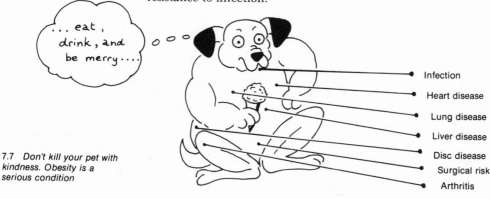

7.7 *Don't kill your pet with kindness. Obesity is a serious condition*

The problem which the vet faces is often to convince the owner that there *is* a problem. Frequently we are told, "But he only has one meal a day," or, "he must have something wrong with his glands." Certainly the overweight dog should be examined to rule out any possibility of such a condition before any weight reduction is started.

> Most dogs are fat because they eat too much.

Why does a dog eat too much and so get fat? In the wild, a dog gorges its food in times of plenty and stores the excess food eaten as fat to be used when prey is scarce. Domesticated dogs still have the same eating instincts as their wild forebears and so tend to overeat if given the opportunity. Unfortunately this is the start of a vicious cycle—the fatter a dog becomes the lazier he gets and is disinclined to run about and burn up the food he has eaten. Unless food intake is restricted the dog will become increasingly obese.

Are pure-breeds more likely to get fat than cross-breeds?

Some breeds, such as the Labrador Retriever, Cocker Spaniel and Collie, appear to have more obesity problems than others. However, breed type alone does not cause obesity—you just have to be more careful with some breeds and make sure that they do not overeat.

Does neutering cause obesity?

In a word, no, although in females the sudden reduction of hormones called estrogens may stimulate the appetite, so do not overfeed. In males there may be a reduction in activity, so once again do not overfeed. With both males and females there need be no weight increase if you manage the diet carefully.

Are some people more likely to have an overweight dog than others?

Yes, middle-aged and elderly people because they tend to spend more time at home and are more likely to give treats or snacks to their dogs. Overweight owners tend to have overweight dogs.

HOW TO REDUCE YOUR DOG'S WEIGHT

Reducing the daily diet can result in deficiencies, so a nutritionally balanced diet is essential. Most weight reducing programs fail in the first ten days, mainly because the dog becomes extremely hungry and looks for food elsewhere. So stop your dog from scavenging garbage and stop yourself from feeling sorry for him and giving him snacks.

The main aim of a reducing diet is to reduce the intake by removing high calorie foods such as carbohydrates and fat from the diet and replacing them with bulk to fill the dog.

However, before you commence a reducing diet it is wise for the dog to have a thorough veterinary check-up to ensure that there are no underlying disorders.

Find out what weight your dog should be and then work out from the table the calories needed for a dog for that weight, and feed him 60 percent of those calories.

Energy requirement of dogs on reducing diet

Target weight (lb.)	Approximate daily requirements (oz.)	60 per cent of daily requirement (k-cal)	Approximate quantity of tinned food needed (g)
11	10	270	270
22	17	450	450
33	21	600	600
44	26	750	750
55	32	900	900
66	36	1020	1020
77	40	1140	1140
88	44	1260	1260
99	48	1380	1380
110	53	1500	1500

As given by 'Nutrient Requirements of Dogs' National Research Council, National Academy of Sciences, USA, 1974.

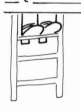

7.8 *A veterinary check prior to starting a reducing diet is advisable*

A reducing diet below for those of you who like to cook for your dog:

125g lean meat (lightly cooked, with any fat drained off)
50g cottage cheese

200g carrots (cooked)
200g green beans (cooked)
2 teaspoons calcium carbonate

This diet contains less that 700k-cal per kg. Work out from the chart above how much you need. To this diet you should add a balanced vitamin/mineral supplement and a teaspoon of good quality vegetable oil. Alternatively feed a nutritionally complete canned dog food which provides around 100k-cal per 100g of weight of food. Remember that with nutritionally complete food you do not need supplementation.
Do not feed chocolate to a dog, it can be very harmful.

SOME MORE QUESTIONS ABOUT DIETING

My dog keeps begging and I cannot resist him (or perhaps feel sorry for him?)

If treats, snacks or rewards are necessary, feed pieces of raw carrot or other vegetables, clean bones or rawhide chews, *never* chocolates or biscuits.

How fast should my dog lose weight?

Most dogs can be reduced to their optimal weight in 8-10 weeks, but if grossly obese it may take longer.

If my dog is not losing weight should I reduce the diet further?

No. Consult your vet.

Should water be restricted as well?

No, always allow plenty of fresh water. But do not feed milk as it contains calories. Water contains no calories at all.

8. Teeth, mouth and throat

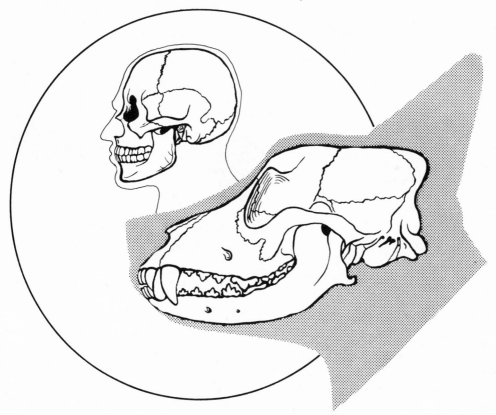

TEETHING IN PUPPIES

Most pups are born without teeth. By 3 or 4 weeks of age, the first of the pups' temporary teeth (or "milk" teeth) emerge, and by 6 weeks most of the 28 baby teeth have emerged.

The permanent teeth start to emerge at 4 or 5 months of age, starting with the incisors (teeth at the front of the mouth, Fig. 8:3). Teething takes about two months. The pup may experience occasional soreness of the gums, accompanied by drooling of saliva and a reluctance to eat. Overall, the effects are mild, and teething in pups is far less traumatic than in babies and children.

Retained baby teeth

The temporary teeth should be displaced by permanent teeth. In some cases this fails to happen and temporary teeth are retained. This is especially common with the *canine* teeth. The temporary canine tooth is retained alongside the much larger permanent canine tooth. The teeth most likely

*, **, *** indicate increasing likelihood of a particular trait or problem occurring.

to cause trouble are retained temporary *incisors*. If the temporary incisor teeth are retained, they may prevent permanent incisors from emerging in their correct site and this can result in an uneven bite. A correct bite (Fig. 8:2) is particularly important in show dogs.

Retained temporary teeth not only interfere with correct alignment of permanent teeth, but also trap food debris and can be a site of gum infection and inflammation. You should inspect growing pups' teeth weekly. If temporary teeth are being retained when the permanent are emerging, consider extraction of the temporary teeth.

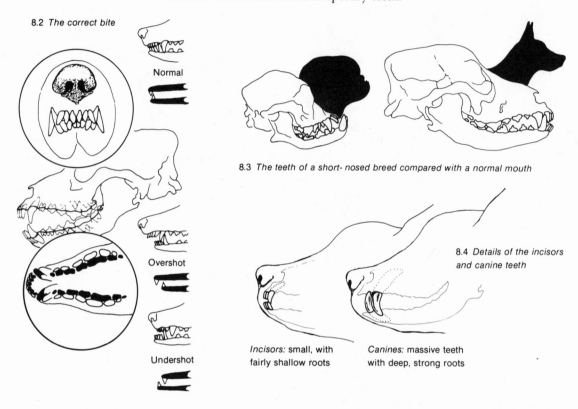

8.2 *The correct bite*

Normal

Overshot

Undershot

8.3 *The teeth of a short- nosed breed compared with a normal mouth*

8.4 *Details of the incisors and canine teeth*

Incisors: small, with fairly shallow roots

Canines: massive teeth with deep, strong roots

Teeth and age

Type of teeth	Use	Age at which they erupt
Incisors	Small; are at the front of the mouth. Used for tearing meat off the prey.	2-5 months
Canines	The huge "wolf" teeth which have a very large root. Designed to hold the prey.	5-6 months
Molars	Molars crush and break up food. (Molars of dogs do not grind the food as do the molars of grass eaters, such as horses, cows and man).	4-7 months

TELLING THE AGE BY THE TEETH

Although there are subtle changes with age, these vary so much with the diet and the general health of the dog that one cannot be sure of the age of a dog by his teeth. (Horses' teeth, on the other hand, have quite distinctive changes with age.)

8.5 *The Collie has an "overshot" mouth and this is considered normal for the breed. The Boxer has an "undershot" jaw, resulting in crowding of the teeth, yet this is considered normal for the breed*

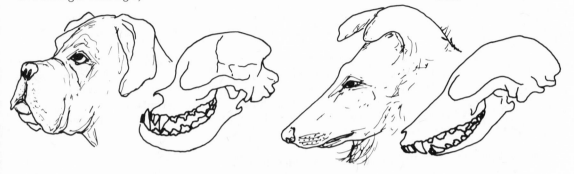

OVERSHOT AND UNDERSHOT MOUTHS

Overshot mouth (when the upper jaw is longer than the lower jaw) is common in some breeds, such as the Collie.

Undershot mouth (when the lower jaw projects beyond the upper) is considered normal in some breeds, e.g.: Boxer, Boston Terrier, Bulldog.

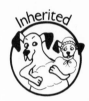

INFLAMMATION OF THE GUMS (GINGIVITIS)

In pups, inflammation of the gums is usually associated with teething, and so is seen most commonly between 4 and 6 months of age. This inflammation is transient and rarely requires treatment.

In adults, inflammation of the gums is most commonly associated with the build-up of a hard mineral deposit on the teeth called *tartar*. Gingivitis can also be a sign of kidney or liver disease and is seen occasionally in other wasting diseases.

TARTAR: WHY IT FORMS AND WHAT TO DO ABOUT IT

Tartar, or dental calculus, builds up slowly on teeth. It starts with the formation of dental plaque, an invisible film on the teeth. Gradually this plaque becomes stained, and minerals, salts, and food particles build up on the plaque to form hard concretions on the sides of the teeth. These masses of tartar form slowly at first but can become very large. Tartar can push back the gums allowing infection to develop between the gums and the teeth. The teeth may become loose in their sockets and fall out as a result.

Signs of tartar

The owner usually first notices a dreadful smell on the dog's breath due to rotting food debris and bacteria breeding among the tartar.

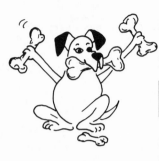

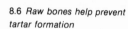

8.6 *Raw bones help prevent tartar formation*

If you look into the mouth, gum inflammation appears first as a thin red line at the junction of the teeth and gums. If neglected the gums can become painfully swollen and ulcerated.

Prevention of tartar formation

> A faulty diet is the most common cause of dental tartar.

Soft, processed foods that require no chewing leave the teeth without the natural exercise they need to remain healthy. Food debris remains instead of being flushed away by chewing and the flow of saliva this stimulates.

The dog's diet should include foods that encourage chewing. Give him strips of meat (do not chop meat into small pieces) plus hard biscuits, raw bones or dog "chews."

Treatment once tartar has formed

If the build-up is small and gum inflammation is mild, then a change of diet to encourage chewing may be enough.

If tartar has already formed, a thorough teeth clean under a general anesthetic may be needed. The tartar is removed with special instruments or an ultrasonic scaler. At the same time, loose, cracked or infected teeth are removed.

> A dog keeps his mouth healthy by chewing.

KEEPING YOUR DOG'S TEETH CLEAN

Diet

The aim is to reduce or eliminate the need to clean your dog's teeth by exercising the teeth and gums. Give firm foods that require chewing, raw bones, rawhide chews, toy bones or other hard mouth exercisers. Dry food stimulates the mouth and dogs fed on dry food tend to form less plaque and tartar on their teeth.

Teeth cleaning

If tartar or plaque still builds up despite the diet, teeth cleaning is necessary. If your dog is unco-operative or you cannot manage, then routine cleaning by a vet may be needed every 6-18 months.

Many dogs will allow their master to clean their teeth. If this is the case with your pet, then use a very soft toothbrush or a soft cloth with a paste of baking soda and salt in a 3:1 ratio, or hydrogen peroxide diluted to a 3 per cent solution. There have been some toothpastes designed specifically for dogs, but human toothpastes are not recommended as dogs do not like the powerful taste.

It is usually better to concentrate on cleaning one or two teeth at a time and leave the others for another day—*daily* cleaning is unnecessary. Monthly to six monthly cleanings will usually suffice.

OTHER CONDITIONS OF THE MOUTH AND TEETH

Dental abscess

Dogs have a huge molar tooth used for crushing bones. This is called the *carnassial* tooth. It has three long roots holding it firmly in the jaw bone. If the carnassial tooth is cracked or if there is excessive tartar build-up on the tooth, infection can spread to the roots, and a condition termed "dental abscess" follows.

The root of this massive tooth projects close to a sinus, or cavity of the skull (Fig. 8:7). Infection can spread from the root of the carnassial tooth into this sinus and ultimately a discharge of pus erupts just below the dog's eye.

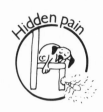

8.7 *Dental abscess: the first sign of a dental abscess may be pus discharging from a hole just below the eye*

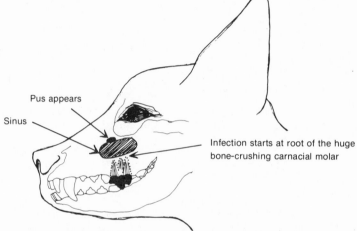

Pus appears

Sinus

Infection starts at root of the huge bone-crushing carnacial molar

Antibiotics may temporarily control the infection, but it is usually necessary to remove the tooth and drain the infected sinus. Without extraction, infection tends to flare up again after the course of antibiotics is finished.

Thrush

Thrush is a common complaint in children and adults but is not common in dogs. It is a fungal infection of the mouth and is most commonly seen in young dogs that have been given a long course of antibiotics for some other problem.

The tongue becomes covered with soft, white areas which may eventually cover the whole tongue. Ulcers often develop.

Treatment of thrush

Drugs that are effective against fungal and yeast infections are required. The most commonly used is Nystatin, but because some dogs suffer side-effects to the drug, treatment must be given under veterinary supervision.

TRENCH MOUTH

Signs of trench mouth

The dog has red inflamed gums which bleed easily. The dog drools saliva

93

which is discolored brown or reddish and has a putrid odor. Owners often notice this condition because of the rancid smell and because the mouth and front legs become stained with the discharge. The dog suffers a lot of discomfort and usually will not eat.

Treatment of trench mouth

Antibiotics will usually control the infection. Attention should be paid to the teeth, which should be cleaned if necessary.

WARTS IN THE MOUTH

Warts in the mouth are cauliflower-like in shape and can become quite large and numerous. The cause is a virus and it is mainly young dogs that are affected. In some cases there may be vast numbers of these warts so that the dog has difficulty in eating.

Treatment of warts in the mouth

The warts usually spontaneously disappear after 6-8 weeks. In cases where the dog cannot eat properly or where the warts are not spontaneously clearing, surgery may be considered.

EPULIS

An epulis is a small, hard, elevated area where the gums have thickened to form firm nodules which cluster around the teeth, in some cases even covering them.

This condition is most commonly seen in short-nosed breeds where the teeth are crowded together. The Boxer** is the most commonly affected breed.

Treatment of epulis

Epulis is *not* a cancerous condition and in most cases does not cause the dog any discomfort. In advanced cases, where there are many large growths and eating is affected, surgical removal may be attempted. Treatment is difficult and recurrence of the epulis after removal is quite common.

CLEFT PALATE

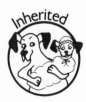

When cleft palate is present a defect exists along the center line of the roof of the mouth. This means that the mouth is not sealed off from the nose and food can get into the nose and, in a young puppy, into the lungs. It is impossible for a pup with a cleft palate to suckle unless the defect is very small. Cleft palate may be hereditary, so do not breed with affected animals.

Cleft palate may also be caused by stress to the pregnant bitch, an excess of Vitamin A during pregnancy, or occasionally by administration of corticosteroids during pregnancy.

Even when non-inherited causes are suspected, the affected pup should *not* be bred. It is not possible to be certain that the cleft palate is due to non-hereditary factors.

Treatment of cleft palate

If the pup is so severely affected that it cannot suck then it should be euthanized. In mild cases the pup can drink well and will grow and thrive. Surgical treatment is possible, but difficult.

SOFT PALATE PROBLEMS

Overlong soft palate

If you explore the roof of your mouth with your tongue, you will discover that at the front the roof is hard (the "hard palate"), but toward the rear it is soft. This soft part is termed simply the "soft palate."

In some dogs, this soft palate protrudes too far to the rear and can cause difficulty in breathing if the soft palate falls around the air intake (or larynx). A "snorting" breathing results (sometimes called "reverse sneezing").

Examples of this condition are seen in the Pug* and Boston Terrier*, and occasionally in other breeds, even in dogs with normally shaped heads.

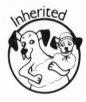

> Breeding dogs for a short snout can cause an overlong soft palate with resultant serious breathing difficulties.

Treatment of overlong soft palates

Surgical correction is the only permanently effective treatment for an overlong soft palate.

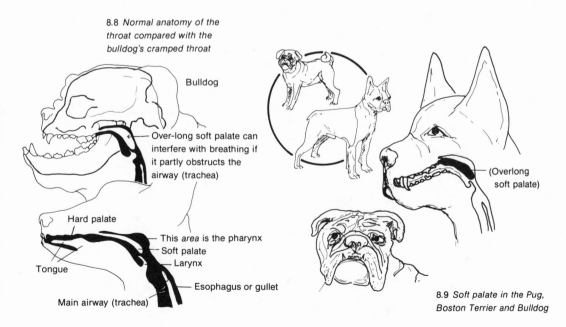

8.8 *Normal anatomy of the throat compared with the bulldog's cramped throat*

Bulldog

Over-long soft palate can interfere with breathing if it partly obstructs the airway (trachea)

Hard palate

This *area* is the pharynx
Soft palate
Larynx

Tongue

Esophagus or gullet

Main airway (trachea)

(Overlong soft palate)

8.9 *Soft palate in the Pug, Boston Terrier and Bulldog*

HARE LIP

A hare lip is a deformed upper lip in the area under the nose. Hare lip is often associated with a cleft palate and is most common in toy breeds* and English Bulldogs*.

The defect is mainly a cosmetic problem and treatment is plastic surgery.

Dogs affected by hare lip should not be used for breeding as the defect may be hereditary.

SORE THROAT (pharyngitis)

Signs: coughing and gagging

It often appears that the dog may have something caught in his throat, but on examination the throat is seen to be red and inflamed and no foreign object is present.

The dog may have difficulty swallowing, drool saliva and have his mouth slightly open.

Cause of sore throats

Sore throat is often caused by viral infection (see Kennel cough, p. 71-2) but the condition is very common and can be caused by many different factors—eating hot food, chewing sticks, infection by bacteria or virus.

Treatment of sore throats

Restrict exercise if your dog has a sore throat. Mild cases do not require additional treatment. If the dog is constantly coughing and gagging or retching, antibiotics and cough suppressants may be required.

A children's cough syrup is useful if the throat is merely inflamed. Do *not* use adult syrups or tablets as these can make the dog very drowsy and in some cases may be toxic.

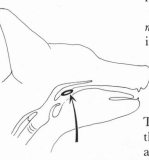

8.10 *The tonsils lie at the rear of the mouth — one on either side. They normally sit almost hidden in their crypts, but when inflamed, stand out as reddened, bean-shaped swellings*

TONSILLITIS

The tonsils are two little bean-shaped structures that lie near the back of the throat (Fig. 8:10). They are composed of specialized cells and the tonsils are designed to meet any bacteria or other germs that invade the mouth and prevent them spreading further.

When the tonsils are actively engaged in countering infections, they may swell and—especially in young dogs—become inflamed. This condition is termed tonsillitis.

Signs of tonsillitis

Depending on the severity of the swelling, the signs vary from a vague lack of appetite to a high fever. The severely affected dog will not eat, swallows painfully and may drool saliva from the mouth. The tonsils are not normally visible but when inflamed they swell out of their crypts and look like elongated red beans.

Can tonsillitis spread to other dogs?

Some forms *are* infectious (tonsillitis may be caused by many different bacteria and viruses). Tonsillitis may be part of a more serious disease—for example, distemper or kennel cough.

Pups

Pups are especially at risk as their immune system is not yet well developed. Some pups will get recurring episodes of tonsillitis. As they get older many will overcome this tendency.

Treatment

Mild cases may need no treatment other than rest and a soft diet for a few days.

If the tonsillitis is troubling the dog, treatment may include antibiotics and analgesics (pain suppressors) such as aspirin.

If the tonsillitis is severe and frequently recurs, removal of the tonsils may be recommended.

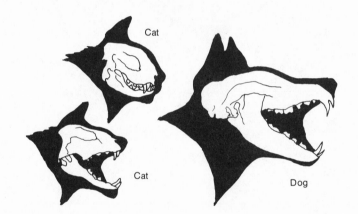

8.11 *Difference between jaws of the dog and cat*

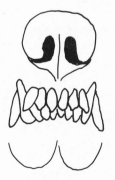
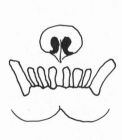
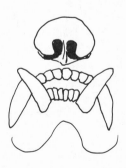

Difference between 'bites' of some dogs

Normal

Pekingese: lower jaw juts out and does not meet with the upper incisor teeth

Bulldog: crowding of the teeth as a result of breeding for a short snout

97

9. The gut

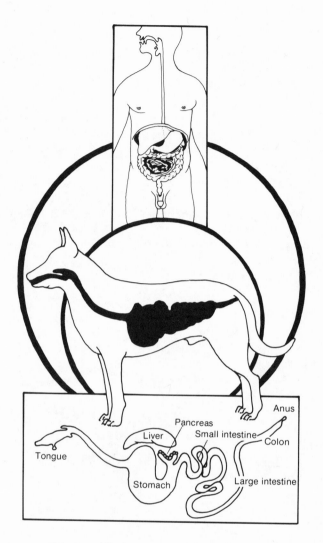

9.1 *The digestive system of the dog has much the same organs as man, although there are differences in their digestive capabilities*

DIARRHEA (very loose or fluid bowel motions)

All dogs at some time in their life will experience a bout of diarrhea. Diarrhea is not a disease in itself, but is a sign of bowel disorder. Some of the conditions that may result in diarrhea are:

Indigestion
This is by far the most common cause of mild diarrhea. If the dog eats foods that are indigestible, too rich, or foods that irritate the bowel, diarrhea may result. An excessive amount of food or feeding of foods that the dog is not used to can also result in diarrhea.

Enteritis
Enteritis is a disease of the bowel due to infection by bacteria (e.g., salmonella); or a virus (e.g., parvovirus); irritation from chemical poisons, foreign bodies or by an allergy to some food matter. In general, enteritis is more severe than diarrhea and there may be blood, mucus and/or gas in the fluid motions.

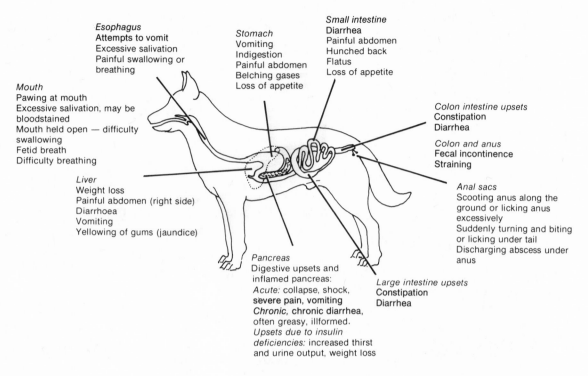

Esophagus
Attempts to vomit
Excessive salivation
Painful swallowing or
breathing

Stomach
Vomiting
Indigestion
Painful abdomen
Belching gases
Loss of appetite

Small intestine
Diarrhea
Painful abdomen
Hunched back
Flatus
Loss of appetite

Mouth
Pawing at mouth
Excessive salivation, may be
bloodstained
Mouth held open — difficulty
swallowing
Fetid breath
Difficulty breathing

Colon intestine upsets
Constipation
Diarrhea

Colon and anus
Fecal incontinence
Straining

Liver
Weight loss
Painful abdomen (right side)
Diarrhoea
Vomiting
Yellowing of gums (jaundice)

Anal sacs
Scooting anus along the
ground or licking anus
excessively
Suddenly turning and biting
or licking under tail
Discharging abscess under
anus

Pancreas
Digestive upsets and
inflamed pancreas:
Acute: collapse, shock,
severe pain, vomiting
Chronic, chronic diarrhea,
often greasy, illformed.
*Upsets due to insulin
deficiencies:* increased thirst
and urine output, weight loss

Large intestine upsets
Constipation
Diarrhea

9.2 *Signs of digestive system
upsets:* these signs are a
guide only. For more detail
refer to the text. One or
more of the signs listed may
occur together

Parasites

Worm parasites of the gut can irritate the bowel and cause diarrhea. (See p. 108-14.)

Liver disease

The liver is a key organ in digestion. Liver diseases can result in diarrhea if the liver is not producing enough bile and digestive enzymes.

Pancreas disease

The pancreas is the center of fat and carbohydrate digestion. If the pancreas is producing insufficient enzymes (essential to digestion) diarrhea will result (see p. 105-6).

Poisoning
See p. 252-9.

Obstructions

Surprisingly, one of the first signs of an obstruction in the intestine can be diarrhoea. This diarrhoea is usually transient and followed by no bowel movements at all.

Treatment of mild diarrhea (due to overeating unsuitable foods)

To allow healing of the affected bowel, provide only foods that are easily digested.

• Withhold all food for 24 hours (in the case of puppies withhold for 8-12 hours only).

• Withdraw all milk and instead provide plenty of fresh, clean water.

• Feed small amounts of a soft, bland food.

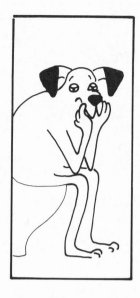

The object of this diet is to provide easily digestible foods without milk protein, low in fats and low in indigestible fiber.

Diet for dogs with diarrhea

Remember: No food for the first 24 hours. After that feed cooked, minced white meats plus boiled rice or potatoes, which are a good source of digestible carbohydrates, and cottage cheese. The diet need not be balanced since it usually will only be fed for a short time.

A daily diet for a 12 kg dog could be made by boiling one cup of dry rice in two cups of water and then adding either 155 g of cottage cheese or 115 g of cooked lean meat. Feed small amounts frequently, up to 5-6 times daily.

In cases of vomiting and diarrhea, withhold food and water for 24-48 hours. After that small amounts of the above diet every few hours for two or three days will control most cases.

Once diarrhea is controlled, *gradually* change back to a normal diet over the next few days. Do not feed anything the bowel may be affected by, such as sweets or "treats."

If you want to feed milk, dilute it with 50 per cent water and only gradually revert to 100 per cent milk.

If diarrhea persists, consult your vet.

Drugs useful in aiding the treatment of mild diarrhea

Activated charcoal tablets (available from pharmacist)
    Small dogs: ½ tablet   Give three times daily or at
    Medium dogs: 1 tablet   each loose motion.
    Large dogs: 2 or more tablets
Kaomagma (aluminium hydroxide gel)
    Toy dogs: ½-1 teaspoon   Give three times daily or at
    Medium dogs: 1 dessertspoon   each loose motion.
    Large dogs: 1 tablespoon

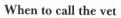

When to call the vet

- If the dog is depressed or very lethargic.
- If there is blood in the motion.
- If diarrhea is accompanied by vomiting.
- If diarrhea persists or recurs after treatment.

CONSTIPATION

Constipation is the infrequent passage of feces (bowel motions). As a result, feces become dry and difficult and painful to pass.

Signs of constipation:

- Difficulty passing motions.
- Dry, hard feces, sometimes slightly blood streaked.
- Frequent attempts to pass motions *(straining)* with little or no success.

When your dog squats and strains look to see if the motion is passed.

Constipation can be insidious in onset and at first the dog shows few

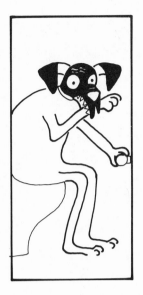

signs. If neglected, the condition can result in a very sick dog which is not eating, losing weight and perhaps vomiting.

A warning: Occasionally we are presented with a dog passing a very fluid motion but still straining. What happens in some cases is that a mass of hard faeces is sitting immovable in the rectum (usually just at the entrance of the pelvic canal. Fig. 9:6) and the dog is straining and passing fluid *around* the mass, giving the owner a false impression of diarrhea when in fact the dog has an obstruction.

The causes of constipation

The following are important factors:

Diet
Some foods lacking in fiber, such as bones and dry food, tend to produce a dry motion, and this leads to constipation in *some* dogs.

Inactive dogs are more liable to constipation.

Age
Older dogs have less muscle "tone" in their bowel and this may lead to constipation.

Obstructions
Eating indigestible matter can cause temporary slowing of the bowel and even a complete blockage. This is more common in pups and dogs who are liable to eat rubbish such as fruit stones, plastic bags, socks and underwear and toys. Rubbish eating is common in some breeds, such as the Basset and Labrador.

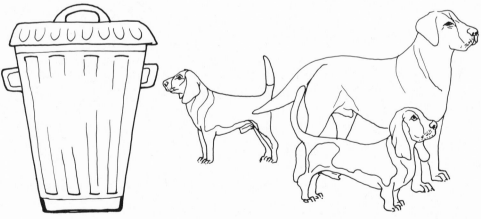

9.5 *Notorious rubbish eaters: Bassets, Beagles and Labradors. Any dog that invades rubbish bins runs a risk of obstructions or gastroenteritis developing*

Enlarged prostate
Male dogs have a gland near the brim of the pelvis (Fig. 9:6). If this becomes enlarged it may become painful to pass feces and the dog may become constipated. An enlarged prostate is more common in older dogs.

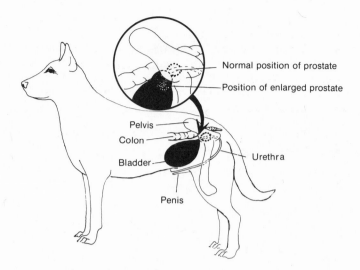

9.6 *Prostatitis: the prostate gland normally lies in the position marked by the dotted line. When enlarged it may drop back into the abdomen and can interface with both bowel movements and urinating*

Normal position of prostate

Position of enlarged prostate

Pelvis

Colon

Bladder

Urethra

Penis

Treatment for constipation

The aim of the treatment is to either lubricate the bowel and so allow easier passage of the stool, or to try and soften the hard mass that is blocking the bowel.

You may find some of the following treatments useful:

Liquid paraffin (paraffin oil is a lubricant, buy it from a chemist *not* a service station)
Dose: Small dogs: 5 ml twice daily.
    Medium dogs: 10-20 ml twice daily.
    Large dogs: 15-30 ml twice daily.

Oil emulsions (e.g., Agarol (Warner))
Dose: 5-30 ml daily according to size.

Olive oil is mildly laxative.
Dose: 5-30 ml daily.
(*Note:* These oil preparations should not be used continuously as they interfere with some vitamins and digestion over a long period. Do not use more frequently than twice weekly.)

Bulk producers (cereals and natural bran)
Breakfast cereals and natural bran designed to avoid constipation in man can be very helpful in dogs liable to constipation. Simply add a tablespoon or so daily to the food and increase or decrease the amount according to effect.

Methyl cellulose tablets (e.g., Cellulose, give 1-3 tablets daily) are available from chemists and may be given continuously.

Fecal softeners

There are tablets available which will soften hard bowel motions. Try Coloxyl 50 mg tablets and give 1-3 tablets daily.

Castor oil

Castor oil is not recommended as it can eventually constipate, although at first it will cause loosening of the bowel motions.

Cascara sagrada
Dose: Liquid: 2-5 ml.
Granules (e.g. Senokot): ½-1 teaspoon daily.

Enemas
Enemas (a soapy water infusion inserted into the rectum to loosen feces) must be administered with great care. They are extremely useful in the hands of a competent person.

Suppositories
These are capsules inserted into the rectum. They are useful in human sufferers but dogs usually eject them before they have had time to work.

If home treatments are not successful after one day, do not leave your dog in unnecessary discomfort, but consult your vet.

Preventing constipation

You should, at all times, try to determine the cause of the constipation and prevent it occurring again, e.g., you may have to stop giving your dog bones.

If you know your dog is liable to constipation, then watch for regular bowel movements. Early treatment is not only easier but avoids unnecessary discomfort for your dog.

My dog passes a lot of wind. Can I stop this?

Some gas production in the gut is normal. Most gas is absorbed into the blood stream and eventually eliminated, mainly through the lung as CO_2.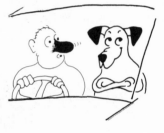

Sometimes, however, too much gas is produced and is released as a foul-smelling wind. Some foods tend to produce more gas, especially those containing uncooked carbohydrates, slightly "off" meat and some vegetables (p. 81). Older dogs have less muscle tone (strength) in their bowel than younger dogs and are therefore more likely to suffer from this problem than younger dogs.

The following may help to reduce gas formation (farting):
• Feed only **cooked** carbohydrates.
• Avoid legumes (beans and peas).
• Feed small amounts frequently rather than one large meal a day as this allows for easier digestion.
• Activated charcoal tablets may help. Give 1-3 tablets 3 times a day.

SWALLOWED OBJECTS

Dogs, especially pups, love to chew. It is one of their ways of investigating new things. If they swallow large or dangerous objects trouble may follow.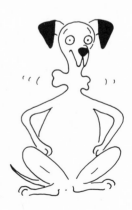

Some objects such as golf or squash balls can be swallowed by larger dogs. Stones, thrown for your dog to catch, may accidentally go straight down a dog's throat.

How does the intestine become obstructed?

Obstruction may occur in many ways. Eating indigestible material such as socks, stockings, balls, stones, toys, is a common cause.

The obstruction may also arise as a result of the gut twisting or telescoping into itself. In pups heavy roundworm infection may cause a blockage.

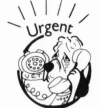

Signs of an obstructed intestine

A twisted bowel results in an acute emergency with the dog becoming very shocked, extremely depressed and often in a lot of pain. Early diagnosis is important. If the *stomach* is involved, a large swollen gas and fluid filled stomach bloats the abdomen.

Beware: If the obstruction is blocking the bowel near its lower end (in the large intestine or colon) then signs are not so spectacular and it is very easy to mistake the condition for constipation.

The signs of obstruction are very variable, so home diagnosis is difficult.

If you suspect your dog has swallowed a foreign body,
seek advice from your vet immediately.

Signs of obstruction

High obstructions (near the start of the gut) may cause vomiting, depression, a tense abdomen, and even collapse, due to shock.

Low obstructions (closer to the end of the gut) may be harder to pick. Vomiting of fecal matter and a foul breath, gradual depression, blood and mucus in the droppings, abdominal discomfort and dehydration may be seen.

There are several places where foreign objects are liable to get stuck:

Stuck in the mouth: Usually a foreign body can be gently prised out. If sharp edges are involved *do not* attempt to dislodge it, leave it for your vet to remove under anesthetic.

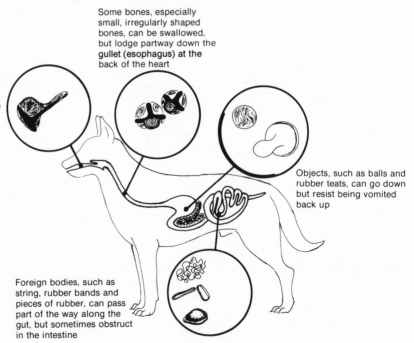

9.9 *Places where foreign objects are likely to become stuck*

Some bones, especially small, irregularly shaped bones, can be swallowed, but lodge partway down the **gullet (esophagus) at the** back of the heart

Bones, especially when cooked, may splinter and lodge around the teeth or the roof of the mouth or the throat

Objects, such as balls and rubber teats, can go down but resist being vomited back up

Foreign bodies, such as string, rubber bands and pieces of rubber, can pass part of the way along the gut, but sometimes obstruct in the intestine

Stuck "half-way down": The gullet (esophagus) has a bend in it (as it goes around the heart). Sometimes objects get stuck in the bend. If they are irregular in shape, they may be wedged there. Chop bones stuck there are especially dangerous. If not surgically removed they will lead to death.

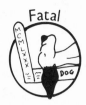

Stuck in the stomach: Both authors have removed a great number of objects from dogs' stomachs, including a gorilla (a rubber toy one of course). Objects stuck in the stomach cause indigestion with some vomiting and diarrhea.

Examples of foreign bodies the authors have removed include nails, golf balls, rocks, underwear, clothes pegs, peach stones, rubber door stopper, teats from baby's bottle and in one case five 10 dollar notes.

Stuck in the bowel: Some objects can get part of the way through the intestine before getting stuck. If the bowel is blocked then this is an emergency case. The closer this blockage is to the stomach, the more acute the emergency. Rough or sharp edges on a foreign body create even further hazards as they may puncture the intestine and cause peritonitis—a severe infection produced by leakage of gut contents into the abdomen.

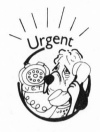

> When a foreign object is swallowed, it may be dangerous to
> try to induce vomiting. Always seek veterinary advice.

Can a foreign object pass through the gut?

This depends on the size and shape of the object. Seeds, nuts, fruit stones and small glass marbles are objects commonly swallowed that usually produce no problems. Sharp bones may be digested before they cause trouble, but sometimes they do cause blockages.

> Avoid feeding small bones or cooked bones.
> Both can cause bowel blockages.

How to avoid foreign objects being swallowed

If your dog has a tendency to eat foreign objects, move potentially dangerous items out of reach. *Never* throw stones or short sticks for dogs to catch as these can be accidentally swallowed. Take special care on garbage collection days to keep your dog from wandering. Keep stockings, small plastic toys, golf balls out of reach, especially from the young, chewing pup.

PANCREATITIS

The pancreas is a small but vital organ that sits near the stomach. It has two functions. One is to produce insulin which is necessary to control the blood sugar level. The second is to produce chemicals called enzymes which are essential in the digestion of the food.

Sudden inflammation of the pancreas produces a serious and very painful condition termed *Acute Pancreatitis*. The cause may be infection or

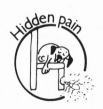

105

tumor, although most cases are of unknown cause. Digestive enzymes released from the inflamed pancreas begin to digest the pancreas itself and death can be the result.

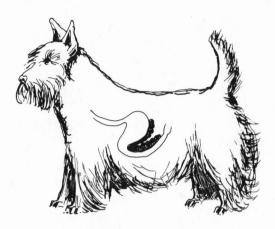
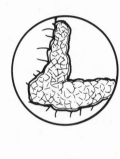

9.10 *The pancreas is situated around the stomach and start of the small intestine*

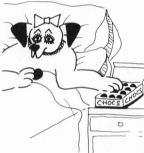

9.11 *Overweight, lazy females are particularly prone to pancreatitis*

Signs of acute pancreatitis

Fat, middle-aged female dogs are more likely to be affected, but acute pancreatitis can occur in any dog.

The dog usually has very painful abdomen (shown by a tense, hunched back and a disinclination to move). He will be depressed and usually will not eat and may vomit. In severe cases he may collapse.

Other conditions can also produce these signs and diagnosis requires a careful examination, laboratory tests and perhaps X-rays.

Chronic pancreatitis

When production of the pancreas' enzymes is inadequate, some types of foods (protein, fat and some starches) are not digested properly.

Signs of chronic pancreatitis

The dog may show a gradual loss of weight and yellowy, greasy droppings are suggestive. If subtle changes are present then laboratory examination of the droppings may provide a diagnosis.

Treatment of chronic pancreatitis

Supplementary pancreas enzymes are given prior to feeding or mixed with the food, to allow digestion of fats and protein.

LIVER PROBLEMS (hepatitis)

The liver is the power house of the body. It produces and stores foods, breaks down toxins and poisons, manufactures essential chemicals to digest food stuffs, stores and filters blood, stores vitamins and iron and converts food to energy.

Signs of liver disease

Because it is such a complex organ, signs of liver disease vary considerably with the nature of the condition and are often insidious in onset. (See Infectious Canine Hepatitis, p. 69-70).

Signs include lack of appetite, abdominal pain—especially on the right side behind the ribs, yellowing (jaundice) of the gums, anemia and build-up of fluid in the abdomen.

These signs are not exclusive to liver disease and laboratory tests of blood and urine are usually required before a diagnosis is made.

DIABETES

There are two types of diabetes:

Diabetes insipidus

The waste products of the body are normally concentrated in the urine and excreted. In *Diabetes insipidus* the kidneys cannot concentrate the urine and so large volumes of dilute urine are passed.

Signs of Diabetes insipidus

- Increased thirst.
- Increased volume of urine output.
- Increased frequency of urine output.

Diagnosis of Diabetes insipidus

Diagnosis is made by veterinary examination of the urine.

Causes of Diabetes insipidus

Complex and vary from compulsive water drinking to hormone disturbances.

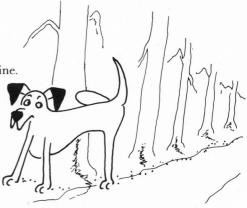

Treatment of Diabetes insipidus

Often unrewarding.

Diabetes mellitus

Was first discovered by the Greeks, who noted that sufferers had "sweet" urine. Is also called "sugar" diabetes. It is caused by a lack of sufficient *insulin* in the blood stream. Insulin is normally produced by an organ in the abdomen (the pancreas) and is essential for the body to be able to use the sugars in the blood stream. If insulin is not present it is very like an engine without spark plugs: no matter how much gas is pumped in, unless the spark plugs are there, nothing can happen. Similarly, unless insulin is present, the cells of the body cannot "fire" their normal fuel, which is glucose. Not realizing the problem, the cells call for more glucose to be released to them and so the glucose levels in the blood stream rise. But, without insulin, the body cells cannot use the glucose, so, a lot of the glucose spills out in the urine, taking fluids with it.

9.12 *Diabetes: one of the common early signs of diabetes is increased urine output*

Signs of Diabetes mellitus

- Increased urine output.
- Increased thirst.

• Weight loss.
• Increased hunger.
• Cataracts occur in 10-15 per cent of diabetic dogs (see Eye Diseases, p. 183-4).

Diagnosis of Diabetes mellitus

Veterinary diagnosis is made by finding abnormally high glucose levels in urine and blood.

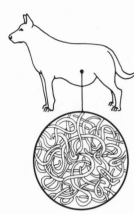

Insulin treatment

Insulin may be provided by daily injections, which dogs tolerate very well. An observant owner can maintain his pet in a happy state for the rest of his life by regularly using a dip stick to measure urine glucose.

For successful therapy a good liaison with your vet is essential. Any problems should be discussed as they arise.

You will need to keep a strict watch on both diet and the amount of exercise the dog gets as both must be strictly regulated to a specific amount per day.

Caring for a diabetic dog will involve you in a lot of effort. Be certain you are willing to make this effort before you accept the responsibility for the care of a diabetic dog.

WORMS

Worms are parasites that live in the intestines. There are several types.

Roundworms

Roundworms are quite large; the males can grow up to 10 cm and females to 18 cm long. Roundworms belong to the family Ascaridae, of the genera *Toxocara canis* and *Toxocaris leonina*.

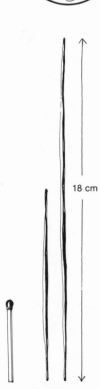

18 cm

Roundworms are the most common worm parasites of the puppy. All pups should be routinely checked for roundworms.

What harm do worms do?

Because of their life cycle, the developing roundworm can cause inflammation of the lungs, stomach and intestine. The severely affected pup is typically "pot bellied."

The adult worms live in the pups' intestines and can cause indigestion, diarrhea, pain and, in very severe cases, death.

Life cycle

Pups can be infected by eating hatched eggs from around the mother's nipples; from contamination of food or soil; by the mother's droppings; and by eating infected rodents, insects and birds.

Immature worms in the mother are stimulated to move into her womb (Fig. 9.15) to infect the unborn pups.

Pups can be infected with roundworms before they are born.

9.13 *Roundworms: severely affected dogs can be infested with massive numbers of worms, some of which grow to 18 cm long*

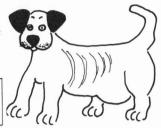

Diagnosis of roundworm
This is done by a laboratory examination of the puppy droppings. Multiple stool samples should be run to be sure your pet is free of parasites.

> Roundworms are a possible human health hazard.
> ard. Keep untested young pups away from thumb-sucking children.

9.14 *Pups severely affected by roundworm have a typically pot bellied appearance and are thin and poorly developed*

Treatment of roundworm
If the lab test reveals roundworms, your veterinarian can treat your puppy with a variety of drugs. Another stool sample should then be run at three weeks to be sure that the worms are eliminated.

Adult dogs
Adult dogs can get worms, too, although they are less common after puppyhood. Have a stool sample checked every six months for the life of the dog.

9.15 *The lifecycle of roundworms*

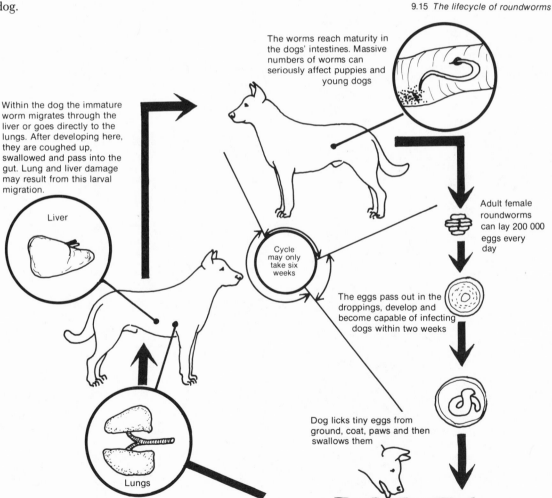

The worms reach maturity in the dogs' intestines. Massive numbers of worms can seriously affect puppies and young dogs

Within the dog the immature worm migrates through the liver or goes directly to the lungs. After developing here, they are coughed up, swallowed and pass into the gut. Lung and liver damage may result from this larval migration.

Liver

Cycle may only take six weeks

Lungs

Adult female roundworms can lay 200 000 eggs every day

The eggs pass out in the droppings, develop and become capable of infecting dogs within two weeks

Dog licks tiny eggs from ground, coat, paws and then swallows them

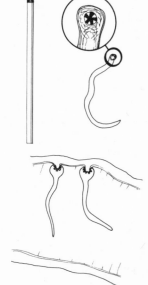

How to avoid roundworms

Assume your pups are affected. Treat them routinely without waiting for a positive diagnosis. Female pups treated correctly at 28 days, 35 days, 42 days and 2 months of age may *not* subsequently infect their pups when they mature and are bred.

Public health: a warning

If people (usually children) eat canine roundworm eggs severe disease may result. This is mainly in dirt eating children or children who may pick up pups' droppings and subsequently suck their thumbs.

- Children should be told to wash their hands after handling pups.
- All droppings should be removed as soon as possible.
- Treat your pup regularly for roundworm.

Hookworms (scientific names: *Ancylostoma* species, *Uncinaria* species)

One or two cms long, hookworms have one end bent into a hook (Fig. 9:16).

These worms have teeth or "cutting plates" and are common invaders of the intestine, causing inflammation of the gut and anemia.

How dogs are infected

- Sometimes by the larvae (immature worms) burrowing through the skin (and thereby causing skin inflammation). The most common method is infection by mouth via contaminated grass or food.
- From the milk of the mother. Some infection can occur in the uterus (womb) before the pups are born. The life cycle of these worms helps to explain the damage they do.

9.16 *Hookworm possess teeth or cutting plates which can severely damage the lining of the gut*

9.17 *The lifecycle of the hookworm: hookworm affects dogs of all ages. Infection occurs by hookworm larvae penetrating the skin, or by being swallowed. Pups can be infected by ingesting larvae along with the bitch's milk*

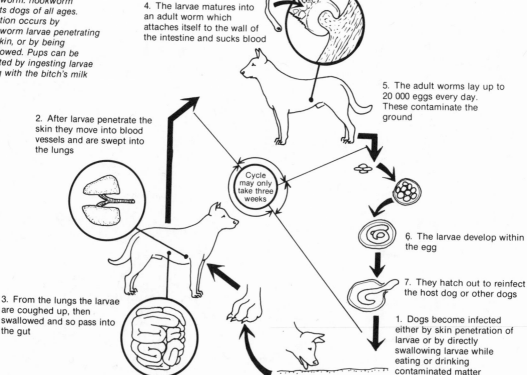

4. The larvae matures into an adult worm which attaches itself to the wall of the intestine and sucks blood

5. The adult worms lay up to 20 000 eggs every day. These contaminate the ground

2. After larvae penetrate the skin they move into blood vessels and are swept into the lungs

Cycle may only take three weeks

6. The larvae develop within the egg

7. They hatch out to reinfect the host dog or other dogs

3. From the lungs the larvae are coughed up, then swallowed and so pass into the gut

1. Dogs become infected either by skin penetration of larvae or by directly swallowing larvae while eating or drinking contaminated matter

Enormous numbers of eggs can be produced. These eggs can survive for years on the ground.

The young hookworms move to the intestines, grow, and start to burrow into the gut wall. Blood loss can be severe, especially in pups. Diarrhea reduces food absorption and wasting of the body follows.

Diagnosis of hookworm
Weight loss, diarrhea, blood in the droppings, and skin inflammation (especially around the paws). Pups are much more likely to be seriously affected than adult dogs. A small sample of the feces (droppings) examined by a vet provides a positive diagnosis.

Treatment of hookworm
The aim is to:
• Kill the worm.
• Correct the anemia and malnutrition, if present.

Treat the dog at intervals to prevent any new worms from developing to troublesome adults (more worms are picked up from eggs previously dropped). Each female adult worm can produce 500-800 eggs per gram of feces *per day.*

Note that "worm tablets" from the pet shop may not kill all types of worms and in many cases are not effective against hookworm.

Some drugs used: Canex-plus (Pfizer), Task (Shell), Canopar, Telmintic and Vermiplex

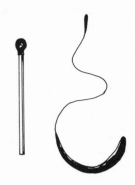

9.18 *The whipworm is small but dangerous. The thin front section is buried deep into the gut wall to suck blood and large numbers of worms can cause serious disease*

> Repeated treatment at regular intervals is necessary for
> hookworm-infected dogs.

Whipworm (scientific name *Trichuris* species.)

Shaped with a very thin, long front part and a relatively thicker tail the "whip" worm does resemble a whip. When feeding, the whipworm sticks the front part deep into the lining of the intestine and sucks.

Signs of whipworm infestation
Diarrhea, bloody droppings (usually very dark, almost tarry in severe cases). Poor coat, weight loss. Sometimes there is dehydration and pain in the abdomen.

Life cycle
The adult female passes her eggs out in the droppings. These eggs are very hardy and can survive for up to five years, although one year will allow most eggs to hatch and develop to the infective larvae (young, immature worms).

The larvae are eaten and grow and develop as they slowly pass down the gut. Adult worms are found towards the lower portions of the gut (the cecum and colon).

Diagnostic aid
Fecal samples can be regularly examined by your vet.

Treatment of whipworm
Effective drugs, such as a Canex-plus, Task, Telmintic are available. Because of reinfection due to eggs hatching out, repeated treatments are advisable.

9.19 *The lifecycle of the whipworm*

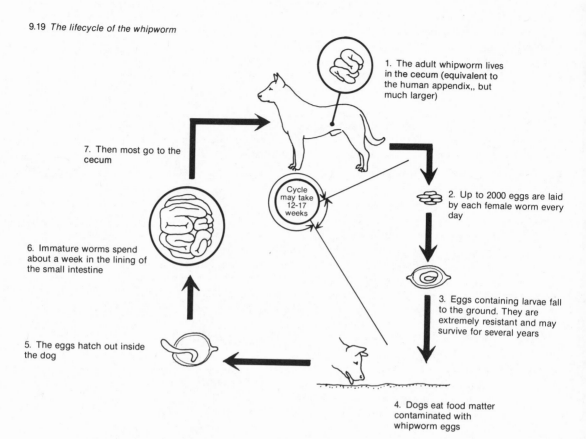

1. The adult whipworm lives in the cecum (equivalent to the human appendix,, but much larger)

7. Then most go to the cecum

Cycle may take 12-17 weeks

2. Up to 2000 eggs are laid by each female worm every day

6. Immature worms spend about a week in the lining of the small intestine

3. Eggs containing larvae fall to the ground. They are extremely resistant and may survive for several years

5. The eggs hatch out inside the dog

4. Dogs eat food matter contaminated with whipworm eggs

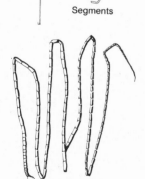

Segments

Head of tapeworm

9.20 *Tapeworms can be extremely long and are composed of many barrel-shaped segments. The rear-most segments which break off and pass out with the dogs feces are actually capsules stuffed full of eggs*

Remove droppings from the garden, kennel or run every day to prevent build up of parasite eggs.

Tapeworm

There are many different types of tapeworm. The most important to humans is the *Hydatid* tapeworm. *Apart from hydatids, dog tapeworms cannot be transmitted to man.*

The tapeworm can be very long (a meter or more). It consists of a head which is attached to the wall of the intestine and a body made up of many segments (Fig. 9:20). The hindmost segments can be shed in the droppings and segments contain thousands of eggs.

Signs of tapeworm
Tapeworms are usually diagnosed by seeing the segments in the droppings. 0.63-1.27 cm long and pinkish white to yellow, these segments can be seen to expand and contract and they move about. When the segments have dried they resemble grains of rice. They can stick to the dog's coat especially around the anus, sometimes causing an itch and rubbing results. Contrary to popular belief tapeworms rarely cause much discomfort to the dog. They may occasionally cause abdominal pain and it is rare if they ever block the gut. In very young, old or sick dogs they can weaken the dog and cause weight loss.

Diagnosis of tapeworm
Seeing the segments in the droppings.

In the case of hydatid tapeworm (see below) diagnosis is made by purging the dog and examining the excreta for the worm.

Treatment of tapeworm
Treat with pragiquantel (Doncit) or other drugs

How to avoid tapeworms
• Treat the dog with the appropriate drugs or bunamidine (Scoloban)
• Control fleas (to prevent reinfection).
• Avoid possibility of your dog eating small rodents or raw offal. If this is not possible, regular dosing may be required every 3 months.

When to see the vet
• If segments are still seen after treatment.
• If vomiting or diarrhea occurs after treatment.
• If weight loss persists after treatment.

Do tapeworms go from dog to dog?

Tapeworms are *not* passed directly from dog to dog. Their life cycle needs an intermediate host, such as fleas, mice, lizards, rabbits, and sometimes fish.

The hydatid tapeworm

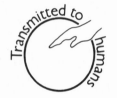

The hydatid tapeworm deserves special consideration because of the public health significance. The dog can be infected by eating *raw* infected sheep offal. Most important of all, *man can be infected by the dog*. Fortunately hydatid tapeworm is controlled readily.

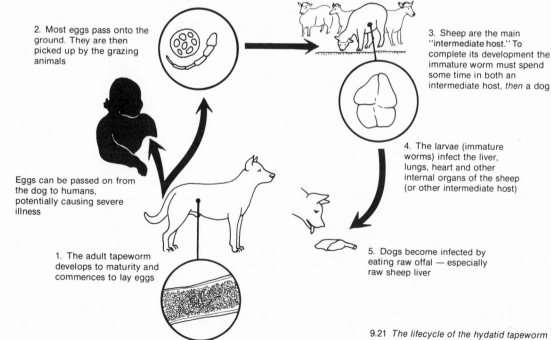

2. Most eggs pass onto the ground. They are then picked up by the grazing animals

3. Sheep are the main "intermediate host." To complete its development the immature worm must spend some time in both an intermediate host, *then* a dog

4. The larvae (immature worms) infect the liver, lungs, heart and other internal organs of the sheep (or other intermediate host)

Eggs can be passed on from the dog to humans, potentially causing severe illness

1. The adult tapeworm develops to maturity and commences to lay eggs

5. Dogs become infected by eating raw offal — especially raw sheep liver

9.21 *The lifecycle of the hydatid tapeworm*

113

The adult hydatid tapeworm is very small—only 4-6 mm long. This tapeworm only infects dogs (including the dingo). Each adult lays about 1000 eggs a fortnight. These eggs are picked up by sheep, cattle, pigs, goats, kangaroos and wallabies. It is the sheep-to-dog cycle that is by far the most important.

How to avoid hydatids

> To avoid parasites, cook any meat scraps given to your dog.
> Avoid any access to sheep carcasses.

Always boil sheep's livers for 40 minutes before feeding them to your dog. Other measures to take include disposing of all sheep, goat or pig carcasses away from all dogs; reducing or controlling all roaming dogs and tying up country dogs at killing time.

In some farm areas, dogs can pick up this parasite by eating the carcasses of sheep and cattle.

> Country children should not be allowed to play
> with untreated dogs.

Signs of hydatid tapeworms
The dog usually shows no signs of infection by the hydatid tapeworm.

Diagnosis of hydatid tapeworms
Diagnosis is achieved by identification of the worm in the feces.

In the sheep, the immature form of the tapeworm moves from the gut and invades the liver and also (but less commonly) the lungs, bones and other organs. Large cysts develop, within which hundreds of thousands of young worms start to develop.

ANAL SACS AND GLANDS

Dogs have two small sacs close to their anus, one on either side. They are also known as "scent glands" as they contain a foul-smelling fluid, a little of which is expressed when the dog has a bowel motion. It is thought that their function is to mark the droppings with the dog's individual scent. The modern dog does not need anal sacs.

Problems arise when the duct through which these sacs empty becomes blocked. Secretions within the sac build up and the subsequent swollen sac causes discomfort to the dog.

Signs of anal gland impaction

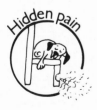

The dog tries to relieve the pain by rubbing or licking around the area of the anus. The dog may suddenly sit down, turn around and look at the base of his tail or scoot on his bottom along the ground.

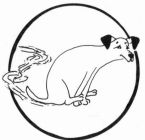

> If your dog is scooting on his rear end along the ground it usually means that his anal glands are itching.

If infection develops, the area will become swollen and very sensitive to touch. The dog may become constipated due to his reluctance to strain and the pain of passing a motion.

Infection of a swollen gland may lead to an abscess developing. This is seen as a red swollen area at the side of the anus. These abscesses usually burst and you will then see a ragged opening discharging a little pus or blood-stained fluid.

Treatment of anal sac impaction:

The sacs may be expressed (or emptied) by squeezing them. Although this can be done at home, have your vet show you the correct method first.

Beware: The secretions may be ejected at quite a velocity and are extremely foul smelling. It is advisable not to wear your favorite shirt when squeezing anal sacs!

Method
Take the tail in one hand and lift it high. Wear a rubber or plastic glove. Put thumb and forefinger around the anus at the 4 o'clock and 8 o'clock position (Fig: 9.22). Squeeze firmly but gently upwards and slightly inwards. The sacs should empty out around the edge of the anus. If the sacs are swollen and infected, veterinary treatment is advisable. It may be necessary to give antibiotics or to pack the gland with ointment.

In severe or recurring anal sac problems your vet may advise surgical removal of the glands. As they have no useful function, the dog suffers no handicap from their loss.

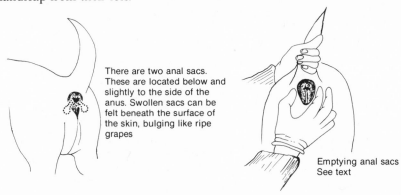

There are two anal sacs. These are located below and slightly to the side of the anus. Swollen sacs can be felt beneath the surface of the skin, bulging like ripe grapes

Emptying anal sacs
See text

9.22 *Anal sacs: dogs with swollen anal sacs frequently scoot their bottom along the ground or lick frantically beneath their tail*

ANAL FURUNCULOSIS
(open ulcerated or discharging areas around the anus).

It is thought that German Shepherds are more prone to this condition as many carry their tails pulled down over the rectum, thus making conditions more favorable for infection to develop.

Treatment may involve extensive surgery if washes, lotions and antibiotics are ineffective.

PERINEAL HERNIA

This condition occurs when intestines or other abdominal organs are no longer in their correct position in the abdomen, but are pushed back through the pelvis and are seen bulging out near the anus.

9.23 *Perineal hernia*

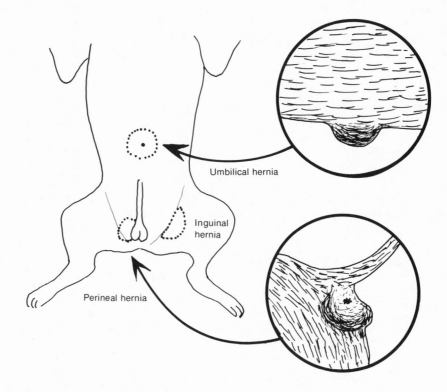

Umbilical hernia

Inguinal hernia

Perineal hernia

Signs of perineal hernia

Perineal hernia occurs mainly, but not exclusively, in male dogs of 8 years and over. The most common sign is *straining*, associated with a swelling near the anus. This swelling is soft and is not the tight, hot and tense swelling of an abscess or infection. This swelling may be on one or both sides of the rectum.

Treatment of perineal hernia

Surgical treatment may be necessary.

10. Kidney and bladder

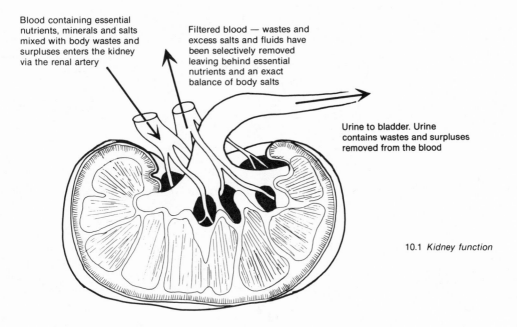

Blood containing essential nutrients, minerals and salts mixed with body wastes and surpluses enters the kidney via the renal artery

Filtered blood — wastes and excess salts and fluids have been selectively removed leaving behind essential nutrients and an exact balance of body salts

Urine to bladder. Urine contains wastes and surpluses removed from the blood

10.1 *Kidney function*

KIDNEY DISEASE

The dog has two kidneys which filter the blood and remove body wastes which would otherwise build up and "poison" the system. If the kidneys are damaged, wastes may not be effectively removed, resulting in illness. There are two main groups of kidney disease—chronic and acute kidney disease.

10.2 *The urinary organs*

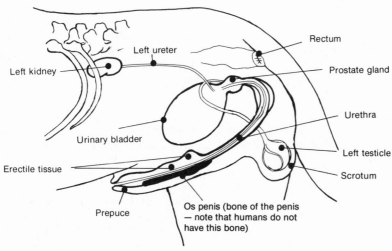

Left ureter

Left kidney

Rectum

Prostate gland

Urethra

Urinary bladder

Left testicle

Scrotum

Erectile tissue

Prepuce

Os penis (bone of the penis — note that humans do not have this bone)

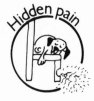

Chronic kidney disease

In chronic kidney disease there is a slow destruction of the kidney which may take months or years. This may be caused by low grade infection (by bacteria, virus or parasite), by poisons, chemicals, or physical damage such as a car accident. In most cases the cause is not determined.

Signs of disease are not seen until two-thirds of both kidneys are destroyed, because until then the remaining healthy kidney tissue manages to cope. Once the two-thirds mark is passed signs of chronic kidney disease start—often suddenly.

Signs of chronic kidney disease
Signs are not specific for chronic kidney disease but may include:
- Depression.
- Lack of appetite.
- Vomiting and diarrhoea.
- Mouth ulcers.
- Changes in the amount and nature of urine. (Usually larger quantities of dilute urine are passed.)
- Weight loss.

10.3 *Kidney disease: kidneys can suffer damage in many ways: by disease, infection or drugs Early detection of kidney disease is essential to minimize damage, but the warning signs are not always obvious and can be overlooked*

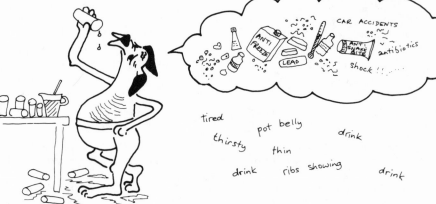

Veterinary care
Urine and blood tests will show if the kidneys are working properly. The most common test determines the amount of urea in the blood. Urea is a substance that is normally present only in small quantities in the blood. Increased urea in the blood is a sign that the kidneys are not adequately filtering excess urea out of the blood stream.

Treatment of chronic kidney disease
Treatment is aimed at reducing further damage and easing the "work load" on the kidneys. There is no cure and the damage is permanent, but often treatment can make the dog comfortable and greatly prolong his life.

Diet for chronic kidney disease
The average dog's diet has four times the amount of protein he needs. When kidney disease exists you must reduce the amount of protein fed so that the kidney has to eliminate less wastes. The protein given should be high quality, such as is found in lean meat, cottage cheese and eggs. White

meats such as chicken, veal and tripe are preferable to red meats such as beef.

A 13 kg dog would get enough protein from 120 g white meat plus one egg daily. He also needs other foods to balance his diet. Other foods that may be given include:

• Potatoes.
• Rice.
• Cooked vegetables (e.g., green beans, carrots).
• Bread (preferably wholemeal).
• Multivitamin/mineral supplement.

Several companies manufacture special balanced low-protein diets in canned moist, semi-moist, and dry forms.

Two low protein diets*

Recipe No. 1:

Cook as a stew:

460 g minced white meat or fish	450 g dry rice
1 large can (850 g) tomatoes	2 cups water
6 large potatoes	Juice 4 cans of green beans
2 large onions (optional)	Juice of 2 cans carrots
1 cup macaroni	Add the green beans and carrots from the cans.

This makes about 10 liters of food. Feed 1 liter per 18 kg bodyweight daily.

Recipe No. 2

120 g cooked white meat or fish
1 egg, hardboiled and finely chopped
0.5 cup dry rice, boiled
2 teaspoons dicalcium phosphate
3 slices bread, crumbled
Balanced vitamin-mineral supplement in a quantity sufficient to provide the daily requirement for each vitamin and mineral.

Mix all ingredients together thoroughly. This makes about 600 g food, which is the correct amount for a 13 kg dog. The mixture is dry and palatability may be improved by adding a little water (not milk).

Water

Always allow access to plenty of fresh, clean drinking water. Do not restrict the dog's water intake.

Vitamins

Some vitamins are lost in chronic kidney disease, so supplements, especially in the Vitamin B group and Vitamin C, are useful.

Minerals

Calcium supplements are an advantage. Examples are calcium carbonate, calcium gluconate, calcium lactate.

Salts

Sodium may be lost by a failing kidney and replacement is desirable. Common table salt contains sodium and could be used. Bicarbonate of soda (sodium bicarbonate) could also be used. Because of potential problems in

*Australian Veterinary Practitioner 7 (2), June 1971

dogs with heart conditions, leave the decision regarding sodium supplement to your vet.

If a low protein diet is given before kidney failure occurs will this prevent the problem?

No, although you may slow the onset of the problem. Diet does not *cause* the disease.

How common is chronic kidney disease in dogs?

It is the most common chronic condition in older dogs (i.e., over 8 years).

Are kidney transplants possible?

In theory, yes. In practice they are usually not considered.

Acute (sudden) kidney disease

Acute kidney disease (actually a group of conditions) differs from the chronic type in two main respects:
- The sudden onset of signs following damage to the kidneys.
- If the disease is halted quickly enough the outlook for the patient can be good and recovery complete.

Causes of acute kidney disease
There are many, and damage by agents listed below may not always result in kidney damage. In some diseases (for example, Infectious Canine Hepatitis) the kidney is not the main organ affected.
- Infection by bacteria, for example, Leptospirosis (see p. 76).
- Infection by a virus, for example Infectious Canine Hepatitis.
- Damage by chemicals such as: antifreeze (ethylene glycol), lead, carbon tetrachloride, mercury, some antibiotics.
- As a sequel to some venomous snake bites.
- Shock (see p. 17) from any cause can produce a reduction in the blood supply to the kidney and damage may result. The most common example is following a severe motor car accident.

When should you call the vet?

The signs are not specific for acute kidney disease, but may include the following:
- Vomiting.
- Appetite loss.
- Depression.
- Pain in the mid-back (lumbar) area.
- Change in urine output—may be more or less.
- Change in urine—discolored, or have clots, or cause pain in passing.
- Dehydration (shown as inelasticity of the skin).

Kidney disease presents itself with a variety of symptoms.

The absence of some of these signs does not rule out the possibility of kidney disease.

Diagnosis of acute kidney disease
Diagnosis is made by blood and urine tests and in some cases a sample of the kidney is taken (a renal biopsy) and examined microscopically by a pathologist.

DRIBBLING URINE (incontinence)

A dog that is dribbling urine is said to be "incontinent." This situation is often first noted by the owner as a wet patch on the floor where the dog has been lying or sleeping.

What is the most common cause?

The most common cause of dribbling urine in older dogs is a lack of muscle strength, or tone, in the bladder. It is especially common in older spayed females. Fortunately, effective treatment is simple and straightforward.

Why does dribbling occur?

The bladder sphincter is a ring of muscle which tightens to stop urine leaving the bladder. If this sphincter cannot tighten, urine leaks out and dribbling results.

Treatment of incontinence
The muscle of the sphincter will strengthen and tighten to seal the bladder under the influence of hormones of the estrogen type. These can be given by injection or in tablet form.

It is usually necessary to continue the estrogen supplement for many weeks and perhaps for the life of the dog, but weekly treatment is often enough to maintain the sphincter's tone once dribbling ceases.

What other problems cause dribbling urine?

• Birth defects: especially where the tube bringing urine from the kidneys does not empty into the bladder as it should, but elsewhere along the urinary tract (termed ectopic ureter).
• Hormone imbalances.
• Nerve damage or disease.
• Bladder inflammation.
• Paralysed bladder.
• Bladder stones, strictures or growths.

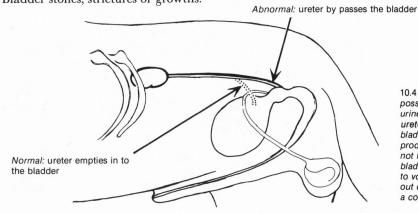

Abnormal: ureter by passes the bladder

Normal: ureter empties in to the bladder

10.4 *Ectopic ureter: a possible cause of dribbling urine. In this situation, the ureter "by passes" the bladder, so that urine produced by the kidney is not held in storage in the bladder until the dog is ready to void, but instead dribbles out of the penis (or vulva) in a constant slow drip*

121

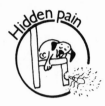

Kidney stones and bladder stones

Stones (uroliths) may form in the kidneys or bladder. The bladder is the more common site in the dog. These vary in size from tiny grains to large plum-sized stones.

What age is usually affected?

Any age dog can be affected but the middle-aged (about 6 years old) is most commonly affected.

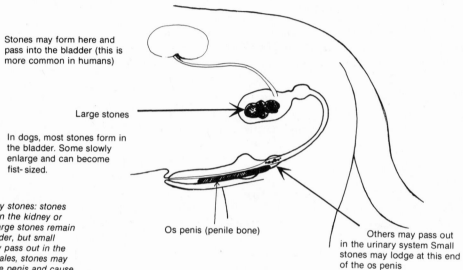

Stones may form here and pass into the bladder (this is more common in humans)

Large stones

In dogs, most stones form in the bladder. Some slowly enlarge and can become fist- sized.

Os penis (penile bone)

Others may pass out in the urinary system Small stones may lodge at this end of the os penis

10.5 *Kidney stones: stones may form in the kidney or bladder. Large stones remain in the bladder, but small stones may pass out in the urine. In males, stones may lodge in the penis and cause obstructions*

Signs of kidney stones
The signs vary; there may be some or any of the following:
- No urine at all (a blockage—this is an emergency).
- Difficulty or pain in passing urine.
- Increased frequency of urinating.
- A swollen, tense and sore abdomen.
- (Sometimes) dribbling of urine.

Diagnosis of kidney stones/ bladder stones
A diagnosis of stones in the urinary tract is helped by several aids. These include:
- Feeling the stones in the bladder through the wall of the abdomen.
- X-ray.
- Urine examination.
- Blood tests.
- Catheterization. This involves passing a special tube into the bladder through the urethra (see diagram).

Treatment of stones
In the same way that cheeses vary there are many different types of stones—some are hard, some soft, some large, some small. Surgery may be needed to remove the stones but medications and diet restrictions may be sufficient for others.

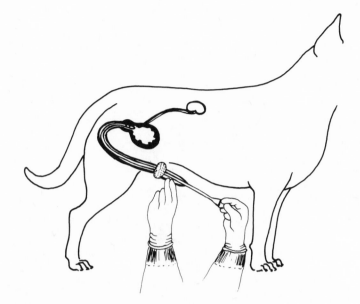

10.6 Catheterizing the bladder: *the vet may insert a thin rubber tube into the dog's urethra in order to clear a blockage, or to help in diagnosis of urinary tract disease by obtaining samples, or prior to x-raying the bladder*

Can you avoid a recurrence of stones?

This depends on the type of stone involved. Usually by strictly watching the diet and perhaps by using some medication you can greatly reduce the chance of more stones forming.

When to call the vet
If your dog
> • Has difficulty urinating or has blood in the urine.
> • Urinates in spurts and dribbles.
> • Cannot urinate. Beware—this condition requires urgent attention.
> • Has a swollen abdomen—see your vet immediately.

Diet restrictions (for dogs recovering from stones in bladder)
> • Avoid foods that tend to concentrate the urine, such as dry foods.
> • Always allow plenty of water.
> • Always allow your dog to eliminate all bodily wastes.
> • Avoid foods specified by your vet—these will vary according to type of stone involved.

Your vet may advise you to add some items to the diet. These include, in some cases, salt and Vitamin C.

Cystitis
Cystitis means inflammation of the bladder wall. The affected dog may strain after urinating as if the bladder were still full, and may pass a few drops of blood-stained urine. The cause is usually a bacterial infection. Caution: a blocked bladder and cystitis can be confused—call the vet.

11. Heart and lungs

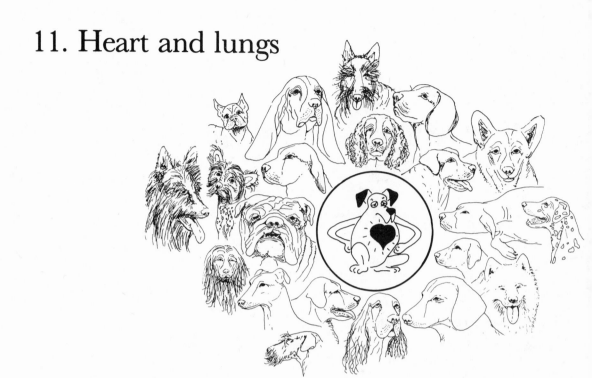

HEARTWORM

Heartworms are worms that live in the chambers of the heart and in some of the major blood vessels near the heart.

The worms are thin and long and when mature vary in length from 12-30 cm. It is quite common for infected dogs to have between 50 and several hundred worms living in or near the heart (Fig. 11:2).

11.2 *Heartworm: masses of heartworm coil together in the heart chambers and major blood vessels*

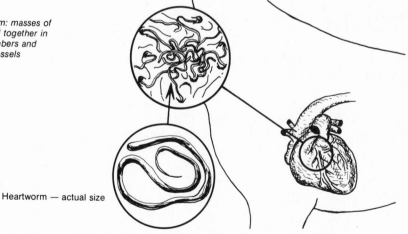

Heartworm — actual size

*, **, *** indicate increasing likelihood of a particular trait or problem occurring.

The signs of heartworm infection

At first, the signs are not dramatic, but as the worms grow and the numbers increase, heartworms damage the heart and reduce its effectiveness in pumping blood around the body. Other vital organs, such as the liver and kidney, are also handicapped by the poor blood supply. The signs at first are often of a general malaise—the dog is just "unwell."

Signs of heartworm infection may include:
- A cough (usually persistent or chronic).
- Gradual weight loss (in spite of good appetite—this is often overlooked at first).
- Lack of stamina—the dog tires easily.
- Fluids may build up in the abdomen, causing a swollen or pot-bellied appearance.
- Anemia.

In what areas are dogs liable to become infected with heartworm?

Heartworm is spreading. In the past, heartworm was confined to areas of high humidity and high temperature—such as the southern states of the USA, Africa, South America, Italy, Spain and Portugal and the northern states of Australia. For reasons that are not clear, the disease has become far more widespread recently. In North America, for example, even places such as Ontario, Canada (which has snow in winter and a relatively short summer) are experiencing heartworm cases.

It may be that new strains of mosquitoes and of heartworm that can survive prolonged cold periods are allowing this spread. The great increase in the numbers of dogs moving around and between countries is probably also important. Your local vet is the best source of information for the current situation in your area.

How does a dog become infected with heartworm?

The adult heartworm lies in the heart and lays enormous numbers of larvae called microfilaria. These microfilaria circulate in the blood stream and are picked up by feeding mosquitoes. The microfilaria continue their development within the mosquito and after about 14-21 days they are ready to invade a new host dog. When the mosquito bites a dog, the immature heartworms are transferred into the dog and continue their development in this new host.

About three months later, the heartworm larvae have developed to almost maturity and move into the heart where, after another three months or more, they begin to lay microfilaria for mosquitoes to pick up and continue the cycle.

Mosquitoes carry heartworms from dog to dog.

What happens after the heartworms reach the heart?

The worms gradually develop in the heart, some growing up to 30 cm long. They reach maturity after living in the heart for 2-3 months and start producing their own young, which are in turn picked up by feeding mosquitoes to infect other dogs.

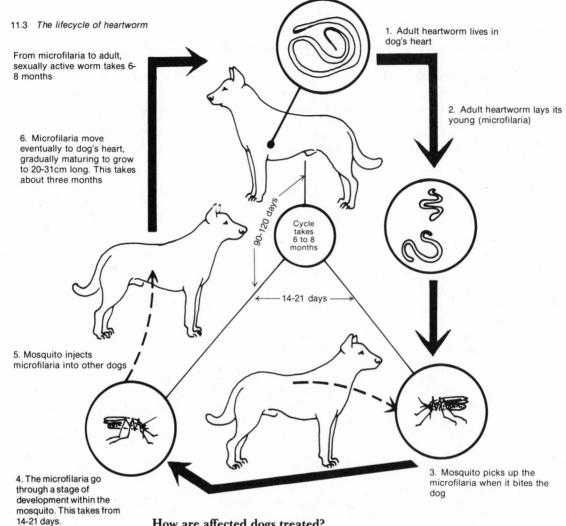

11.3   *The lifecycle of heartworm*

From microfilaria to adult, sexually active worm takes 6-8 months

1. Adult heartworm lives in dog's heart

2. Adult heartworm lays its young (microfilaria)

6. Microfilaria move eventually to dog's heart, gradually maturing to grow to 20-31cm long. This takes about three months

90-120 days

Cycle takes 6 to 8 months

14-21 days

5. Mosquito injects microfilaria into other dogs

4. The microfilaria go through a stage of development within the mosquito. This takes from 14-21 days.

3. Mosquito picks up the microfilaria when it bites the dog

How are affected dogs treated?

Heartworms can be successfully treated but because of the dangers involved in treating affected dogs they are often hospitalized during treatment.

An intravenous injection of a drug such as sodium carparsolate will kill the adult worm; *but* this may result in dead worms being swept out of the heart to lodge in the lungs and this can cause severe lung damage.

Follow-up treatment is essential, as the dogs will still carry immature worms for up to three years after the adults have been killed. Drugs presently used include Levamisole and dithiazine iodide but not DEC (diethylcarbamazine citrate). DEC is used only in prevention.

In order to avoid the dangers of infection, it is far better to put your dog on a preventive program.

How to prevent your dog from becoming infected

Prevention is the best way to handle the heartworm problem. If you live in an area known to be a "heartworm area," or if you are visiting or travelling through such an area, you can prevent heartworm developing in your dog by daily administration of drugs to kill the mosquito-borne heartworm (immature forms) *before* they develop into adults.

The drug most widely used at present is DEC (diethylcarbamazine citrate) at a dose of 6.25 mg per kg weight.

By giving small doses of DEC daily the microfilaria (immature heartworms) injected into the dog by mosquitoes are destroyed before they can mature into harmful adults.

> Use DEC drugs to prevent infection if your dog is travelling through heartworm country. DEC prophylaxis must be started 2 weeks before travelling and continued for 60-80 days after leaving endemic area.

Diagnosis of heartworm

If your vet suspects heartworm he will usually take one or more blood samples to look for microfilaria in the blood stream. As blood samples alone may not be enough to determine the severity of the condition, X-rays of the heart may be taken. ECGs and further blood tests to detect damage in other organs may also be useful.

> Have your dog checked every six months if you live in a heartworm area.

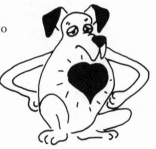

11.4 *Congestive heart failure: the heart beat speeds up in an attempt to push the required blood through the body*

Can humans be infected by heartworm?

The worms cannot mature in humans but there are reports of damage to the lungs by microfilaria in man.

When should you start to treat pups if you live in a heartworm danger area?

Start as soon as the pups take solid food—as early as 4-6 weeks of age.

HEART FAILURE

Heart disease can strike at any age, but chronic heart disease becomes more common with advancing age.

11.5 *Congestive heart failure: the heart gradually enlarges in size as the heart muscle stretches in its struggle to pump more*

Congestive heart failure (CHF)

Is the most comon heart condition of old dogs*** and occurs when the heart cannot pump blood fast enough around the body. Because of a decrease in the efficiency of the heart, several things happen:

• The heartbeat speeds up in an attempt to push the required blood through the body.

• The heart gradually enlarges in size as the heart muscle stretches in its struggle to pump more.

• Fluid builds up in the lungs or in the abdomen; sometimes in both.

• As the heart fails to keep blood moving in sufficient volume through the body, you will begin to notice changes in your dog.

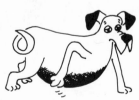

11.6 *Congestive heart failure: fluid builds up in the lungs or in the abdomen; sometimes in both*

127

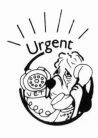

Warning signs of (congestive) heart failure:

• Reduced exercise tolerance: the dog tires easily, he goes for shorter walks and puffs and pants more. Note that when resting, the dog may show no signs until the disease is well advanced.

• A cough or retching may develop: often it is especially noticeable when the dog rises in the morning.

• Breathing becomes more frequent and labored. In advanced cases the dog's gums may be pale or even bluish tinged.

Treatment of heart failure

Exercise should be limited to *below* the level that provokes signs of discomfort.

In the early stages of CHF it may be enough to stop long periods of vigorous exercise and games. Later, activities such as long walks or stair climbing may have to be stopped. Gradually less and less exercise stimulates distress.

Eventually some dogs need to be restricted to a cage until treatment relieves the heart failure.

Diet

Once congestive heart failure has been diagnosed, the vet may recommend that salt in the dog's food be restricted or avoided. This is because salt increases the amount of fluid retained in the body and may increase congestion in the lungs or abdomen.

Salt does *not* cause congestive heart disease, but once the disease is present, excessive salt intake can make things worse.

Foods which are high in salt and should be avoided:

• Processed meats (e.g., meat blocks, frankfurts, sausage, ham, bacon). NB: Note that most commercial canned and dry foods are high in salt as it improves palatability.
  • Cheese.
  • Bread.
  • Cereals.
  • Carrots.
  • Spinach.
  • Heart, kidney and liver.
  • Dairy foods: butter, margarine, cream, ice cream, yoghurt.
  • Shellfish.
  • Canned or frozen vegetables, vegetable relishes.
  • Dried fruits.
  • Salted biscuits, potato chips, pretzels.

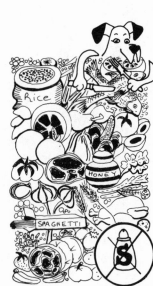

11.7 *The correct diet is important for the dog who has been diagnosed with congestive heart failure*

Foods which are low in salt and recommendable for heart patients:

• Rice, corn, oatmeal.
• Fish (freshwater).
• Chicken, rabbit, beef, lamb and horsemeat.
• Egg yolk.
• Most fresh vegetables.
• Fresh fruits.
• Macaroni, spaghetti.

• Unsalted butter, unsalted nuts.
• Honey.
• Garlic.
• Salad oils.

Sedatives

In general, sedatives are used only in the case of excitable dogs, and then only in moderation. They may be useful for dogs with heart disease that become very excited during thunderstorms or car travel.

Heart drugs/diuretics

Drugs such as Digoxin or Digitalis may be used to increase the power of the heart muscle. Veterinary supervision of these drugs is essential as they can be dangerous.

Drugs (e.g., Lasix) that reduce the amount of fluids accumulated in the chest and/or abdomen may be useful. (These drugs are termed Diuretics.)

Other drugs may be used according to individual cases. These include a drug to dilate the small air passages—a bronchodilator (e.g., Millophylline, Elixophylline, Neophylline).

Valve defects/leaking heart valves

A common cause of CHF in dogs is a leaking heart valve.

There are two main valves in the heart whose function is to seal a heart chamber while it pumps blood out into the major blood vessels.

If the valve is leaking, the heart "beat" loses some of its effect and so the efficiency of the heart is reduced.

What causes the valves to leak?

The valve's leakage is due to the formation of nodules on the valve's surface, preventing them from sealing effectively.

The treatment of leaking valves

There is no treatment which stops the growths forming on the surface of the valves. Many dogs have some valve leakage but show little or no ill effects. It is only in severe cases that treatment for heart failure becomes necessary. If the valves' efficiency is greatly reduced then congestive heart failure may result. The treatment of CHF is described on p. 127-8.

PNEUMONIA

Pneumonia is inflammation of the lungs.

The signs of pneumonia

The signs include some or all of the following:

• A deep, moist cough. This cough brings up exudate or fluid and mucus from the lungs. Usually exudate is swallowed but occasionally is coughed out or vomited up. A small amount may be discharged through the nose.
• Harsh breathing sounds.

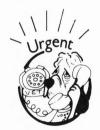

11.8 *The dog's lungs occupy most of the chest. They are sealed from the abdominal cavity by a muscular diaphragm and protected from injury by the ribs*

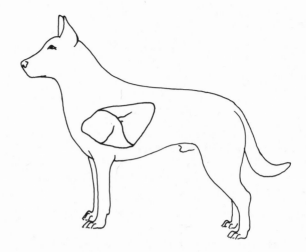

• A rumbling or bubbling sound in the chest (termed "rales"). These sounds are heard readily through a stethoscope, but you may hear them by putting your ear to the dog's chest.

• Dog tires easily and is reluctant to run or move about.

There are many terms used to describe infections of the airways, some of these terms are:

Bronchitis
Inflammation is mainly in the major air passages (or bronchi) and not in the lung tissue itself. The bronchi conduct air from the windpipe to the lung tissue.

Bronchopneumonia
The inflammation involves the lung tissue as well as the air passages.

Tracheobronchitis
Inflammation involving the windpipe (the trachea) and the bronchi.

Double pneumonia
Both lungs are affected.

The causes of pneumonia

Anything that invades the lungs to irritate the delicate airways can lead to pneumonia. Agents that overcome the body's defences include:

• Viruses: e.g., Distemper***, canine influenza virus and Herpes virus.

• Bacteria: Bacteria complicate other illness.

• Fungus or yeasts: In certain geographic areas, e.g., histoplasmosis, blastomycosis**, nocardiosis, cryptococcosis**.

• Inhalation of foreign matter, such as vomit, water or food.

• Parasites: some worms (e.g., the roundworm, which is very common in pups***) have a life cycle where the immature worms (or larvae) burrow through the lungs.

• Gases or fumes: e.g., car exhausts containing carbon monoxide.

• Allergic reactions: Allergic reactions involving the lungs are not common in dogs.

The treatment of pneumonia

The cause of the pneumonia must be established and eliminated if possible.

Pneumonia is a serious condition. Do *not* attempt home treatment and call your vet immediately. Delay may be fatal.

> Absolute rest is vital if pneumonia is suspected.

PLEURISY

The inside of the chest walls and the lungs are coated with a very thin membrane called the pleura (Fig. 11:9). If this membrane becomes inflamed, for example through infection, it often produces excess fluid which fills up the chest and pushes the lungs away from the chest wall. This condition is termed "Pleurisy."

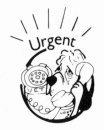

Signs:

These may be very gradual in onset and only noticed late in the course of the condition.
- Fever.
- Painful breathing.
- Labored breathing.
- Occasional coughing.

> If breathing is difficult, veterinary attention is urgent.

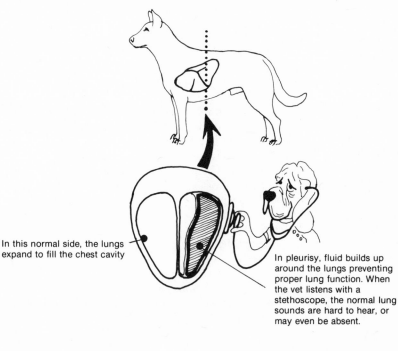

In this normal side, the lungs expand to fill the chest cavity

In pleurisy, fluid builds up around the lungs preventing proper lung function. When the vet listens with a stethoscope, the normal lung sounds are hard to hear, or may even be absent.

11.9 *Pleurisy: diagram of cross section through the chest showing one normal lung in comparison with one severely affected by pleurisy*

131

12. Skin and coat

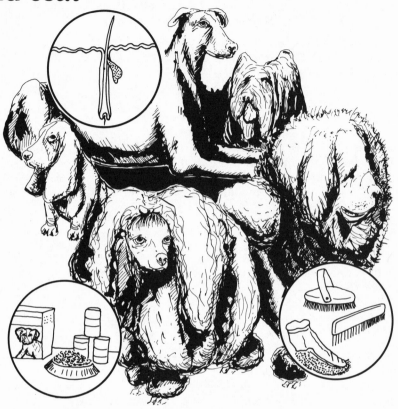

GROOMING

The dog's coat

A dog's hair is periodically shed, unlike human hair which grows continuously and therefore has to be cut. Dogs' hair grows in cycles: a short period of growth, a resting phase and then the shedding phase.

The average dog's coat takes four months to regrow, but there is a wide variation according to the breed. Long-haired breeds, such as Old English Sheepdog and Afghan, take up to eighteen months to regrow after shaving.

The rate at which hair regrows varies with many factors. Hormones have a profound effect on hair growth—for example, the coat of a bitch in heat will grow more slowly (as estrogen slows growth). A dog lacking thyroid hormone will have a dull, rough and slow-growing coat. A good diet is also essential for a healthy coat, so vitamin or other deficiencies are reflected by a poor coat, as are parasite infestations or ill-health.

> If your dog's coat is poor, suspect his general health.
> A general check-up may be wise.

*, **, *** indicate increasing likelihood of a particular trait or problem occurring.

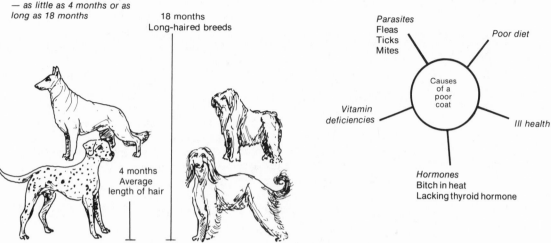

12.2 *The time taken for a dog's coat to grow back after shaving varies dramatically — as little as 4 months or as long as 18 months*

18 months
Long-haired breeds

4 months
Average
length of hair

12.3 *Causes of a poor coat*

Parasites
Fleas
Ticks
Mites

Poor diet

Causes
of a
poor
coat

Vitamin
deficiencies

Ill health

Hormones
Bitch in heat
Lacking thyroid hormone

Shedding hair

In the wild, dogs have a general shedding of their coat in spring and autumn. It was thought that temperature change was the main influence on coat shedding, but research has proved that it is the change in hours of light per day that is the most important influence. This is why house dogs, exposed to long hours of artificial light, shed throughout the year.

Most dogs have a general routine shedding of the coat once a year, although other factors can influence shedding. Bitches shed more after heat, during pregnancy and especially while nursing pups.

12.4 *Detail of a hair follicle of a German Shepherd*

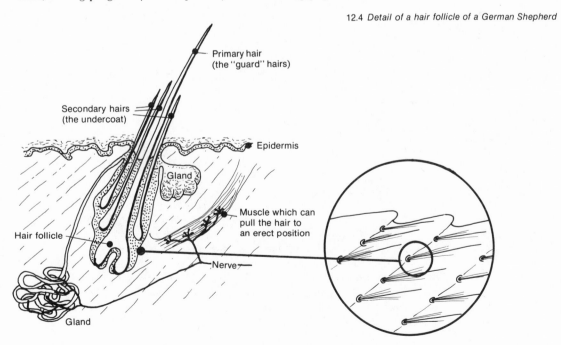

Primary hair
(the "guard" hairs)

Secondary hairs
(the undercoat)

Epidermis

Gland

Muscle which can
pull the hair to
an erect position

Hair follicle

Nerve

Gland

When dogs such as the German Shepherd, which has a "double coat" (coarse long hairs with an undercoat of short fine hairs), begin to shed, the inner coat is shed in tufts and this can give the appearance of a skin disease.

When shedding begins, daily brushing or grooming is advisable as dead hair next to the skin is irritating to the dog and may lead to excessive scratching and self-mutilation. A bath will help to loosen the hair which is then removed by thorough brushing.

Care of the skin and coat

(*Note:* This section is not intended to be a discussion of the cosmetic aspects of the coat, such as trimming, cutting and styling.)

The condition of the coat often reflects the general health of the dog. If the dog has a dry, lifeless coat the problem may be more than skin deep. Coat health depends on good health, good diet (including fat, p. 81) and regular grooming.

Grooming

Encourage regular grooming habits as early as possible when the dog is a pup, especially in long-coated breeds such as Old English Sheepdogs, Afghans, Pekingese and Maltese Terriers. A dog that enjoys and co-operates with grooming is so much easier to manage.

12.5 *Grooming aids*

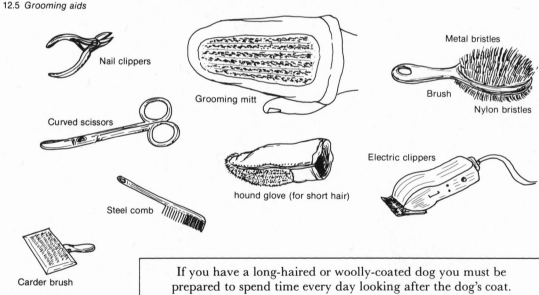

Nail clippers

Grooming mitt

Metal bristles

Brush

Nylon bristles

Curved scissors

Steel comb

hound glove (for short hair)

Electric clippers

Carder brush

Rake

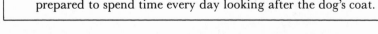

If you have a long-haired or woolly-coated dog you must be prepared to spend time every day looking after the dog's coat.

If you cannot spare the time every day, then select a smooth short-coated breed. Fluffy pups look cute, but when they grow into long-haired adults they need constant attention to keep them comfortable.

While long-coated dogs should not need more than 15 minutes spent on their grooming if it is done every day, the emphasis is on *every* day.

Brush the coat vigorously, parting long hair down to the skin. Pay special attention to the ears, tail and between the toes. All grass seeds must be removed daily in the summer.

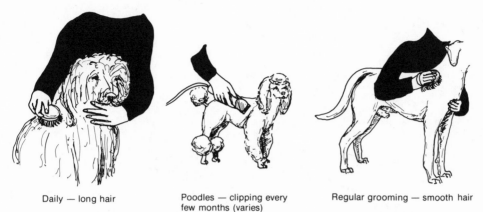

12.6 *Grooming*

Daily — long hair

Poodles — clipping every few months (varies)

Regular grooming — smooth hair

A number of dogs have an undercoat, especially those breeds which originated in the colder climates, and this must be teased out with a comb—brushing it is a waste of time because it is more like cotton wool than hair. Some dogs lose this undercoat when they become adults but others retain it permanently; Scotch Collies are an example. A steel comb is more effective than the plastic variety as the teeth penetrate better and are not too sharp.

Ears

Comb all long-haired ears daily to ensure knots do not occur. Ears which are heavily weighted with hair block off the ear canal and induce disease inside the ear (Fig. 12:8). If you are too busy for daily combing then clip *all* hair off the ears and keep the ear hair short.

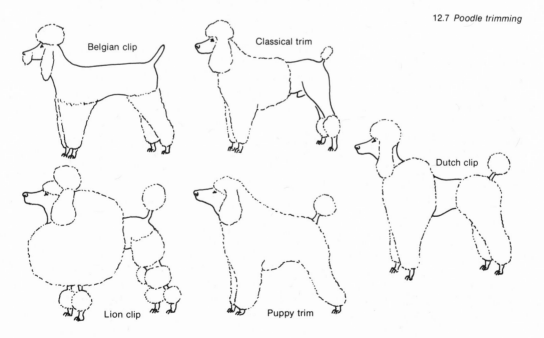

12.7 *Poodle trimming*

Belgian clip

Classical trim

Dutch clip

Lion clip

Puppy trim

135

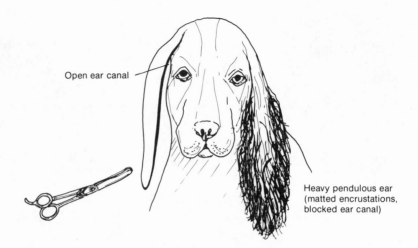

12.8 *Clipping ears: if the ear flap becomes excessively matted and hairy it becomes uncomfortable and can lead to an ear disease. Such ears should be groomed regularly*

Open ear canal

Heavy pendulous ear (matted encrustations, blocked ear canal)

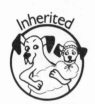

Groom under the ear flaps whenever your dog has been in tall grass, weeds, and brush. Foreign material, particularly grass seeds, can enter the ear canal after clinging to the hair near the outer opening.

The best breeds are hair-free inside the ears; however, if the canals are hairy pluck the hair inside the ears rather than cut it. Very few dogs object to this and it makes it easier to apply drops or ointment if and when that is needed. If scissors are used they should be the blunt-nosed type as no dog appreciates being pricked.

Bathing

In general, your dog should be bathed as little as possible. A lot of oil is lost from the dog's skin and coat during bathing and excessive bathing may lead to a dry skin and poor coat. As a rule, bath no more than once a month, unless for specific purposes, such as treatment of skin parasites.

12.9 *Bathing do's and don'ts*

Use a pure unscented soap and rinse all soap residue off before drying. Medicated or other special shampoos are not needed for the healthy coat. Baby shampoos are useful in dogs which normally struggle when the lather gets close to the face as they are very mild and do not irritate the skin and

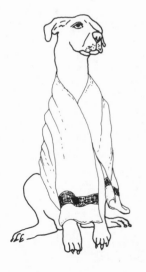

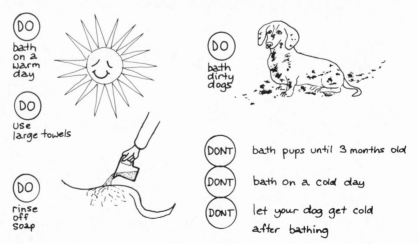

DO bath on a warm day

DO use large towels

DO rinse off soap

DO bath dirty dogs

DONT bath pups until 3 months old

DONT bath on a cold day

DONT let your dog get cold after bathing

apparently cause no irritation in the eyes. If one side of the face is lathered and rinsed, allowing one eye to be open to see what is going on, the dog will then let you lather the other side without any qualms. Generally washing the coat in winter is not desirable unless thorough drying is immediate. Envelop the wet dog in a warm towel (or towels) until the towel has soaked up most of the moisture. A good brisk rub with another dry towel seems to cope with whatever dampness is left.

Soap causes conjunctivitis, so keep it out of the eyes. Have a 10 ml syringe full of clean tap water handy in case you have to rinse out soap which gets in the eye. Eye ointment placed in the eyes before washing offers no real protection and may trap irritating soap, so prolonging eye inflammation.

What to use
Use soaps and shampoos designed specifically for use on dogs. Avoid using your personal hair shampoos or conditioners, as the dog has a much more sensitive skin than we do and many human products are quite unsuitable for dogs.

"Pure" soaps or mild coconut oil shampoos are safe and effective. Avoid products containing "phenols."

Do's and don'ts in bathing dogs
• DO choose a warm, windless day if possible
• DO use many large towels and avoid draughts, especially when the dog is drying off.
• DO thoroughly rinse off any detergents or soaps from the coat.
• DO bath your dog only when he is dirty and not because it is Sunday.
• DON'T bath pups until they are at least 3 months and be careful to avoid chills. Keep dogs warm after a bath.
• DON'T use soap near the eyes.

Matted hair

Regular grooming will prevent mats developing and this is the best way to handle this problem.

Once the hair has matted, approach the problem as follows:
• Tease the mat apart using one or two teeth of a comb. If necessary, cut the mat to produce smaller mats which can be teased out more readily.
• Some mats can be cut off with scissors but be *very* careful as it is easy to accidentally cut the skin. Use curved scissors if possible.
• In severe cases of extensive matting a complete clip may be necessary, sometimes under general anesthetic.

Removal of paint from the coat

Allow the paint to harden, then cut off the paint and hair. *Never* use thinners or solvents on or near a dog's skin as they can cause severe skin damage.

Removal of crude (e.g., sump) oil from the coat

• Wash the dog in vegetable oil several times. Vegetable oil joins chemically to sump oil far better than detergents do.
• When most of the sump oil is removed, wash off with warm, soapy water.
• Rinse thoroughly.

Removal of skunk oil

• Soak area in tomato juice.
• Thoroughly bath in warm soapy water.
• A dilute solution of ammonia can be used if the first two steps are not effective. Rinse thoroughly after using the dilute ammonia solution.

THE NAILS

Should I clip my dog's nails?

Natural wearing down of the nails by walking on firm surfaces is the best way to control nail length. Most dogs never need their nails cut. If the toenails have not been worn down, they should be filed or trimmed. Pay special attention to the front and rear dew claws if they are present. As these claws do not touch the ground, they are not worn down and may grow back into the pads or leg if neglected.

Clipping nails

Before you clip your dog's nails, identify the pink part of the nail (the quick). Avoid cutting into the quick as it contains nerves and blood vessels. Should the nail bleed, hold pressure over it with a cotton ball. The blood will usually clot in a few minutes. If bleeding persists, a styptic pencil (such as used for shaving) can be used.

It is easier to trim the nails (see p. 136) straight after the bath while they are still soft. Dogs do not like their front paws being handled and the clipping should be done quickly with a sharp pair of clippers.

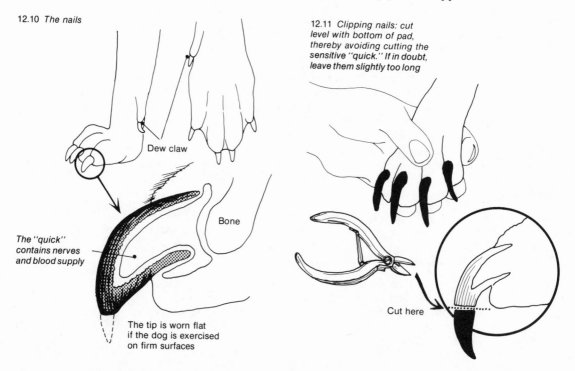

12.10 *The nails*

Dew claw

Bone

The "quick" contains nerves and blood supply

The tip is worn flat if the dog is exercised on firm surfaces

12.11 *Clipping nails: cut level with bottom of pad, thereby avoiding cutting the sensitive "quick." If in doubt, leave them slightly too long*

Cut here

Infections of the nails

Infection can localize in the nail fold (see p. 139) and often this infection is chronic.

Treatment of nail infection

Treatment in severe cases consists of removing the nail under general anesthetic to allow the infected area to drain. The treatment depends on the nature of the infection. Mild cases may respond to antiseptic soaks or painting with gentian violet or acriflavine.

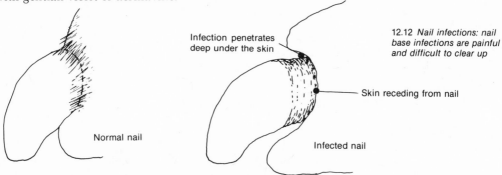

Infection penetrates deep under the skin

12.12 *Nail infections: nail base infections are painful and difficult to clear up*

Skin receding from nail

Normal nail

Infected nail

Drug treatment

Bacterial infection: Antibiotics may be prescribed.
Fungal infection: Griseofulvin (given by mouth) is needed. (*Note:* This antibiotic is very effective but can take some weeks to exert its full effect.)
Yeast infection: Antibacterials such as Nystatin are used.

In most cases, when the infection is cured, the nail will grow back normally.

FLEAS AND FLEA ALLERGY

Fleas cause more skin problems in dogs than all other causes put together.

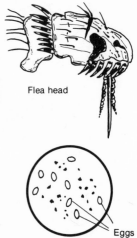

Flea head

Fleas are fiendishly cunning at finding and infesting dogs, so *every* dog owner should read this section.

Signs of fleas

Fleas are quick moving and shy of light, so spotting them can be difficult. Instead, look for the evidence they leave—*flea dirt.* "Flea dirt" is, in fact, fleas' droppings and consists mainly of digested blood. The droppings appear as small, black specks within the coat.

Look especially on the dog's back near the base of the tail and around his neck.

Eggs

Flea droppings

Flea dirt is seen by brushing the dog's hair back against the way it lies and looking for black specks near the base of the hairs.

12.13 *Small, black flea droppings are readily seen deep in the dog's coat. Flea eggs, being small and white, are harder to see*

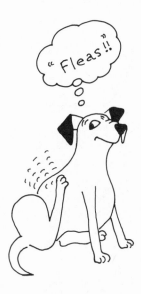

The life of a flea

Most of the life cycle of the flea is spent *off* the dog. This means that *when trying to control a flea infestation you must deal not only with the dog but with his bedding and surroundings as well.*

The growth from egg to adult takes at least 20 days, and in cooler weather, far longer. Newly emerged fleas can live for many weeks without feeding—just lying in wait for a dog to pass. Both these facts mean that after you have dealt with the fleas *on* your dog you must prevent reinfestation.

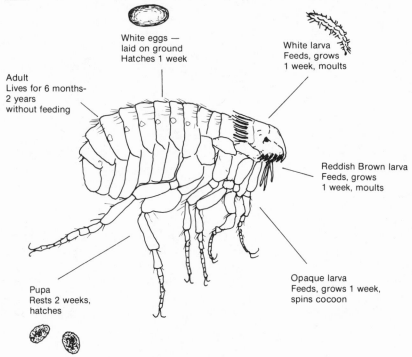

White eggs —
laid on ground
Hatches 1 week

White larva
Feeds, grows
1 week, moults

Adult
Lives for 6 months-
2 years
without feeding

Reddish Brown larva
Feeds, grows
1 week, moults

Opaque larva
Feeds, grows 1 week,
spins cocoon

Pupa
Rests 2 weeks,
hatches

12.14 *The lifecycle of a flea (21 days): the flea may spend as little as 10 minutes a week on the dog. A single cat can support as many as 15 000 fleas*

How many eggs do fleas lay?

Each female lays one or two hundred eggs. Cats have been documented as supporting 10,000 fleas, and dogs presumably support similar numbers. The flea-infested dog leaves enormous numbers of eggs in his wake daily.

What do flea eggs look like?

Flea eggs are pin-point sized, white and oval shaped. They are very hard to see with the naked eye and are resistant to insecticides.

What damage do fleas do?

Fleas are a double danger. Firstly, they can carry disease and parasites—especially the dog tapeworm.

Secondly, fleas are extremely irritating skin parasites, which cause intense itching. The itchy dog can damage the skin from vigorous scratching. Some dogs become so distracted that they cannot rest, their appetite wanes and they lose weight.

Flea allergy (Summer eczema)

Some dogs become allergic to flea bites. In these cases subsequent flea bites reactivate previous bites thus causing a generalized severe itch. By scratching and biting at himself the dog damages his skin, causes further irritation, and so sets up a vicious cycle, itch, scratch, itch, scratch, etc.

This condition (also called 'summer eczema') becomes self-perpetuating. Even after the fleas are killed the itch persists and further medication (usually cortisone) is needed to control this irritation.

The degree of skin damage may be out of all proportion to the number of fleas present as most of the damage is produced by self-mutilation by the dog.

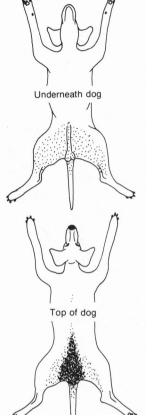

Underneath dog

Top of dog

> A single flea can trigger off an attack of summer eczema.

To prevent any flea bite when flea allergy is present you must keep the dog unattractive to fleas.

How to control fleas and repel future infestations

Dealing with the fleas on the dog:
The aim is not only to kill the fleas but to repel other fleas.

Flea powders
A wide range is available and most are effective, but they must be applied frequently—usually twice weekly to give continued protection.

Sprays
These are effective, but dogs often do not like being sprayed. *Beware:* Do not spray in or around the eyes, mouth or nose. Flea larvae and eggs can now be destroyed by a spray named Siphotrol plus, made by Vet-Kem.

Flea rinses (e.g., malathion)
These are generally effective and are longer lasting than either powder or spray. *Warning:* Rinses can be dangerous if not used properly. When using a rinse, read the instructions very carefully and follow dilution rates exactly.

Flea collars
Many types are available. Some produce an insecticidal vapour and these should be used with caution as the skin and eyes of some dogs are very

12.15 *Fleas are especially fond of biting the dog in these areas.*
As a result, the dog may develop an allergic skin condition that is most severe in these same areas.This is the 'distribution pattern' of a typical case of 'flea allergy dermatitis' or summer eczema'

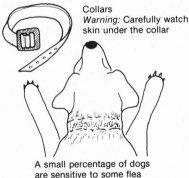

Collars
Warning: Carefully watch skin under the collar

A small percentage of dogs are sensitive to some flea collars and may develop a severe rash

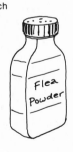

Flea powders
Twice weekly

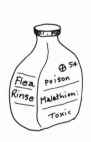

Rinses
Warning: Follow instructions carefully

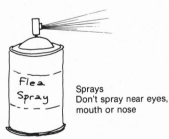

Sprays
Don't spray near eyes, mouth or nose

12.16 *Flea control*

sensitive and a severe rash may develop. Other collars have microfine particles of insecticide that gradually work their way through the coat. These can be very effective and have fewer side-effects than the vapor collars.

When you first put on an insecticidal flea collar, you should carefully watch the skin under the collar, especially for the first week. If the skin becomes reddened and inflamed, the collar should be removed. If inflammation is severe, or persists, or if the dog is unwell, consult your vet.

Oral drugs

If the situation warrants, and a vet recommends it, an oral drug, Proban, may be given once a week for one month. Nothing else should be used with this medication.

Treatment of the bedding

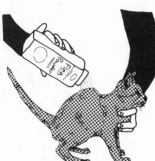

12.17 *Treat all pets for fleas, not just the itchy dog, and don't forget to treat bedding and kennels too*

As well as treating the dog himself it is essential to treat the bedding, surroundings and any other animals in the house. Cats are a common source of fleas. They may show no signs of skin irritation themselves, yet act as a reservoir of fleas. Treat cats with powders or collars. Vacuum the house thoroughly paying special attention to cracks and crevices. Fleas love to breed in these dusty areas. Burn the contents of the vacuum cleaner when you have finished. House bombs are available to take care of flea eggs in the house.

Control of flea allergy (summer eczema)

Long-term control of flea allergy is best achieved by controlling the fleas not only on the dog but in his environment.

To relieve the itch, a small cortisone dose given for a short time is very effective. *Cortisone treatment should always be under strict veterinary supervision.* The drugs have side-effects if used in excessive doses or for long periods. Some side-effects noted by owners include increased thirst and urination, lethargy and increased hunger.

Are flea collars harmful to the eye?

In rare cases flea collars cause a severe allergic reaction and marked eye inflammation. When the eye is inflamed it is wise to remove the flea collar. Flea collars contain a poison and if the eyes have been sick, a strong reason (e.g., flea allergy) is needed to justify placing a poison continuously near the eyes. Remove the flea collar if the eye is receiving glaucoma drops (Tosmilen, Phospholine-iodide).

LICE

Lice occur rarely but are seen mainly in neglected, run-down dogs.

Biting lice cause irritation. Sucking lice feed on blood and cause anemia.

Signs of lice

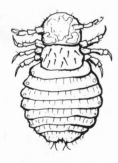

12.18 *Biting lice — lifecycle 14-21 days.*

Irritation, bare spots where the hair has been rubbed off. Lice are seen as small (2 or 3 mm long) white bodies under matted hair, and around the head, ears, neck, shoulders and anus. Lice lay eggs called "nits," which are attached to hair and look similar to sand or dandruff.

Treatment of lice

Cut off matted hair. Dip the animal once a week in a flea wash until no further scratching sign is seen.

Lice do not live for long off the dog, but infected bedding should be destroyed and sleeping quarters disinfected. Anemic dogs need a high protein diet, iron, vitamins (and, rarely, a blood transfusion).

ALLERGIC ECZEMA (ATOPY)

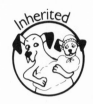

Allergic eczema is a skin condition characterized by severe itch, scratching, paw licking and face rubbing. Some breeds have a hereditary predisposition to allergies, in a similar way that humans have to hay fever and asthma. Dogs are usually 1-3 years old when the condition starts.

What breeds are most commonly affected?

Any breed can be affected, including cross-breeds, but white-haired terriers (especially West Highland White**), Poodles*** and Dalmatians** are especially prone.

Cause of allergic eczema

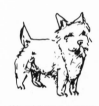

West Highland White

which he is allergic. Such a substance is called an "allergen," and the most common "allergens" include fleas, pollens, house dust, wool, feathers, kapok. The list of potential allergens unfortunately runs into hundreds of substances, so tracking down the offending substances may be exceedingly difficult.

The most common route by which the dog picks up the allergen is through inhalation. In humans, an inhalation allergy usually results in "hay fever"—sneezing and congestion. This is not so in dogs. The usual result in dogs is intensely itchy skin.

Relief (but not cure) can be obtained by using cortisone.

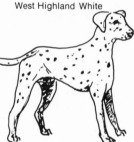

Dalmatian

> The itch produced by an allergic reaction can lead to
> great discomfort and skin mutilation.

Under strict supervision some dogs can be maintained on low doses of cortisone every second or third day for many years.

Treatment

Remove the offending allergen from contact with your dog—if you can. This is easy if it is wool, feathers or kapok, but almost impossible if it is pollens or house dust.

Another cure (not always successful) is a course of injections of antigen hyposensitization aimed at reducing the dog's sensitivity to the offending antigen. Such a course tends to be expensive.

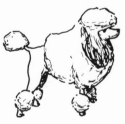

Poodle

12.19 *Allergic eczema (Atopy): these breeds are amongst the most commonly affected*

FOOD ALLERGIES

Food allergies do occur in dogs but are not as common as in humans. Your vet may suggest you avoid feeding your animal anything but dog food.

dairy foods (milk and cheese) and any sugary foods. Instead feed white meats (chicken, rabbit, tripe, fish) and dry foods and rice. Dogs with skin conditions often benefit from such a diet.

HOT SPOT ECZEMA

"Hot spot eczema" is a painful, moist, raw and weeping area of inflammation. It flares up within hours and leaves a hairless area that is usually round in shape.

Why do hot spots occur?

Hot spots may be triggered by fleas, allergy or a sting. The dog scratches vigorously and damages the skin. Bacteria invade the raw skin and turn the area into an acute infection.

Are any breeds more susceptible?

Yes, the dense-coated breeds such as the Labrador**, German Shepherd**, Golden Retriever**, St Bernard** or breeds with a tight, curly coat. (Bacteria like a dark, warm and moist area in which to multiply.)

Do you always see early signs?

No, infection can incubate out of sight, deep in the coat. It is only when the hair falls out that the infection becomes obvious.

Treatment of hot spot eczema

• In severe cases veterinary treatment is advisable, otherwise:
• Clip the hair away. This allows air to dry out the infection. If the affected area is large and painful, a tranquillizer or general anesthetic may be necessary.
• Use an antiseptic wash to clean away the discharge and to leave an antiseptic residue. Be careful to dilute any antiseptic (e.g., Savlon antiseptic liquid) strictly according to the directions. Note that Phisohex (Winthrop) should not be used on pups less than 6 weeks old. Your vet will show you how to clean the wound.
• Dry the area, very gently, by patting with dry towels.
• Apply an antiseptic or antibiotic dressing or cream, e.g., Savlon.
• Note that antibiotics may be required.
• If the dog is worrying the area and causing further damage, cortisone, sedatives or an inverted bucket over the dog's head (see p. 10) may be needed.

FLY BITES ON EARS

The stable fly has a mouth capable of biting and damaging the dog's skin. These flies especially like the ear tips of dogs with erect ears, but also attack the folded ear edges of dogs such as Shelties** and Collies**, and occasionally will bite other parts of the face or body.

The teeth of these flies lacerate the skin causing bleeding, and a crusty,

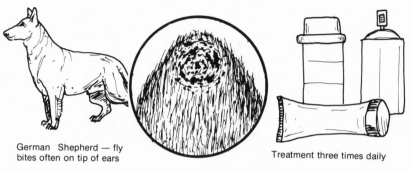

German Shepherd — fly bites often on tip of ears

Treatment three times daily

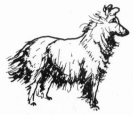

Shetland Sheepdog — fly bites often where the ear folds are

12.20 *Stable fly bites on ears*

inflamed ear results. The dog then further damages the ear by scratching and shaking his head.

Treatment for fly bites

Fly repellents on the ears (gels or sprays) used *frequently* (3 or more times daily) are usually effective.

Remove the breeding grounds of the fly, especially manure, grass clippings and soiled straw, or spray breeding sites with insecticide every 2-3 weeks.

COLLIE NOSE (Sunburned nose—nasal solar dermatitis)

Collies***, Shetland Sheepdogs* and related breeds may lack pigment on the skin of their noses. Because of this they have little protection from sunburn. In dogs living in warm, sunny climates a condition called "Collie nose" can develop. (Fig. 12:21)

The signs of collie nose

"Sunburn" is seen on the nose and sometimes the eyelids and lips. It first appears at the junction where the hair stops and the hairless skin of the nose commences. At first the skin becomes red. Each successive summer the condition becomes worse as repeated exposure causes further damage to the already sensitive area. If untreated, the condition progresses to crusty sores and then to raw, open ulcers and ultimately to skin cancer.

How much sun is safe for my dog with collie nose?

Sunburn is only a problem in areas with many hours of sun, for example, Australia or California. The occasionally sunny day will not cause collie nose.

Once a dog has developed a sensitized nose *any* further sunburn is harmful.

Treatment of collie nose

• Keep the dog out of the sun.
• In mild cases skin creams (especially lanolin based) soothe and promote skin repair. Ultraviolet screening suntan preparations can help. Use a children's "total block-out" sun screen.

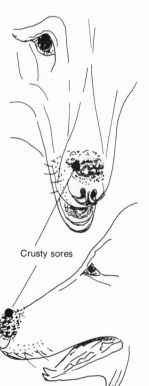

Crusty sores

12.21 *Collie Nose*

145

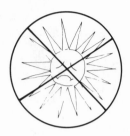

Avoid excessive exposure to sunlight

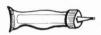

Use a softening, protective balm, such as lanoline

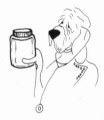

Sometimes drugs, such as cortisone, are prescribed

Black tattooing of nose provides protection. The tattoo substitutes for natural pigments

12.22 *Treatment of Collie Nose*

• Cortisone is sometimes used by vets and can give dramatic relief, but does not prevent future sunburn.

The best long-term treatment is to tattoo the dog's nose black. This requires a general anesthetic and more than one tattooing session may be required.

> For dogs sensitive to the sun avoid exposure to sunlight in the summer months between 10 a.m. and 4 p.m.

MANGE

For centuries, "mange" was a word used to describe almost all skin diseases of dogs.

A "mangy dog" was accepted as being a miserable, run-down, and scrawny animal.

Today, however, mange is known to be a specific skin disease caused by the invasion of the skin by tiny parasites, called *mites*. There are two common types of mites which cause "mange." The two manges are quite different. The two types are:

Demodectic mange and Sarcoptic mange (scabies)

Demodectic mange (caused by the mite *Demodex canis*)

This is the more common form.

Most healthy dogs have this mite present (in small numbers) as a normal inhabitant of their skin and it causes no problems. Only when demodex multiply and populate the skin in their thousands do they cause trouble.

> Most dogs do not "catch" a dose of mange—it *develops* from mites already present.

Diagnosis of demodectic mange is made by a vet taking skin scrapings. If mites are present microscopic examination of the skin scrapings provides a diagnosis.

At what age are dogs affected?

The disease occurs typically in young dogs less than 12 months of age. Exceptions do occur.

The signs of demodectic mange
There are two distinct types. Firstly there is a mild form localized to only a few sites, usually around the head (especially the eyelids) and forelegs. The second type is a severe form widespread over the body, and called "generalized" demodectic mange. This form is a serious problem and may be incurable in some dogs.

Localized (demodectic) mange

Patches of hair loss are seen. There may be slight itching but often the dog is not worried.

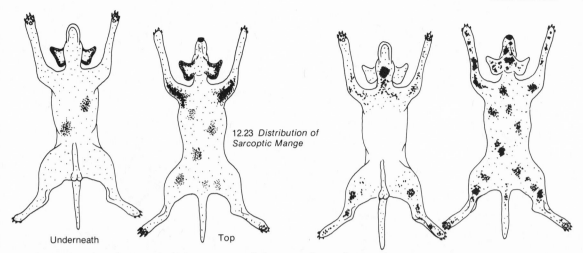

12.23 *Distribution of Sarcoptic Mange*

Underneath

Top

Common sites are around the corners of the mouth, under the jaw, on the forelegs and occasionally on the body. Usually only 1-5 patches are present.

12.24 *Distribution of Demodectic Mange: demodectic mange can become widely distributed over the body, although most cases are mild and restricted to the face and ears*

Treatment of mild cases
Most clear up by themselves within one month. For this reason lots of different treatments have been claimed to produce a cure, but preparations containing benzyl benzoate, malathion, lindane and rotenone seem to be effective.

Generalized (demodectic) mange

When the resistance of the host dog falls demodex mites may breed to produce tens of thousands of mites. Patches of hair loss develop all over the body. This is called generalized mange. Frequently, the skin becomes further infected with bacteria and pustules develop. These may be itchy, causing further damage when the dog scratches itself.

Treatment for generalized mange
Treatment of generalized mange must be supervised by your vet as the drugs used are toxic. Mitaban dip is often prescribed.

In severe cases treatment is prolonged and may be unsuccessful. Many dogs improve with age, however, and the problem clears up once the dog is sexually mature.

Why does mange develop from a simple skin condition to a severe problem?

There is a failure in the dog's immune system to prevent the spread. This may occur in a debilitated dog, or a dog suffering from another generalized disease such as distemper or hepatitis.

Scabies or sarcoptic mange

Scabies is a "mange," caused by a mite called *Sarcoptes scabei.* This mange is very different from demodectic mange (p. 146).

At what age is a dog usually affected?

Dogs of any age may be affected.

The signs of scabies

The dogs develop an intense itch and will rub and scratch vigorously at affected areas.

Scabies is highly contagious to other dogs and may even infect the owners if they are in close contact with the dog.

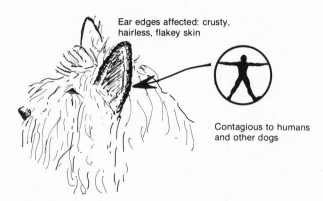

Ear edges affected: crusty, hairless, flakey skin

Contagious to humans and other dogs

What areas are affected by scabies?

The most commonly affected areas are the ears (especially the edge of the ears) and the elbows, although any area of the body may be affected.

The affected areas become red and itchy. Hair usually falls out and the skin becomes flaky and sometimes crusty.

How is scabies diagnosed?

Your vet will take deep skin scrapings—the sarcoptes mite can be very hard to find as very few mites may be present even when scabies is severe and they tend to lie deep in the skin.

Treatment of scabies

Treatment is always necessary. Scabies will not get better by itself and the intense itching causes the dog to mutilate his own skin. Paramite dip is often prescribed.

Ointments containing benzyl benzoate, sulphur and other drugs which kill mites are available from vets and some pharmacists. These can be used if only small areas are affected.

ABSCESS

Localized collection of pus. An abscess is surrounded by a "wall" of thick fibrous tissue.

Abscesses usually take 3-5 days to form after the initiating wound.

Causes of abscesses

Abscesses commonly form after deep bite wounds (for example from a cat); or cuts, splinters, penetration by grass awns (especially between the toes) or other foreign objects.

Should an abscess be opened (lanced)?

Usually, yes, but this is a decision for your vet to make. An abscess is lanced to allow drainage. After lancing, the abscess cavity is flushed with a mild antiseptic solution to clean it out. Antibiotics may be required to prevent the abscess from re-forming.

If an abscess bursts itself, what should you do?

When an abscess bursts, some but not all the pus will escape. Treatment is needed to drain remaining pus.

• Clip all hair around the abscess and clean the area thoroughly with warm mild antiseptic solution, or soapy water.

• Gently massage any remaining pus out through the hole in the abscess. Emptying out the pus may have to be repeated many times over the next 48-72 hours until no more discharge appears.

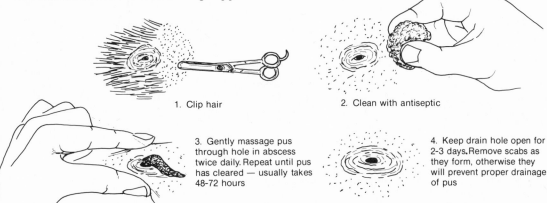

1. Clip hair

2. Clean with antiseptic

3. Gently massage pus through hole in abscess twice daily. Repeat until pus has cleared — usually takes 48-72 hours

4. Keep drain hole open for 2-3 days. Remove scabs as they form, otherwise they will prevent proper drainage of pus

• Aim to keep the draining hole open for 2 or 3 days and gently remove any scab that starts to form. Once the discharge has stopped the draining hole may be allowed to heal over.

12.26 *Burst abscesses*

When to call the vet

It is wise to get early expert attention as a simple abscess may be part of a deeper problem.

LICK SORES (ACRAL TONGUE LICK DERMATITIS)

If your dog persistently licks at any area of skin he will produce a sore— usually on the lower half of the forelegs, near the waist, or on the hind legs. A lick sore frequently escalates from a mild red irritation into a serious problem.

Signs of lick sores

At first, only hair loss is noticed where the dog licks. If licking persists, the skin becomes red and inflamed. The skin eventually is broken and an ulcer forms.

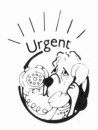

149

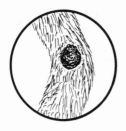

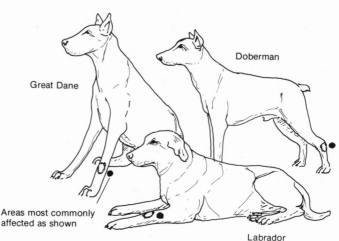

Great Dane

Doberman

Labrador

Areas most commonly affected as shown

12.27 *Lick sores: these are the breeds most susceptible — although any dog may develop lick sores. The ulcer is deep and does not heal as the dog keeps licking at it*

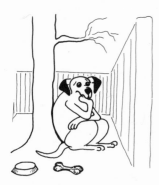

12.28 *Cause of lick sores: boredom can result in many problems including self-mutilation of the skin*

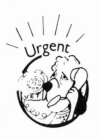

What causes lick sores?

Boredom is the main cause, although some start with a wound or graze. Lick sores often occur in dogs left alone for long periods. Licking starts as a casual habit—a tension release—in much the same way as a child relieves anxiety by sucking its thumb. Constant licking, however, irritates the skin nerves and an itch develops. The dog then licks more—partly to relieve the itch—and eventually the skin is so damaged that an ulcer forms. Constant licking prevents healing and makes the ulcer deeper.

Are some breeds more likely to develop lick sores?

Yes. Dobermans*, Labradors* and Great Danes* seem more susceptible.

Treatment for lick sores

A lick sore can be difficult to clear up. Treat it as early as possible.

In the early stages (when hair loss and skin reddening occur), preventing the dog from licking may be curative. Bandaging the wound is usually not enough. Most dogs find bandages an easy challenge and soon have them off. A bucket over the head is often the best idea (see p. 10).

Try to relieve the boredom by distracting the dog with more exercise, a toy, a bone or a companion dog.

Veterinary treatment

Cortisone is often used to relieve the itch and to reduce the dog's desire to constantly lick—so allowing the skin to heal. Cortisone injections may be given directly around the sore. Fairly drastic treatments such as putting a cast over the leg, or surgically excising the offending area of skin, may be resorted to if all else fails.

Once cured, how do you prevent the lick sores from recurring?

The initial cause (boredom) must be resolved. Some ideas are as follows:
- More walks and human company.
- More canine company—another dog.

- Avoid close confinement—allow as large an exercise area as possible.
- Give chews, bones or toys to divert the dog's attention.

CALLUS

A callus is an area of thickened skin. Calluses usually form where there is pressure on the skin, such as on the elbows, side of the knees or hocks and on the chest. They are especially common in large or overweight dogs. The callus acts as a cushion, reducing wear and tear on these pressure areas.

Do you need to treat callus?

A callus can become a problem only if it becomes hard and cracked, or infected. Otherwise, it performs a useful function in cushioning pressure areas.

How to treat a callus

Lanolin based creams can be used to soften a hard, cracked callus. Give the patient a soft surface on which to lie (a sheep's fleece is excellent). Padded bedding allows the callus to "calm down." You may also need to reduce your dog's weight.

ACNE

Acne is quite common in young dogs of short-coated breeds and shows as small pustules in the skin, especially around the chin and face. Some breeds are especially susceptible: Boxers**, Bulldogs***, Dobermans** and Great Danes*.

What areas are affected?

Mainly the face, especially chin and lips. Other areas less commonly affected are armpits, elbows and between the hind legs where the skin pores become plugged.

Treatment for acne

- Clean the fats and oils from the affected skin with washes such as Pragmatar (Smith Kline), Seleen (Abbott Lab), Phisohex (Winthrop), Sebbafoam.
- Repeat this wash at least once daily until cleared, then once or twice weekly to prevent recurrence.
- If the infection is not clearing, antibiotics may be necessary.

SKIN FOLD INFECTIONS

Including:
- Lip fold.
- Facial fold.
- Vulval fold.
- Tail fold (Screw tail).
- Infection between the toes.

Some breeds are especially prone:

Lip folds: Spaniels**, Bulldogs, Boxers, Newfoundlands, Setters.

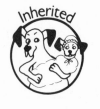

12.29 *Skin fold infections*

Face folds: Pekingese***, Pug**, Bulldogs**, Boxers, Boston Terriers.
Vulval folds: Overweight, spayed bitches**. (The vulvas of spayed bitches are smaller and therefore tend to recede into folds of fat where urine can scald.)
Screw tail folds: Pugs*, Bulldogs*, Boston Terriers.
Infection between toes: Hairy-footed breeds*** (e.g., Spaniels, Schnauzers).

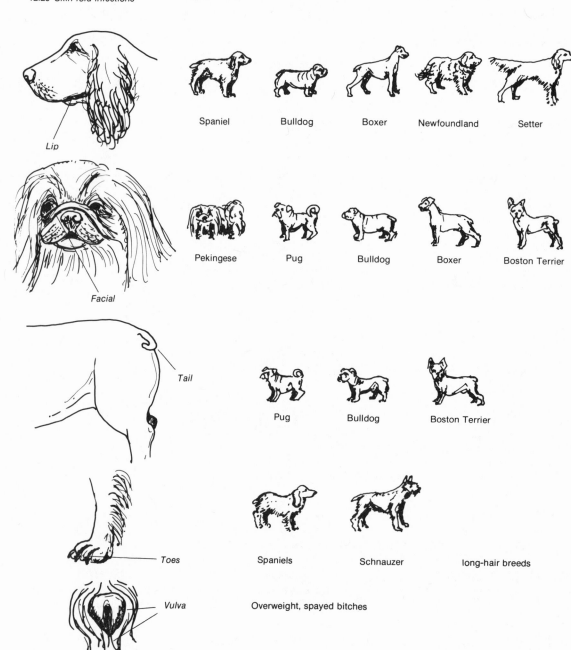

Lip

Spaniel   Bulldog   Boxer   Newfoundland   Setter

Facial

Pekingese   Pug   Bulldog   Boxer   Boston Terrier

Tail

Pug   Bulldog   Boston Terrier

Toes

Spaniels   Schnauzer   long-hair breeds

Vulva

Overweight, spayed bitches

Why do folds in the skin lead to infection?

Moisture—saliva running in lip folds or urine trapped in folds around the vulva—encourages normal skin bacteria to multiply into abnormal numbers.

Moisture accumulates where the skin folds and infection follows.

Treatment of skin fold infections

• Clip hair away to allow air drying of the moist skin.

• Clean away discharges using a mild soap or antiseptic cleanser. Dry the skin well after this treatment.

• Keep the area clean and—especially—*keep it dry*. Moisture is the major enemy.

• Use an astringent (drying) antiseptic lotion to control mild infections. Ask your vet to recommend one.

Surgical treatment

In severe cases and to prevent recurrences (infections in skin folds may recur again and again, despite your best efforts) surgery is the only effective long-term treatment. Surgery eliminates the folds and therefore the infection.

RINGWORM

"Ringworm" is an unfortunate name as this skin condition is not caused by a worm at all, but by a fungus. Originally, it was believed that the characteristic round ringworm sore was caused by a worm burrowing around in circles under the skin. In fact, the reason many ringworm sores are round is because, like the ripples produced when a pebble is thrown into a pond, it starts in one spot and spreads in all directions at once.

The incidence of ringworm is highest in hot, humid climates, such as Southern America, Northern Australia, Spain and North Africa, but it is seen in most areas of the world.

Signs of ringworm

The 'textbook' case of ringworm is a round, hairless area of dry, crusty skin. The borders of the sore are slightly raised. Variations are frequently seen and irregularly shaped ringworm sores are common.

Areas of the body most commonly affected are the face—especially around the ears and nose—and the limbs. In some cases large areas of the body can be affected, but usually only a few sores are present.

Ringworm is quite itchy in man, but this is generally not so in dogs.

Diagnosis of ringworm

The vet may shine an ultraviolet light (called a "Woods lamp") onto the suspected area, as some ringworm fungi fluoresce. A sample of the affected skin can be sent to a laboratory for examination and perhaps to try to grow the fungus. Sometimes the vet may be confident of the characteristic appearance of the ringworm and treat accordingly without actual laboratory confirmation of the diagnosis.

Treatment of ringworm

Many mild cases are self-limiting and will clear up without any help from you.

In some cases, lotions, ointments or washes are effective in clearing the fungal invasion and there are many non-toxic, effective preparations on the market. Ask your vet for advice and remember that because of the dog's habit of licking off ointments, it is better not to try human preparations without consulting your vet first.

In extensive cases, or in cases that are not clearing, a drug called Griseofulvin is used and is given by mouth for 3-6 weeks. It is highly effective, but must be used under veterinary supervision and never given to pregnant bitches.

Can humans contract ringworm from dogs?

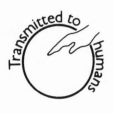

Yes, although the most common source of infection is from cats, and the infection can be picked up from many species of animals or directly from the soil.

Children are especially at risk, but humans of any age can be affected.

Ringworm is usually not a severe condition in humans and responds quickly to ointments and lotions. In some cases it can become deep-seated or spread rapidly. Don't take chances, see your physician for advice.

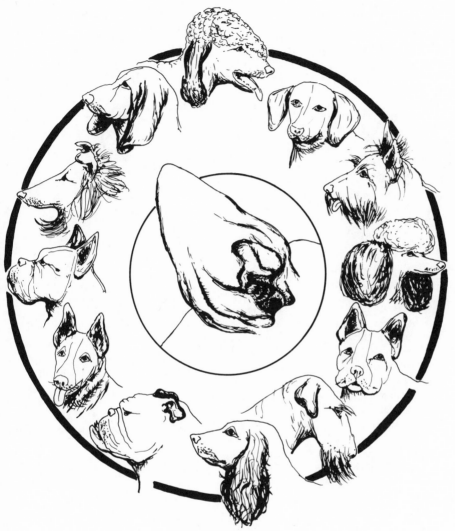

13. Ears

EAR DISEASES

Breeding

Dogs with drooping ears or very hairy ear canals have a greater tendency to ear infections than dogs with erect, hair-free ears. Ear infections thrive on warm, moist conditions. Aim to prevent these conditions by regularly clearing the ear canal of any excessive wax build-up.

It is essential not to neglect your dog's ears when grooming. The ear canal and the ear drum are delicate structures so care must be taken when cleaning them.

> The ear is sensitive. Be gentle when grooming or you
> risk damaging the ear.

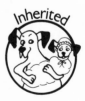

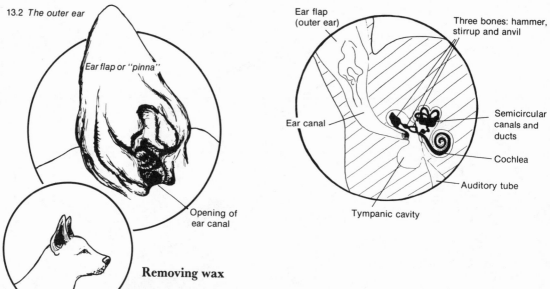

13.2 *The outer ear*

Ear flap or "pinna"

Opening of
ear canal

Ear flap
(outer ear)

Three bones: hammer,
stirrup and anvil

Ear canal

Semicircular
canals and
ducts

Cochlea

Auditory tube

Tympanic cavity

Removing wax

A few drops of mineral oil or baby oil will soften the wax to allow easier removal, or use a special wax solvent available from the chemist or your vet (e.g., Ceramol or Waxsol). Seventy per cent Isopropyl alcohol may be used **if** the ear is not inflamed, but it stings if the ear is raw or inflamed.

It is preferable to use wicks of cotton wool or small damp balls of cotton wool to pick up the wax. They are gentle and will not damage the ear. If you use cotton buds or similar products be careful not to push wax deeper into the ear. Then thoroughly dry the ear, removing all fluid from the ear canal.

If the ear is clear (i.e., there is not a wax build-up) and the ear is clean, then *leave it alone.*

It is an advantage to know the normal smell of an ear canal. Any change, particularly to a "rancid" odor, may indicate infection.

13.3 *Ear care: avoid putting cotton swabs into the ear. Often all you achieve is to pack wax and debris deeper into the ear, rather like loading a cannon!*

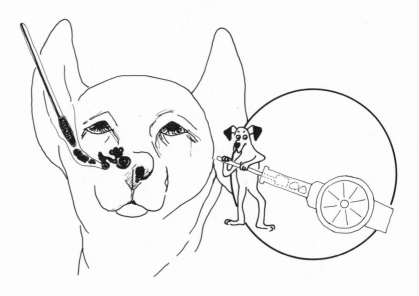

Plucking hair

Some breeds, notably Poodles, have excessive hair in the ears due to faulty breeding and this must be removed from their ear canals.

Examine your dog's ears and if they are hairy seek your vet's advice as to whether they need plucking.

Why should my dog's ear canal be plucked?

Freeing the canal of hair allows better air circulation, reduces wax build-up and the chance of infection.

Professional dog groomers will clear the ears as a routine part of the service.

Plucking is very easy to do: merely grasp a *few* hairs at a time, with fingers or tweezers, and pull them out. This does not hurt the dog unless you grab a large tuft.

It is necessary to repeat plucking as the hairs regrow. This should be done monthly or quarterly depending on the dog.

Infected ear canal (Otitis externa)

Conditions which lead to ear infections include:
- Matted hair.
- Narrow and excessively hairy ear canals (due to faulty breeding).
- Accumulated wax, dried blood or other discharges.
- Mites (tiny parasites that live in the ear).
- Foreign objects (such as grass seeds).

Many people will diagnose your dog's ear soreness merely as "canker." We try to avoid using this term as the infection could be any of the following conditions:

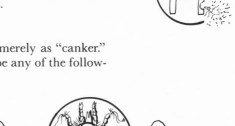

- Grass seed (or similar foreign object) in ear.
- Bacterial infection.
- Mite or parasite in the ear.
- Yeast or fungal infection.
- Injury to the ear.
- Ulcers in the canal or even a growth in the canal (although these are not common).

The ear becomes inflamed (red and sore). There may be a discharge visible but more often than not the discharge and inflammation are visible only when the ear is examined by a vet with an instrument called an otoscope.

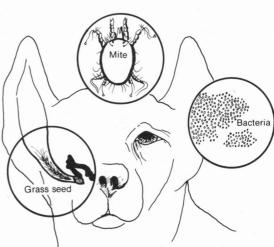

13.4 *Infections of the ear canal can be due to foreign bodies such as grass seeds, parasites such as ear mites, or to bacterial or fungal invasion*

Signs of an infected ear canal

The dog will show some or all of the following signs:
- Head shaking.
- Head tilted to one side.
- Rubbing ear on ground.
- Scratching vigorously at ear.
- A discharge which may be smelly, very dark and thick, pus, or blood-stained fluid.

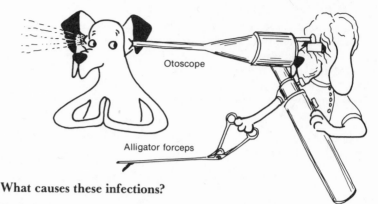

13.5 *Using an otoscope, the vet can look deep into the ear canal. Instruments such as the alligator forceps shown are used to remove grass seed or other foreign bodies from deep in the ear*

Otoscope

Alligator forceps

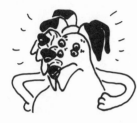

13.6 *Signs of ear diseases: head shaking*

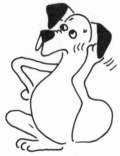

13.7 *Signs of ear diseases: scratching at ears*

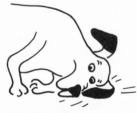

13.8 *Signs of ear diseases: rubbing ear along the ground*

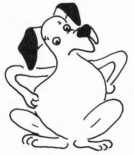

13.9 *Signs of ear diseases: carrying head to one side*

What causes these infections?

Probably there is a combination of factors, but the most important are:

• **Ear mites:** These are tiny pin-point size mites that can infect the ears of both dogs and cats. They are transmissible between animals and cause irritation in the ear which results in the build-up of large amounts of black wax. Mites avoid light and therefore are difficult to see without an otoscope. Ear mites are most commonly a problem in pups.

• **Excessive moisture** due to poor drainage or poor air circulation in the ear canal. Excess moisture may also be due to introduction of water when swimming, or even by the owner when cleaning the ear.

• **Trauma:** that is, bumps and bites to the ear. Also vigorous scratching, possibly due to tangled hair, fleas or other skin irritations will inflame the ear.

• **Faulty breeding:** Poor breeding may produce excessively narrow, tortuous or hairy ear canals, especially in Poodles, Spaniels, Bassets.

Are bacteria involved?

Bacteria are a common cause of infection when warmth, lack of circulating air and lack of drainage lead to moisture build-up.

Are bacteria always involved?

No. Frequently, fungi or yeasts infect the canal. Your vet may want a swab of the ear canal to determine the exact type of infection.

Treatment of ear infections

The ear is too delicate and precious to experiment with home treatment without professional advice.

How to avoid ear infections

Keep the canals clean and free of wax, hair, moisture and foreign bodies and try to avoid trauma to the ear.

Breed to improve ear design, especially in Poodles, Pugs and Pekingese. Breed for open ears and avoid floppy, hairy ears such as in Cockers.

When to call the vet

Take your dog to the vet if he is:
• Shaking his head.

- Hanging his head to one side.
- Has a discharge from the ear.

Should I use powder in a sore ear?

Do not try "canker powders" or similar remedies. Do your dog a favor and get a professional diagnosis and the correct treatment.

Grass seeds or foreign bodies in the ear

"Foreign bodies" include any object that should not be there. Children are sometimes responsible for pushing sticks, hairpins, sweets, chewing gum and even marbles into dogs' ears.

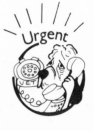

One of the most common causes of ear pain in some areas are grass seeds, or awns or "foxtails" which get into the ear canal then work their way deep into the ear, even through the eardrum.

Grass seeds are designed to travel forwards. Once in the ear they must be removed as they will not come out by themselves.

If you cannot immediately get to a vet, try softening the seeds with a few drops of mineral or baby oil. An anesthetic is sometimes essential to allow removal without pain.

Blood blister of the ear flap

A thick, fluctuating swelling of the ear flap is termed an "aural hematoma." It is an accumulation of blood or serum between the skin of the ear flap and its cartilage. Some cases are caused by the dog vigorously shaking his head. This has a whip-lash effect on tiny blood vessels in the ear flap and may cause them to rupture and bleed into the ear flap. Or the dog may have a blood clotting disorder (as in rat-bait poisoning) or a knock may have caused the bleeding—in some cases we don't know what has started the bleeding.

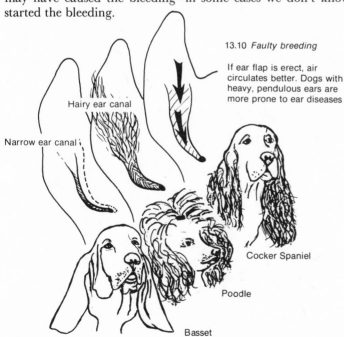

13.10 *Faulty breeding*

If ear flap is erect, air circulates better. Dogs with heavy, pendulous ears are more prone to ear diseases

Hairy ear canal

Narrow ear canal

Cocker Spaniel

Poodle

Basset

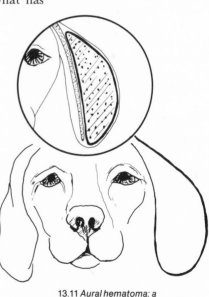

13.11 *Aural hematoma: a swollen, bulging ear flap often means a blood clot beneath the skin—termed an aural hematoma*

Treatment of a blood blister of the ear flap

It is usually necessary to anesthetize the dog and drain the swelling. To prevent swelling occurring again the ear is stitched.

Sometimes buttons, pieces of tubing, or a stiff material such as X-ray film, is sutured on to prevent the stitches biting into the skin. The stitches are removed in 7-10 days time.

Some vets prefer to bandage the ear, either back across the head or incorporating some round object to roll the ear round.

CHRONIC INFECTIONS

Surgical treatment (lateral ear resection)

Some dogs have continual trouble with ear infections and these are often due to poor drainage and airflow. The ear canal may be too narrow, or blocked by excess flaps of cartilage at the opening of the canal.

The vet may recommend an operation to "open up" the ear canal.

EAR CROPPING

Some breeds have their ears "cropped" for cosmetic purposes causing the ears to stand erect and pricked up. Surgery for fashion, however, is not desirable!

The age at which the operation is performed is usually 9-12 weeks for the larger breeds, when the head is fully developed. Other breeds vary—for example, the Boston Terrier is done at 4 months or later.

DEAFNESS

A partial hearing loss can often occur due to ear infection. Treatment of the infection and clearing of the ear canal will restore hearing in these cases.

Some dogs suffer permanent, partial or complete deafness due to a birth defect from faulty breeding. For example, white cats are sometimes deaf and the same is true of other white animals, e.g., Dalmatians.

Old dogs may lose their hearing gradually, especially dogs with a history of chronic ear infections.

My puppy's ear does not stand up as it should. Is treatment necessary?

With time and increase in the strength of the ear muscles, the ear may stand up straight. Surgery has been used to correct some floppy ears which should stand erect.

14. Eyes

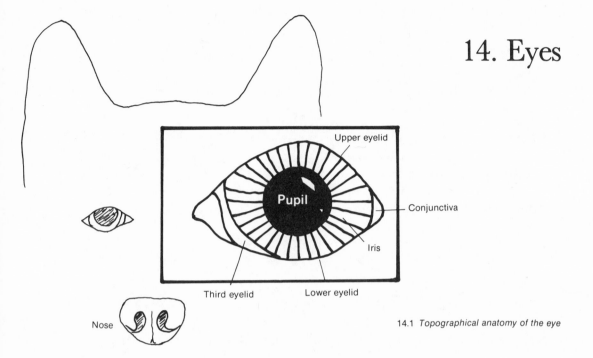

14.1 *Topographical anatomy of the eye*

EYE DISEASE IN THE DOG

Overlooking serious eye disease in the dog is all too easy, especially as warning signs are usually subtle. Early detection of these signs, however, gives a far better chance for treatment to minimize eye damage.

In contrast with man, inherited eye disease is of great significance in the dog. More than 100 breeds are affected. There are about 40 inherited eye diseases and the incidence is increasing rapidly. Fashionable trends in dog breed, especially in altering the shape of a dog's head, have had an unfortunate influence on eye diseases. Ignoring eye disease in the quest for fashionable "good" looks has allowed inherited diseases to increase.

How important are hereditary (due to genes) eye diseases?

At least 100 breeds of dogs have inherited eye diseases (p. 161). In one study in Great Britain 40 per cent of 2374 eye disease cases in the dog were classified as hereditary.*

Signs of eye disease:

- Watery eye.
- Red eye.
- Eye has pus discharging.
- Blue, cloudy eye.

*Barnett, K. C. "Comparative aspects of canine hereditary eye disease," *Adv. Vet. Sci. Comp. Med. No. 20*, p. 39, 1976.

*, **, *** indicate increasing likelihood of a particular trait or problem occurring.

• Winking/squinting eye.
• Rubbing at the eye.
• Dog sticks close to you at night, misses a thrown ball or stick, bumps into things.
• The working or racing dog does not perform well, or performs erratically.
• The young pup does not run around freely.
• Some eye diseases cause the patient to be depressed, lethargic, "not himself."

Note: After *all* physical injuries to the head or eye, seek veterinary advice.

14.2 *Cross-section of the eye*

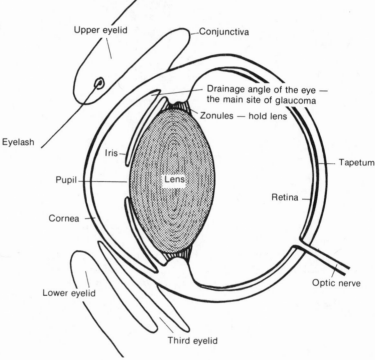

Before you buy or import stock, or start to breed, check with
your vet to find out what eye diseases the breed is predisposed
to and how to avoid them.

The structure of the dog's eye compared with man's

• The cornea and lens are larger than man's to give a wider field of vision
• There is a third eyelid which lies in the inner corner of the eye and can sometimes be seen partly covering the eye
• Immediately behind the eye lies not bone (as in the human eye) but the huge jaw muscles the dog needs for catching and crushing food
• The dog has fewer color receptors than man—the dog mostly sees shades of grey.
• A reflective shield behind the eye shows as a green eye shine at night. It improves night vision

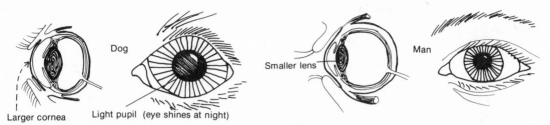

Larger cornea   Light pupil (eye shines at night)

Smaller lens

Man

14.3 *Difference in the eyes of man and dog*

Some common questions on dog's eyes

Why does my dog's eye shine green at night?

Reflection from headlights or a torch is due to a fluorescent reflective layer (the tapetum) at the back of the eyeball. In some cases the reflection is red instead of green. This is sometimes called "ruby eye" and it means that these dogs lack this reflecting layer. In theory this may mean that these dogs don't see as well at dusk and after dark as dogs which do have the reflecting layer.

Does bright sunlight cause eye damage?

The main danger of sunlight is to dogs with pink, unpigmented skin around the eyelids. Strong sunlight can cause sunburn and inflamed lids (and can later, perhaps, lead to cancer).

In dogs already suffering from an eye disease, sunlight can make eye inflammation worse.

> If your dog has sore or sick eyes keep him out of the sun.

My dog seems to have healthy eyes—do I need to see a vet?

Usually not. But check the list on p. 38-49 for diseases from which your dog's breed is most likely to suffer.

Is pain evident if a dog has a sore eye?

Winking, squinting of the eye, holding the eye half closed and avoiding light may all indicate eye pain. A sore eye often causes no obvious pain. It is only after the eye is cured that we notice the dog is back to his old self. In severe cases of eye disease the dog may not eat, lies in bed or somewhere dark and may vomit.

How is management of eye diseases different from other parts of the body?

We need to identify *very slight* disease and see danger *before* it happens. The eyeball, even with expert care, never *fully* recovers from serious disease.

What "sleep" and eye discharge is normal, and what is not?

There are glands at the front of the eye which produce a film of tears to keep the eye constantly moist and lubricated. Residue of these tears or "sleep" may accumulate in the corner of the eyes and then dry out. We see this especially in dogs with deep-set eyes such as Dobermans and Setters.

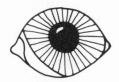

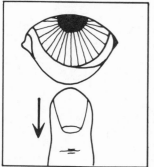

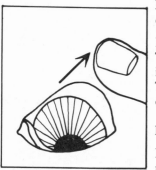

A small amount of creamy or grey discharge is normal in many dogs, but if the discharge becomes copious, or if it starts to stick to the eyeball itself (and this means a *dry eye*) or if the discharge is yellow (which may mean infection) then contact your vet.

My dog has deep-set eyes with a lot of "sleep." What can I do?

Some breeds such as Scotch Collies, Irish Setters, Dobermans, are born with deep-set eyes which collect discharge and may become inflamed. Oversized eye sockets (orbits) in Great Danes***, St Bernards*** and Rottweilers* may allow discharge to collect at the corner of the eye near the nose. You may need to clean the eyes each morning by using saline or artificial tears (Fig. 1:10).

My dog's eye is red—how long do I wait to see the vet?

A bloodshot eye may need veterinary treatment at once—there could be very serious inflammation inside the eyeball! (See Fig. 14:4.)

My dog's face is often stained a brown or rusty color at the corners of his eyes. What is the cause?

Breeds with a white face, such as Miniature and Toy Poodles and Maltese Terriers can have a red-brown stain on the facial hair below the eye. This is due to tears overflowing from the eyelids and running down the face. This chronic wetness plus pigments present in the tears turn the hair a rusty color.

But why do the tears overflow?

Every normal eye is constantly covered with a thin film of tears that keeps the eyeball lubricated, sweeps debris and bacteria from the eye and prevents the cornea from drying out. In most cases, these tears are drained away by the tear ducts (Fig. 14:6). Sometimes these tear ducts become blocked or are too narrow. Instead of being drained away into the nose, the tears spill over onto the face. In other cases, the tear flow may be excessive, overwhelm the capacity of the tear ducts and spill over. Such excessive tear flow can result from chronic irritation to the eyes, for example, from misdirected eyelashes, or entropion (see p. 169).

14.4 *Examining the eye: the inside of the lower lid normally looks pink. Redness inside the lower lid means disease. Pull the upper eyelid back with the fingers firmly applied above the eye. If the white of the eye is pink it means disease*

14.5 *Watery eye is due to irritation or faulty tear drainage*

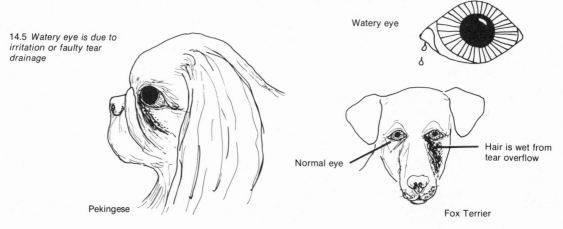

Watery eye

Normal eye

Hair is wet from tear overflow

Pekingese

Fox Terrier

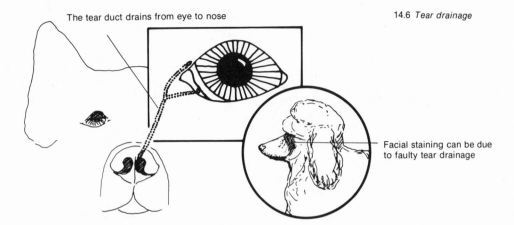

The tear duct drains from eye to nose

14.6 *Tear drainage*

Facial staining can be due to faulty tear drainage

Home care of facial staining from tears

A little vaseline applied below the eyelid (*not* in the eye) may reduce the irritation and scouring effects of chronic wetness. Or use a silicone barrier cream, such as Vasogen. Only use a *tiny* amount and *avoid contact with the eyeball.*

Substances which bleach, such as hydrogen peroxide, have been used in an attempt to take tear stain out of white facial hair. If you use these, take extreme care that none goes in the eye.

Veterinary care of facial staining

A veterinary examination may be helpful in determining the cause of the stain. Antibiotics will decolor facial stain, but they should not be used permanently, systematically, for cosmetic purposes.

Color of the eye

The color of the eye is inherited. The most usual color is dark brown, and this is the best eye color. While one light colored or blue eye is acceptable, *it is a mistake to breed for lack of pigment (color) in the eye as this may lead to more deformed eyes and deafness.*

Light colored eyes do not tolerate strong sunlight as well as dark eyes. The more pigment in the eye the better. Dark eyelids are more resistant to sunburn and cancer.

Wall eye (pearl eye)

Wall eye refers to one blue, white or grey eye. Wall eye is also used to describe a dark eye with a large splash of blue or white. The dog is born with that color. Some wall eyes are a result of disease, such as a white cloud on the cornea, an eye turned out to expose the white of the eye (Fig. 14:7b) and a prominent eye.

Dogs with dappled coats (harlequin dappling)

In some breeds, such as the Great Dane, Dachshund and Scotch Collie***, dogs have been selected for a dappled (or merle) coat. In extreme dappling, where there is lack of pigment in over 50 per cent of the skin, severe eye defects have also shown up. These defects include small eyes, small lenses, and cataracts.

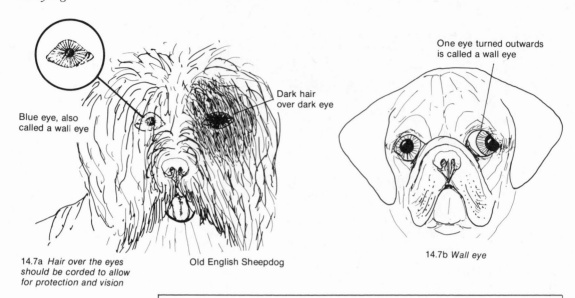

Blue eye, also
called a wall eye

Dark hair
over dark eye

One eye turned outwards
is called a wall eye

14.7a *Hair over the eyes
should be corded to allow
for protection and vision*

Old English Sheepdog

14.7b *Wall eye*

Breeding for dappled coat produces more eye deformities.

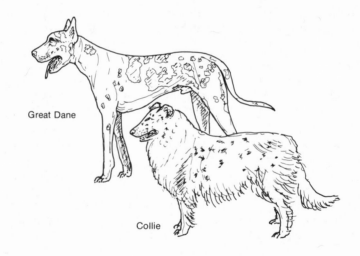

14.8 *Dappled coats
(Harlequin/Merling): dogs
with dapped coats have
more inherited eye disease*

Great Dane

Collie

Blindness in dogs

A dog can be totally blind in one or even both eyes without your being
aware of it; and some slowly progressive diseases of the eye show few or
no external signs.

Vision loss may go unnoticed until well advanced.

Signs of blindness
A blind dog may cope extremely well in his own home. It is difficult to
believe that the dog is nearly or totally blind. It is only when moved to
strange surroundings that he will bump into things. Other signs are seen
when the dog misjudges the flight of a ball, does not move around as much,

does not go outside at night (suggesting night blindness), will go upstairs but not down, and stays very close to the owner.

A high-stepping, hesitant walk is typical and the head may be held low.

> Erratic performances in greyhounds, sheepdogs, field dogs
> or guide dogs may be due to loss of vision.

If you examine the pupils carefully other signs of blindness may be apparent. Two very large pupils, with little or no eye color showing, suggests total loss of sight in both eyes. (Note that light registering in one eye controls the size of both pupils.) Normally, if you shine a torch into the eyes the pupils will contract to shut out excessive light. Try this test on a friend to see the normal reaction, then try it on your dog. If the pupil fails to contract, or does so only poorly, suspect vision loss.

How do I know a young pup in the litter has decreased vision?

Move your hand in front of the litter. The sighted puppies will follow your hand, the pup with poor vision will not.

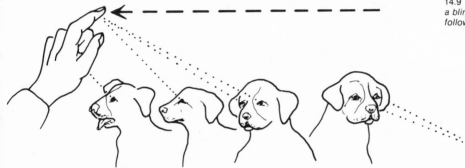

14.9 *Vision tests in puppies: a blind puppy does not follow hand movement*

How does a blind dog cope?

Usually very well, especially if the onset of blindness has been slowly progressive and the sense of smell and hearing are intact. Small dogs kept within a familiar environment cope especially well.

Blind people are described as having "facial vision." For some reason little understood, some blind people are able to "see" objects around them. "What is that object over there?" they will ask, pointing to a large shrub. The dog possesses some *perception*—not vision—from his blind eye and if the eye is removed, may bump into things more often.

Helping a blind dog to cope
A blind dog is helped by:
   • Familiar environment (do not move the furniture).
   • A keen sense of smell and hearing (have his ears checked).
   • Less need of vision than man.
   • Another dog in the household acting as a guide dog (if there is no second dog, he will follow your footsteps).

• A dog has no sense of despair with his disability and accepts life as it is (what a lesson he can offer his master!).

If the dog is moved into a new home or if he suddenly becomes blind there are other ways of helping him.

Some people spray a little very light scented cologne on objects likely to be bumped. Some dogs will avoid obstacles when warned by their owner that there is danger ahead.

Exercising the blind dog
It is wise to use a lead if there is much traffic about, but if you wear a bell on your belt—and keep off busy roads—the dog will learn to follow.

The eyelids

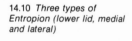

Healthy eyelids are essential for healthy eyes. There are several important conditions of the eyelids that can lead to eye damage and these include:
• Rolled-in eyelids (entropion).
• Excessively large eyelids, or rolled-out eyelids (ectropion).
• Long eyelid hair.
• Excessively long eyelashes.
• Misdirected eyelashes.
• Extra eyelashes.
• Redundant (or excessive) forehead skin.
• Eyelid injuries.
• 'Stye' (small abscess on eyelid edge).
• Inflammation of the eyelids.
• Tumor of the eyelid.

The first seven of these are inherited and must be bred out to save the dog discomfort.

The dog also has a third eyelid (or nictitating membrane). The conditions which affect this are:
• Haws (an excessively prominent third eyelid).
• "Cherry eye"—when a gland at the base of the third eyelid prolapses forward.
• Inflamed third eyelid.
• Deformed third eyelid/oversized third eyelid.

14.10 *Three types of Entropion (lower lid, medial and lateral)*

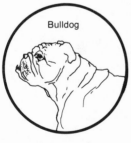 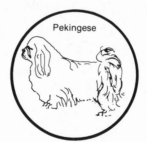 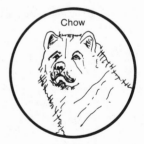

Entropion | Medial entropion | Lateral entropion

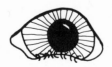 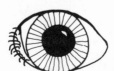 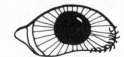

Rolled-in eyelids *(entropion)*

Either the upper or lower lid may be affected. In this condition the eyelid rolls in so that the lashes and hair on the eyelid rub on the front of the eyeball (the cornea). Persistent entropion causes severe corneal damage. Most entropion is inherited, and although *any breed can be affected,* it is a well-documented problem in Chow Chows**, St Bernards, English Bulldogs, Labrador Retrievers, Golden Retrievers, Irish Setters, and Cocker Spaniels.

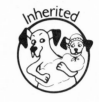

Some entropion is due to oversized eyelid openings. Breeding societies should be aware of entropion and as with all inherited disease *aim to breed it out.* To avoid entropion breed for:

• Correct size of eyelid openings.
• Smooth skin on face (avoid facial wrinkles).
• The outer angle of the eyelid opening should have enough pull to keep the eyelids in their correct position.

Treatment of entropion
The treatment of entropion is surgical. Correction is a fairly simple "plastic surgery" operation and is usually very effective. In severe cases surgery is much more involved. Entropion surgery may have to be repeated to reset the lid edges to their correct alignment.

Droopy or rolled-out lower eyelids (ectropion)

The eyelids may turn out to excessively expose the conjunctiva. This condition is common and hereditary in some breeds such as the Basset**, Bloodhound, American Cocker Spaniel, St Bernard*** and Great Dane***. In very mild cases treatment may not be necessary, but usually ectropion leads to chronic severe conjunctivitis. Ectropion indicates the eyelid opening is too large. In some large breeds of dog the eye socket (orbit) is too large for the eyeball. To reduce the incidence of eye disease when the eyelid opening is too large the eyelid opening is surgically remodelled to the correct size.

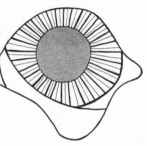

14.11 *Rolled-out eyelids (ectropion): lower lid sags and causes disease*

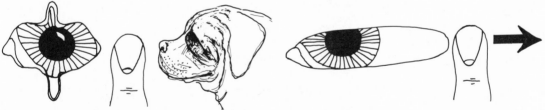

14.11a *Diamond eye (ectropion): a greatly oversized eye opening (diamond eye) leads to eye irritation. Breeding from such dogs must be avoided*

Long eyelid hair

Some dogs have long hair on their upper eyelid which tends to fall on the eye and cause irritation. Breeds affected include Miniature and Toy Poodles**, Cocker Spaniels, Maltese, Welsh and Wire Haired Fox Terriers*. Vaseline applied around the eye *may* help to keep this long hair from falling onto the eyeball. The long-term solution is to discourage breeding from dogs with long hair on the eyelids.

What should I do about long hair over the eyes?

In the natural state, long hair on the forehead "cords" into thick strands which protect the eye from excessive glare with minimum obstruction to sight. This allows dogs like the Old English Sheepdog to work in the snow. Washing an abundant forelock with soap removes its natural oil allowing the hair to cover eyes so much as to seriously restrict vision. In most cases, long forehead hair in front of the eyes is not needed as protection. Uncorded hair over the eyes not only impedes vision, but is a source of irritation to the eye. To improve the vision of your dog (e.g., Old English Sheepdog** or Maltese**) tie the long hair up in a topknot on the forehead or alternatively cut the long hair short—your dog will appreciate it.

My dog gets loose hairs on the eyeball. How do I clean his eyes?

Sweep the eyelids over the eyeball with your fingers to bring any foreign matter to the corner of the eye near the nose (Fig. 1.10).

Excessively long eyelashes

Some Cocker Spaniel*** families have excessively long eyelashes (Fig. 14.13). Long eyelashes on the eyeball cause irritation.

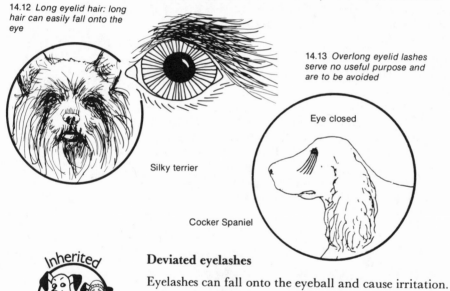

14.12 *Long eyelid hair: long hair can easily fall onto the eye*

Silky terrier

14.13 *Overlong eyelid lashes serve no useful purpose and are to be avoided*

Eye closed

Cocker Spaniel

Deviated eyelashes

Eyelashes can fall onto the eyeball and cause irritation.

Extra eyelashes (distichiasis)

There can be a second row of eyelashes. This extra row may rub onto the cornea and cause problems ranging from mild irritation to severe corneal ulcers.

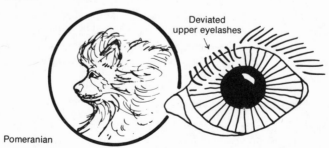

14.14 *Deviated eyelashes can fall onto the eyeball and irritate it*

Deviated upper eyelashes

Pomeranian

Extra lashes can be extremely hard to see without magnification as many are much smaller than the normal eyelashes. Extra lashes usually first cause problems at 4-5 months of age but this may occur at any age. Some dogs have only a few extra lashes, others have dozens. Longer extra lashes are softer and cause less irritation.

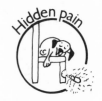

Signs
Short and stubby extra lashes are very painful. Your dog may have red, watery eyes and may wink or squint.

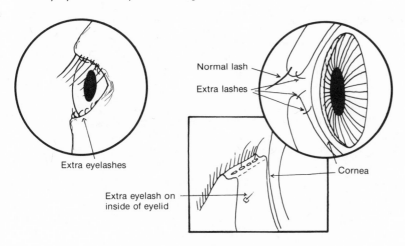

Normal lash
Extra lashes
Extra eyelashes
Extra eyelash on inside of eyelid
Cornea

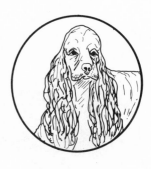

14.15 *Extra eyelashes — a hidden cause of pain.*

> Extra eyelashes are often overlooked as a cause of watery, red eye and winking. A microscope may be necessary for diagnosis.

Some extra lashes grow inside the eyelid and are only seen when the lid is rolled back and examined with magnification.

What breeds are affected?

At least 24 dog breeds can be affected. Breeds include Cocker Spaniel**, Boxer**, English Bulldog***, Pekingese***, Poodle, Shetland Sheepdogs**, Shih Tzu and Weimaraner.

Treatment of extra lashes
The treatment of extra lashes is similar to that for most types of superfluous hair. Plucking out the hair may offer temporary relief but the lashes usually grow back.

The most successful treatment is done under general anesthetic, preferably using a surgical microscope. Sometimes new hairs grow from adjacent (non-operated) sites on the eyelid and follow-up treatments are required.

Redundant (excessive) forehead skin

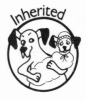

Dogs such as the Bloodhound**, Basset* and Cocker Spaniel*** may have excessively wrinkled forehead skin (see p. 168). This allows the upper eyelids to droop over the eye—especially when the head is lowered. Drooping

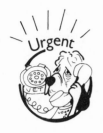

excessive forehead skin can lead to eye disease and blindness. Breeders of such dogs should be aware that this fashion is undesirable and breed for tighter forehead skin.

Eyelid injuries (due to bites, accidents or other trauma)

Most injuries are serious. Very swollen eyelids can hide a badly damaged eyeball. Keep the eyeball moist (see p. 28) while hurrying to the vet. Extensive lid injury may have to be restored by plastic surgery.

How do extensive eyelid injuries harm the eyeball?

When the eyelids cannot cover the eyeball and so sweep tears over the cornea, the eye becomes dry and damage to the eye rapidly occurs. The eyeball also suffers from exposure when the eyeball is too prominent.

> If the eyelids cannot cover the eyeball keep the eye constantly wet while hurrying to the vet.

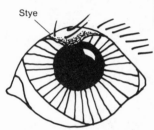

14.16 *Stye*

Stye

A stye is a small boil or abscess at the eyelid edge. It may need to be lanced and drained by your vet. Antibiotics are often needed.

Inflammation of the eyelids

Skin diseases affect eyelid skin. Inflamed eyelids (injury, infection, ringworm) may cause an inflamed eye. Sunlight makes inflammation much worse so keep the patient inside.

Home care
• Skin ointments prescribed to treat the area *around* the eye must not be placed *in* the eye. Protect the eyeball with eye ointment immediately *before* eyelid skin is treated.
• Prevent self-mutilation (see p. 10).
• Keep the patient out of the sun.

Eyelid diseases of newborn pups

The eyelids of the newborn pup remain closed until about the 10th day. Opening of the eyes much before this can lead to later blindness. If the pups' eyes open prematurely you should
• Keep the eyes moist. Artificial tears are ideal but *clean* tap water will do.
• Seek immediate veterinary help. Your vet may have to suture the eyelids together.

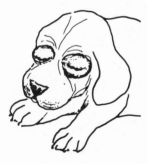

14.17 *Bulging eyelids (neonatal conjunctivitis): when the eyes do not open on time in newborn pups it may be due to very serious infection*

Bulging eyelids

Bulging, closed eyelids in a newborn pup mean eye infection and can lead to loss of the eye. Beware: the infection may not be obvious—showing only as swollen eyelids and a little pus at the corner of the eye.

> Swollen eyelids in the newborn puppy suggest an emergency
> and the eyelids must be surgically opened *at once.*

After opening, apply antibiotic ointment continually to control the infection and keep the eyes lubricated. The eyelids must not be allowed to stick together until the infection has cleared.

The third eyelid

The third eyelid, or nictitating (winking) membrane is a protective "extra" eyelid at the inner corner of each eye, next to the nose. When needed, the third eyelid can sweep across the eyeball, like a windscreen wiper, to help remove debris.

There are several conditions which can affect the third eyelid:

Haws (prominent third eyelid)

The third eyelid can become more prominent due to many causes—some involving the eye—but sometimes due to conditions affecting the whole body such as intestinal worms in pups. The third eyelid appears as a "skin" covering the inner part of the eye, usually about a quarter to a half of the eye being covered. Owners often mistakenly report that their dog has a "growth covering the eye."

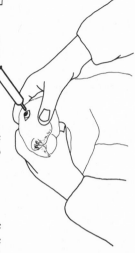

14.18 *Treating a puppy's eyes: lie the pup on a table. Use your fingers to hold the pup's eye open and apply medication*

Treatment
A prominent third eyelid is usually only one sign that there is eye disease or body disease. A veterinary examination determines the cause.

If the third eyelid is persistently prominent, should it be removed surgically?

> The third eyelid is vital for eye health and should *never* be removed.

If the third eyelid is removed, tear production is reduced and later the eye can become dry and very sick.

Pink third eyelid

Lack of dark pigment makes a third eyelid appear prominent as it contrasts with the eyeball behind it. Although tattooing and—alas—removal has been advocated, it is much better to breed the problem out.

Cherry eye

There is a gland at the base of the third eyelid. Normally, this gland is small and tucked well out of our sight. The gland may fall out of position and bulges out at the corner of the eye. This swelling is termed "cherry eye." Breeds predisposed include Cocker Spaniels**, Bassetts and Beagles.

In mild cases of cherry eye the gland of the third eyelid can be returned to its correct position by the owner with the fingers. Surgery is usually needed, however. The gland is stitched back into position and *not* removed, as it is vital for tears.

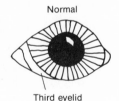

Normal

Third eyelid

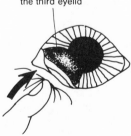

Prolapsed gland of the third eyelid

14.19 *Cherry eye: finger pressure can replace some prolapsed glands of the third eyelid*

The pop-eyed and short-nosed breeds

Pekingese***, Pug**, Lhaso Apso, Shih Tzu, King Charles Spaniel, Chihuahua, Boston Terrier and Boxer all have prominent or bulging eyes, making the eye more susceptible to eye disease. Many breeds also have a fold of skin between the nose and eye (pp. 152, 169). Hair from this fold falls onto the eye and irritates it. In some dogs the eyelids turn in towards the eyeball near the nose (this is medial entropion). Again, irritation from hair results.

14.20 The eyeball of the Pekingese is entirely unprotected by the bony skull and is prone to serious eye disease

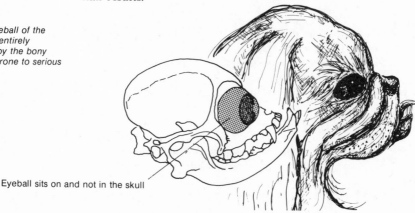

Eyeball sits on and not in the skull

Why is a prominent eye more susceptible to eye disease?

There are two main disadvantages of a bulging eyeball. Firstly, the eyelids are not as efficient at keeping the eyes moist and lubricated. A weak blink reflex of the pop-eyed breeds results in a poorer spread of the tear film. For health the eye must be constantly wet with tears, otherwise serious eye disease will follow. Some Pekingese sleep with their eyes open and this is dangerous, especially if the eye becomes sick. *Not enough tears on the front of the eyeball can cause corneal ulcers and lead to loss of the eye.*

Secondly, the pop-eyed breeds have a very shallow eye-socket in which the eye sits (called the bony "orbit"). This shallow orbit fails to properly protect the eye from accidental injury and makes it far more prone to pop out of its socket (eye prolapse).

My Peke's eye has popped out of its socket, what can I do?

Rush to your vet! Meanwhile, keep the eyeball constantly wet. Tap water is adequate. If there is no water, apply cod liver oil or vaseline onto the eyeball. If no vet is available, pull the eyelids apart by the hairs on the upper and lower lids and try to replace the eyelids over the eyeball.

Do *not* force the eyeball back. Proceed with all haste to the vet.

Why is eyeball dislocation serious?

Without eyelid protection, a dislocated eyeball gets dry. Blood vessels, muscles and the optic nerve can be ruptured. Some loss of vision follows all serious damage and severe dislocation causes blindness.

How to avoid disease in prominent eyes

If your dog's eye is constantly needing attention from the vet for conjuncti-

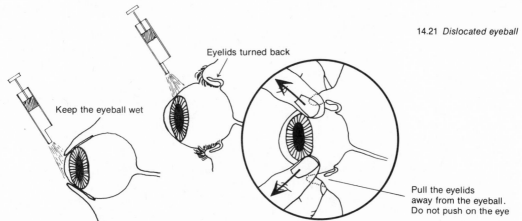

14.21 *Dislocated eyeball*

Eyelids turned back

Keep the eyeball wet

Pull the eyelids away from the eyeball. Do not push on the eye

vitis, ulcers on the eye or other injuries to his prominent eyes, the vet may suggest an operation to narrow the eyelid opening. By making the eyelid opening smaller the tear film becomes more effective and the eyeball is less prone to damage. The eyelid opening is usually reduced on the side next to the nose as this also eliminates irritation:

• From eyelid hair rubbing on the eyeball and
• From hair on the nasal or facial skin fold.

A special note for owners of Pekingese
If the eyelid opening is made smaller by plastic surgery in the young dog before eyelid problems begin you might avoid a lot of eye trouble e.g., ulcers of the cornea.

The short-nosed breeds (such as Pekingese****, Pugs**, Lhaso Apsos, Shih Tzus, Bulldogs) often suffer from a watery eye due to hair irritation from the nasal skin fold.

Moreover, in these and other breeds, eyelids turning inwards alongside the nose cause eyelid hair to rub against the eyeball (medial entropion) and is a quite common but often overlooked condition.

Chronic irritation from these hairs rubbing on the globe may lead to a brown pigment forming on the cornea, or to corneal ulcers starting.

In some breeds, notably the Pekingese and the Pug, the facial skin fold has become accepted as a "desirable" breed characteristic. Veterinary ophthalmologists would strongly disagree with this acceptance. The facial skin fold of these dogs is one of the prime examples of how fashion in breeding has resulted in discomfort for the dog.

Home care
Application of vaseline to the hair of the nasal fold gives *temporary* relief only, but can be used for those dogs which are wanted for the show ring (surgery disqualifies from showing).

DISEASES OF THE OUTSIDE OF THE EYEBALL

Conjunctivitis (inflammation of the conjunctiva)

Many cases are mild and respond readily to treatment, but conjunctivitis can be a severe condition requiring urgent treatment.

The conjunctiva is a thin, moist membrane that covers and protects the white of the eye and lines the eyelids. It is usually transparent but becomes more obvious when it is inflamed.

Conjunctivitis appears as red, runny inflamed eyes.

Common causes of conjunctivitis

Conjunctivitis results when this delicate membrane becomes irritated or infected. Because the eyes are exposed to wind-carrying dust, pollen or other potentially irritating debris, the eyelids have an important role in protecting the eyeball. Dogs with loose or ill-fitting lids, such as Bassets***, Bloodhounds** and Newfoundlands, are prone to chronic conjunctivitis.

Other conditions of the eyelid, such as inturned eyelids, or inflammation of the skin around the eye (leading to the dog rubbing at the eye) can also result in conjunctivitis.

Other common causes of conjunctivitis include:
• Allergies (to grass, pollen, house dust).
• Injury to the eye (hit by a ball; after car accident, pricked by a bush).
• Foreign matter in the eye (grass seed, sand, grit).
• Sun irritation (especially in dogs lacking a dark, protective pigment around the eyes, i.e., dogs with pink or pale eyelids).
• Chemical irritation (due to soap or shampoo or insecticides getting into the eye).
• Distemper (see p. 65-9).

Conjunctivitis may recur. Seek expert advice early.
If a red eye persists, call the vet again.

Treatment of conjunctivitis

Very mild conjunctivitis responds to decongestant drops (e.g., Visine, ⅛ per cent neo-synephrine, Otrivin eye drops). But beware: if redness persists, see your vet. *Be especially suspicious if only one eye is red.* This could mean there is a foreign body within the eye, or perhaps the inflammation is deeper than just the conjunctiva and the delicate inner structures of the eyeball are involved.

Do not treat a bloodshot eye lightly, always seek veterinary advice. Red eyes can be the start of distemper, or be an indication of deeper problems within the eye.

Dry eye

An eye without its covering of tears is called a dry eye (also called keratoconjunctivitis sicca or KCS). Dry eye can easily be overlooked and is a common complication of chronic inflammation. It is a very irritating and potentially blinding disease.

A dry eye looks similar to other inflamed eyes except that the pus is *on* the eyeball rather than in the corners of the eye. If the tear flow was adequate pus could not stick to the eyeball.

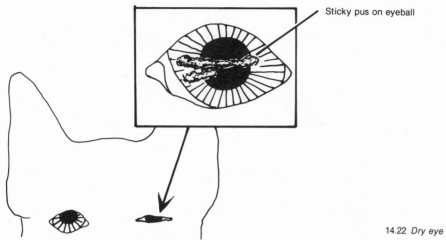

Sticky pus on eyeball

14.22 *Dry eye*

Eye closed when dry eye causes pain

Care of dry eye
The dry eye needs to be kept continually wet and clean. This can often be achieved by applying artificial tears or a special formula supplied by your vet that stimulates tear production as well as lubricating.

Is permanent relief of dry eye possible?

If the condition is severe or non-responsive to treatment, your vet may advise surgery. In this operation, a salivary duct is transplanted from its original opening inside the mouth to the eye, so that the eyeball is kept wet and lubricated with saliva. (This operation is termed a parotid duct transposition.)

Growths on the eye

The most common are:
Dermoid
This is a congenital growth of a hairy skin-like tissue on the eyeball or eyelids. A dermoid is not a cancer but is unsightly and causes severe inflammation. Dermoids are surgically removed.

PKC
Reddish, raised lumps on the cornea and the third eyelid can be a proliferative disease called PKC (proliferative keratoconjunctivitis). It is seen mainly in Rough Collies**. If untreated it can lead to blindness.

Fleshy growth on the eye/pannus
A scientific name for this disease is chronic superficial keratitis or CSK. CSK is a chronic incurable disease of the cornea of German Shepherds ** and German Shepherd crossbred dogs.

Other breeds affected include Greyhound*, Collie, Norwegian Elkhound, Samoyed.

Incidence and severity are much higher in areas of low humidity, high annual sunlight hours and high elevation.

The cause is unknown, but an immune reaction allergy is probably involved. Blindness follows uncontrolled CSK.

CSK/pannus is incurable but can be controlled. If suspected take to vet.

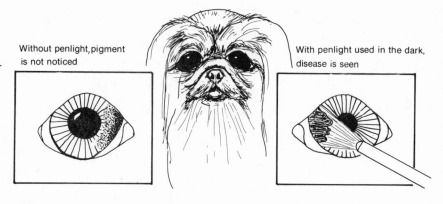

14.23 *Brown pigment on the eyeball: in broad daylight brown pigment on the eyeball is overlooked because it is similar in colour to the iris. In the dark a penlight shone behind the pigment shows up the disease. Pigment on the eyeball is due to irritation*

Brown pigment on the eyeball

Pigment on the eyeball usually follows irritation from hairs. Pigment can gradually spread and cause loss of vision. Among the causes are pop eye (prominent eyeball), extra lashes, and chronic irritation e.g., from hair from the nose, eyelids and nasal fold in Pekingese*** and Pugs**.

Eye worms

In some parts of the world, such as on the West Coast of North America, small (about 1 cm) roundworms live in the eye. Flies feeding on eye discharges transmit the worm from dog to dog. The eye becomes watery, red and irritated. A vet can remove the worms with fine forceps. Eye drops are available which kill the worms.

Blue cloudy cornea

Blue eye

The clear "window" in the front of the eye through which light enters is called the cornea. If it is injured or irritated it may become inflamed and swell with fluid, changing from its normal clear transparency to a bluish color, or appear cloudy or steamy.

(Note: It is *not* a cataract, which involves a deeper structure of the lens, see p. 183.)

> A blue eye (cloudy cornea) indicates serious eye inflammation or increased pressure in the eyeball. Seek immediate advice.

14.24 *Blue cloudy eye: a blue runny eye means serious inflammation*

Blue eye from hepatitis

The virus of infectious canine hepatitis (p. 69-70) causes blue eye, either naturally from infection, or by vaccination with live virus vaccine.

My dog was vaccinated against hepatitis about a week ago and now the eye is blue. Is this urgent?

Yes. See your vet *at once*. There may be serious inflammation in the eyeball.

Glaucoma after hepatitis blue eye

Increased eye pressure (glaucoma) and blindness can occur within a few days of onset of blue eye but typically it is a late rather than an early complication.

How to avoid blue eye after vaccination
  • Some vets prefer a *killed* hepatitis virus vaccine and *not* live vaccine.
  • Early cortisone treatment can stop the patient becoming blind.
Remember—*it is dangerous to use cortisone without veterinary supervision.*

Ulcers on the eye (corneal ulceration)

Corneal ulcers (Fig. 14:25) are a common cause of vision loss. A slow-healing corneal ulcer, corneal erosion (chronic or indolent ulcer, Boxer ulcer) is typical of middle-aged to older Boxer dogs**, Boston Terriers and Welsh Corgis.

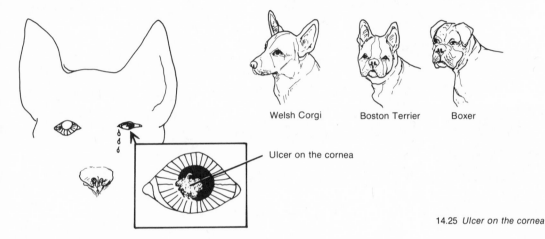

Welsh Corgi   Boston Terrier   Boxer

Ulcer on the cornea

14.25 *Ulcer on the cornea*

Causes of eye ulcers
Injury; inflammation; infection; foreign body; extra lashes; lack of tear film (dry eye); faulty lid function; a prominent eyeball (pop eye).

Signs of eye ulcers
A red, sore, watery eye which may be slightly blue. Half-closed eyelids may hide the ulcer and the dog may wink one eye.

Winking suggests corneal ulcers or a foreign body.

Treatment
Ointments may be sufficient in very mild cases. Otherwise your vet may elect to stitch the third eyelid right across the eye. This "bandages" the eye and is extremely useful in protecting the eye and accelerating healing. This "third eyelid flap" is held in place by one or two stitches, and the vet may use a button or piece of plastic tubing to stop the stitches cutting into the skin.

DISEASES INSIDE THE EYEBALL

Inflammation in the eyeball

Inflammation inside the eye quietly but surely destroys vision. The earlier that inflammation is detected, the better chance there is of reducing the damage. Untreated inflammation becomes very painful.

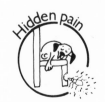

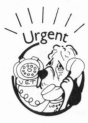

> Slight inflammation in the eyeball is easily overlooked.

Cause of inflammation within the eyeball
- A blow to the eye or head, e.g., following a road injury
- A foreign body (e.g., grass seed, gunshot) within the eyeball
- Following other conditions, such as ulcerated cornea
- As part of general body diseases and *due to immune reactions* such as infectious canine hepatitis
- Cancer of the body or of the eye
- Many cases are of *unknown* cause. Allergies to virus or bacteria are suspected in some cases.

Signs
A red, sore, watery eye. Be especially suspicious if only one eye is involved. Two red, sore, watery eyes could suggest a much less serious disease such as conjunctivitis; but if you are suspicious, seek expert examination.

Blood in the eye *(hyphaema)*

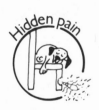

14.26 *Blood in the eye*

Blood within the eyeball itself suggests very serious eye disease. It may occur after car accidents or similar trauma, or it may be apparently spontaneous. In all cases:
- Keep the patient as immobile as possible (in a cage, if necessary) in a quiet, dark room
- *No* exercise at all
- Seek veterinary advice early.

Glaucoma

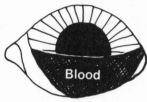

Glaucoma means there is an increase in pressure within the eyeball. The eyeball contains fluid *(aqueous)*. The amount of this fluid, and therefore the pressure it exerts on all parts of the eye, is kept remarkably constant by a fine, sensitive balance between production and drainage of fluid. Reduced drainage means glaucoma. Glaucoma can be very slow and insidious in onset and early cases are difficult to detect. Special instruments (tonometers) are necessary to detect early glaucoma, so diagnosis can be very difficult even for a vet and specialist veterinary ophthalmologist's examination may be required.

Glaucoma is treatable rather than curable: once it is detected, constant treatment and vigilance is required.

> Increased pressure in the eye (glaucoma) is one of the causes of red eye, undetected headache, of the eye turning blue, and *a common cause of blindness.*

There are two types of glaucoma. Both cause vision loss and both require much the same treatment. The significant difference is that one type—primary glaucoma—is inherited and its incidence is increasing.

Type I: (Inherited) primary glaucoma

In some dogs, there is a developmental defect of the drainage structures

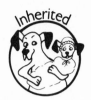

within the eye. This results in inefficient drainage and the eye develops increased pressure—usually in middle age. Primary glaucoma starts in one eye but later always affects both eyes.

What breeds are known to be affected by this hereditary type of glaucoma?

The Basset Hound***, American Cocker Spaniel and English Cocker Spaniel are among the increasing number of breeds affected.

> Before you buy breeds susceptible to inherited glaucoma ask for a veterinary certificate that the family is free.

I have a dog from a breed susceptible to inherited glaucoma. What should I do?

An examination of the angle inside the eye using a special lens on the eyeball (the examination is called gonioscopy) helps to determine the possible risk of glaucoma developing later. A bad angle inside the eyeball means your dog will start eye drops for life—to prevent glaucoma.

My dog is suffering pain from glaucoma. Should the eye be removed?

There are operations which may help. Removal may be easier.

Dogs which have had an eye removed usually manage extremely well. When the hair regrows around the operation site he will look most acceptable and very few problems of after-care ever occur.

Even though the cosmetic appearance of the dog after eye removal is excellent, some owners prefer to have an artificial eye fitted, and this can be done in a suitable patient.

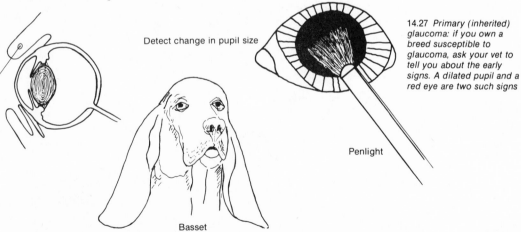

Detect change in pupil size

Penlight

Basset

14.27 *Primary (inherited) glaucoma: if you own a breed susceptible to glaucoma, ask your vet to tell you about the early signs. A dilated pupil and a red eye are two such signs*

Type II: Secondary glaucoma (mostly non-inherited)

If the eye is damaged or diseased, the delicate mechanisms which drain the excess fluid from the globe can be interfered with and partly obstructed. Glaucoma can follow injury and inflammation of the eye (not inherited) or conditions such as lens dislocation (inherited, see p.38-49, 182).

How do you detect glaucoma?

If you own a dog of a breed known to be susceptible to glaucoma, be especially on your guard for these signs:

The eye suffering from glaucoma is usually red and cloudy. The pupil is larger in size than the other eye and does not respond to a light shone on it. (The opening of the normal pupil should quickly contract to a much smaller size when a penlight is shone. Check the suspect eye's reaction to light against that of the other eye.)

A vet can use special instruments to detect the ocular pressure increase of glaucoma.

Treatment

Veterinary (often specialist) treatment can be very successful in *controlling* glaucoma, but it is usually not *curable*. Treatment may include topical, oral medication and surgery. Glaucoma detected too late causes blindness and the eye becomes very large. Glaucoma is painful and the vet might recommend removal of the eye. We are not always as aware of the pain of glaucoma as we should be. It is common for owners to say, "I didn't realize the eye was worrying him so much—he is back to his old bright self now the eye has been removed." In some cases, however, the dog does not appear to be worried by the blinded eye.

Dislocated lens

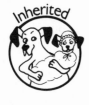

The lens of the eye can become displaced, or dislocated, from its position suspended behind the iris. The incidence of this condition has increased in many breeds and is known to be inherited in Fox Terriers***, Sealyham Terriers***, Welsh Terriers, Jack Russell Terriers, Manchester Terriers, Corgis, Chihuahuas, Bassets, Cocker Spaniels and Tibetan Terriers.

In addition to inherited factors, lens dislocation can also be caused by injury or inflammation in any breed.

The signs are the same as for many deep inflammations of the eye: a winking, squinting eye, the cornea of which is often blue.

If not detected early, lens dislocation leads to glaucoma and blindness.

In breeds susceptible to lens dislocation the other eye is affected, too, usually at a later time.

14.28 *Dislocated lens: inherited dislocation of the lens causes blindness*

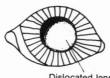

Dislocated lens

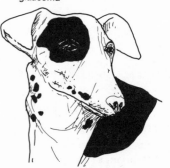

Dislocated lens is inherited in terriers and causes glaucoma

Normal

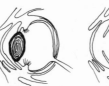

Lens falls forwards

Lens jammed into pupil

Lens falls backwards

Fox Terrier

How to avoid lens dislocation

In breeds which inherit lens dislocation, the loose lens does not occur for some years. Before you buy a susceptible breed, ask for a veterinary certificate that the stud, i.e., the family is free of lens dislocation. Before you breed, select breeding stock free of lens dislocation.

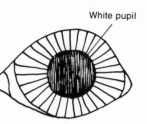

White pupil

Cataracts (white pupil)

A cataract is a cloudy lens and is seen as a hazy eye or white pupil (Fig. 14:29). Light cannot get through the lens to reach the back of the eye. Do not confuse a cataract (white *inside* the eye) with a blue, cloudy cornea at the front of the eye, or a white scar on the eyeball.

What causes cataracts?

Any disturbance to the eye which upsets the lens can cause the lens to become cloudy. A disease in the body (e.g. diabetes); inflammation or disease in the eye; injury; a blow to the head; PRA; can all lead to cataracts. If the bitch has a disease while pregnant, cataracts can form in her pups while they are in her womb. *Some* cataracts are inherited—*most, however, are NOT inherited.*

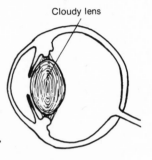

Cloudy lens

14.29 *A cataract is a cloudy lens and turns the pupil white. Small cataracts are not readily detected*

What are the most common inherited cataracts?

Developmental (juvenile) cataracts which appear in dogs under 6 years are the most frequent cataracts in some dog breeds.

Some predisposed breeds

- Afghan Hound
- American Cocker Spaniel
- Beagle
- Boston Terrier
- German Shepherd Dog
- Golden Retriever
- Irish Setter
- Labrador Retriever
- Miniature Schnauzer
- Old English Sheepdog
- Pointer
- Poodle: Toy, Miniature, Standard
- Siberian Husky
- Staffordshire Bull Terrier
- Wirehaired Fox Terrier

Can cataracts be cured medically?

No. In some cases, eye drops that enlarge the pupil can allow some vision past a cloudy lens, but the change within the lens remains. Spontaneous partial disappearance or resorption of cataracts occurs mainly in dogs under 3 years of age.

My old dog has a blue lens. Is this a cataract?

Usually not. The cloudy lens you see in most old dogs is not from disease, but a blue lens due to the hardening of the lens with age.

My dog is getting cataracts—what should I do?

An immediate examination by an eye specialist—before the lens is too cloudy—will tell you whether the back of the eye (beyond the cloudy lens) is healthy. It is vital to learn *early* if surgical removal of the lens is a good idea later on. There is no point in removing a diseased lens if the back of the eye is also diseased.

Cataract surgery

Surgery involves removing the affected lens to allow light to get to the sight-receptors at the back of the eye. Surgery may be considered if there is no disease beyond the cataract or elsewhere in the eye.

Do cataracts always mean an operation?

Certainly not. In most cataracts, surgical extraction is *not* indicated. Most small dogs manage very well in spite of dense cataracts. Surgery in old dogs is not indicated.

My litter of puppies has cataracts. What are some causes?

Cataracts in a litter of puppies may be due to some damage to the young embryo in the mother's womb. Cataracts, even in a whole litter of puppies, do not mean that they are necessarily inherited.

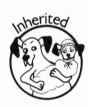

Cataract in the Golden Retriever

Most cataracts in the Golden Retriever—due to an incompletely dominant gene—do not progress to cause blindness, but the control of hereditary cataract in this breed offers an example to all breeders of the results of breeder co-operation.

In 1970, cataracts in the UK affected about half of the best blood lines. The incidence has been dramatically reduced as a result of the British Veterinary Association/Kennel Club Hereditary Cataract Scheme. Dogs with even slight cataracts are not awarded certificates as they can produce progeny with completely cloudy lenses (total cataract).

Most dogs can be certified free by 3 years of age, some, however, develop cataracts between 3 and 6 years, so certificates of freedom are renewed annually until 6 years of age when permanent certification is possible.

Progressive retinal atrophy (PRA)

The retina is at the back of the eye. It is composed of highly specialized nerve cells that receive light impulses. The retina passes on a message to the brain as nerve impulses.

In progressive retinal atrophy, there is a gradually wasting or thinning of the retina, so that sight is lost. (Fig. 14:30) It is an inherited condition and is incurable. Although PRA has been eliminated in some breeds, generally speaking the incidence of PRA is increasing.

The main difficulty with controlling this serious condition is that in some breeds it only becomes apparent when the dog is several years old and by that time the animal may have produced many progeny. In PRA-affected Miniature and Toy Poodles, for example, night blindness is present between 2-4 years of age, and day blindness between about 5-8 years.

What are the signs of progressive retinal atrophy (PRA)?

At first, the dog may be unwilling to go out at night. He may appear to

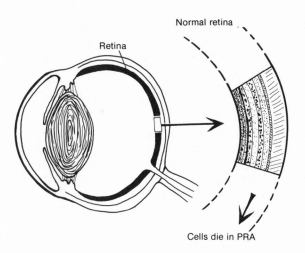

Normal retina

Retina

Cells die in PRA

Reduced layers
of abnormal retina

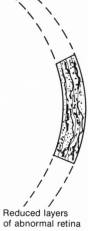

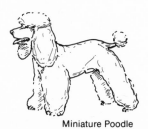

14.30 *PRA (progressive
retinal atrophy) is an
inherited degeneration where
the retina becomes thin*

Miniature Poodle

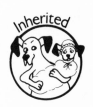

be "afraid" of the dark, stays close to you at night and appears "short-sighted." Little signs such as stumbling while going down stairs, or going much more slowly than before, can be indications of failing sight. In Miniature and Toy Poodles and Irish Setters, sight at night always goes first, progressing to blindness even in the daylight.

All dogs affected by PRA go blind if they live long enough.

Dogs with early PRA appear normal to the owner; loss of vision only becomes evident later.

There is an instrument called an electroretinograph which can be used to detect early PRA before it is otherwise evident and this instrument can be useful in selecting breeding stock.

What breeds are affected?

Any breed can be affected. It is known to be hereditary in many breeds including Border Collie; Welsh Corgi; Dachshund (Miniature and long-haired); Elkhound; Golden Retriever; Irish Setter; Labrador Retriever; Miniature Poodle***; Rough Collie**; Saluki; Shetland Sheepdog; Smooth Collie***; Tibetan Terrier; and Toy Poodle***. See also lists in inherited diseases (see p. 38-49).

At what age can you be sure dogs do not have PRA?

A veterinary ophthalmologist must examine the back of the eye with specialized equipment. The earliest one can be certain with most breeds is 5 years of age, but with some breeds the specialist can certify freedom as early as 3 years (see p. 188).

Is there any treatment for PRA?

No. Sometimes complications such as cataracts and glaucoma set in and they may have to be managed to reduce inflammation or pain.

How can PRA be eliminated?

The only way to eliminate the condition is to avoid breeding from carriers of PRA or from affected dogs. Ideally, suspect carrier dogs should be bred to an affected animal to see if any of the progeny inherit PRA. This takes time and patience—in some breeds you have to wait 4 to 5 years before you can be sure.

Before buying or importing dogs ask for certified PRA-free stock.

PRA *is* eradicable and *can* be prevented by co-operation between breed societies and vets.

Affected dogs must not be used for breeding—but more than that: the *parents* of the affected dogs must not be used and neither should *any* of the offspring.

Inheritance

If the gene causing the condition is autosomal recessive, as it is in this case, the numbers of pups affected are as follows:

Both parents affected → all progeny affected

One parent affected, one carrier parent → 50 per cent affected, 50 per cent carriers

One parent affected, one parent free → all progeny carriers

Both parents carriers → 50 per cent carriers, 25 per cent free, 25 per cent affected

One parent free, one carrier parent → 50 per cent carriers, 50 per cent free

Both parents free → all progeny free

Thus, both the parents and all the progeny of an affected animal must be at least carriers and are not used for breeding.

Central retinal atrophy

Central retinal atrophy (CRA) is another inherited disease of the retina and is different from PRA. CRA causes progressive loss of vision, but the progression may be so slow as to leave your old dog with some sight.

It is mainly seen in the UK in working dogs like the Labrador Retriever**, Border Collie**, Briards, Scotch Collie, Cardigan Corgi, English Setters, English Springer Spaniel, Golden Retrievers, Shetland Sheepdogs.

Collie eye anomaly

Collie eye anomaly (CEA) affects approximately 85-90 per cent of Scotch Collies**and 10 per cent of Shelties in North America. The extent of the disease in Europe, Australia and other countries is also very high. In 160 Collies examined in the Netherlands CEA showed in 41 per cent*†, and in a survey of 120 Shelties in the Netherlands in 1979, CEA occurred in over 48 per cent†.

What is collie eye anomaly?

Anomaly means a "marked abnormality." In CEA there are congenital inherited pathological changes to the choroid, optic nerve and the retina,

*Barnett, K. C., and Stades, F. C., *The Vet Quarterly,* No.3. p.66, 1981
†Barnett, K. C., and Stades, F. C., *J.Sm. Animal Practice,* No.20. p.321, 1979

some of which are severe. The most severe form is where there are pits in the optic nerve, and it is this form that must be avoided by breeders.

The Collie and Shelties are the most severely affected breeds, but other breeds have been reported with collie eye anomaly.

How do I know if my dog has collie eye anomaly?

CEA appears at birth. Mildly affected pups show no signs to the owner and require veterinary examination. Severely affected pups are blind—perhaps only in one eye—and this may be hard for an owner to detect.

Does vision get worse as the pups get older?

Usually not—collie eye anomaly is *not* a progressive condition. In rare cases vision does deteriorate even more with age.

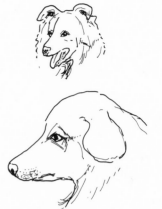

Old type

How do I avoid collie eye anomaly at time of purchase?

Only buy Collies or Shelties which have had a specialist ophthalmoscopic examination before 14 weeks of age. Some signs may be obscured after 14 weeks.

How is collie eye anomaly eliminated?

- Examination of *all* 6 to 14-weeks-old pups to be used for breeding
- *Affected dogs, their parents and progeny should not be used for breeding.* Collie eye anomaly has been reduced in incidence from 97 to 59 per cent in three years by selective breeding in North America. Affected animals, even if showing minimal lesions, cannot be used for breeding

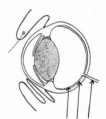

Collie eye anomaly

- *Detection of carriers* is achieved by test-mating to detect carriers and slightly affected dogs. Test-breed to a known affected dog and examine *all* progeny. If even one pup is affected, this condemns the test animal as a carrier. Eight pups free of collie eye anomaly from 2 affected bitches are necessary to prove a stud dog clear at the 99 per cent confidence level.
- *Sire-selection*—breeder co-operation within a breed society—can start progeny tests to select those sires which produce fewest eye defects.

> To reduce the incidence of collie eye anomaly, breed from dogs selected from progeny testing to be *genetically* free of the disease.

Some inherited eye conditions associated with vision loss (common diseases shown with asterisk)

Merling, excessive dappling of the coat, albinism.
Inherited cataracts
*Defects of the drainage angle (leading to glaucoma)
Lens dislocation (leading to glaucoma)
*Collie eye anomaly (severe form)
*PRA
Retinal detachment, faulty retinal development (underdeveloped retina) called *retinal dysplasia*
Small eye (microphthalmia)
Fat (lipid) 'storage diseases' of the brain

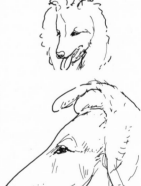

Modern type

14.31 *Collie Eye Anomaly: change in the shape of the head may lead to more inherited eye disease as shown in the Shetland Sheepdog*

Common inherited diseases which do not appear until later in life

PRA
Cataracts (not all cataracts are inherited)
Extra eyelashes
Glaucoma (increased pressure due to abnormal drainage angles, e.g., in the Basset eye)
Lens dislocation

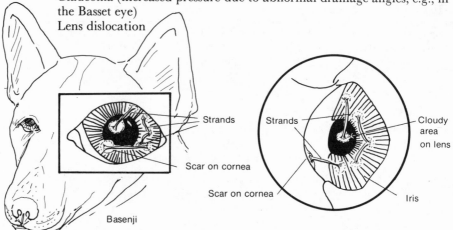

Strands

Scar on cornea

Basenji

Strands

Scar on cornea

Cloudy area on lens

Iris

14.32 *Persistent pupillary membrane (PPM)*

MINIMUM AGES FOR PERMANENT CERTIFICATION

Hereditary Cataract

Breed	*Minimum Age*
Afghan Hound	3 years
American Cocker Spaniel	5 years
Boston Terrier	18 months
Golden Retriever	6 years
Miniature Schnauzer	3 years
Staffordshire Bull Terrier	18 months
All other breeds	5 years

From the Joint British Veterinary Association/Kennel Club Hereditary Cataract Scheme (1977)

Progressive Retinal Atrophy

Border Collie	3 years
Cardigan Welsh Corgi	3 years
Dachshund (Miniature Long-Haired)	3 years
Elkhound	3 years
Golden Retriever	6 years
Irish Setter	3 years
Labrador Retriever	4 years
Pembroke Welsh Corgi	4 years
Rough Collie	3 years
Saluki	3 years
Shetland Sheepdog	3 years
Smooth Collie	3 years
Tibetan Terrier	3 years
Working Trials and Obedience Register: Cross Breed	5 years
Working Trials and Obedience Register: Working Sheepdog	5 years
All other breeds	5 years

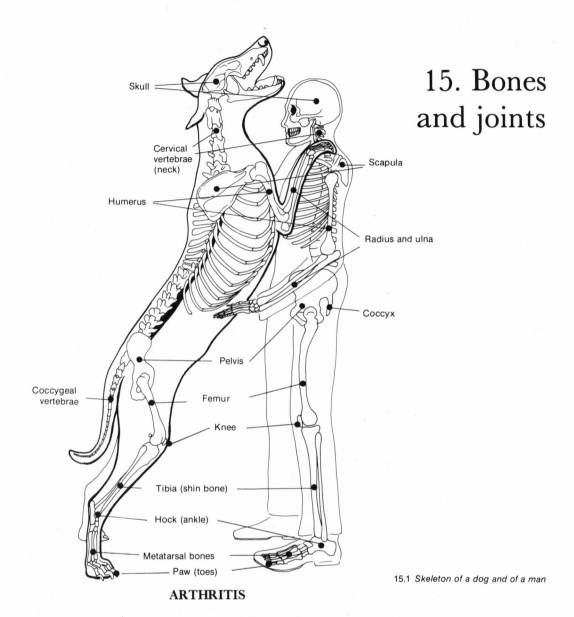

15. Bones and joints

Skull

Cervical vertebrae (neck)

Humerus

Scapula

Radius and ulna

Coccyx

Pelvis

Coccygeal vertebrae

Femur

Knee

Tibia (shin bone)

Hock (ankle)

Metatarsal bones

Paw (toes)

15.1 *Skeleton of a dog and of a man*

ARTHRITIS

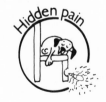

Arthritis is inordinately common in man, yet not quite so common in the dog. For all its familiarity to us there is a lot of misunderstanding. "Arthritis" means inflammation of a joint, usually resulting in pain and a degree of lameness. The causes vary, and an understanding of these causes helps owners to treat a dog suffering from arthritis more effectively. There are three categories of arthritis.

Infectious arthritis

In infectious arthritis the joint is attacked by bacteria or viruses which damage the joints' inner surfaces and destroy the delicate harmony within the joint. The infection may be let in due to an injury, such as a puncture

*, **, *** indicate increasing likelihood of a particular trait or problem occurring.

189

wound from a dog fight, or an open wound from a car accident.

The infection sometimes enters the joint via the blood stream as a part of a disease affecting other parts of the body.

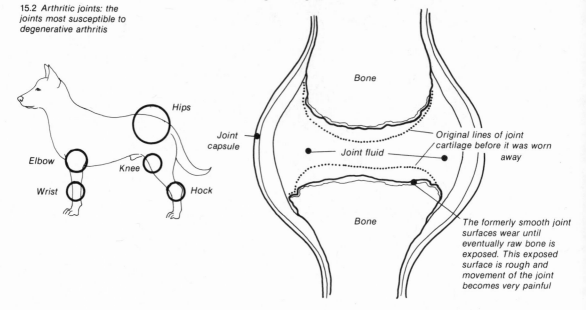

15.2 *Arthritic joints: the joints most susceptible to degenerative arthritis*

Hips

Elbow

Knee

Wrist

Hock

Bone

Joint capsule

Joint fluid

Original lines of joint cartilage before it was worn away

Bone

The formerly smooth joint surfaces wear until eventually raw bone is exposed. This exposed surface is rough and movement of the joint becomes very painful

Auto-immune arthritis (rheumatics)

This is a group of diseases in which the dog may become allergic to parts of his own body. The result is that the dog's own immune system incorrectly identifies some parts of the joint as being "foreign" and so reacts against that part of the joint in the same way it would react against bacteria invading the body. The resulting inflammation produces arthritis. One such disease is rheumatoid arthritis (usually called "rheumatism"). The "auto-immune" form of arthritis usually affects more than one joint, especially the elbows, knees, wrists and hocks.

Degenerative arthritis

Degenerative arthritis occurs where there is instability of the joint, as may occur after ligament damage or in hip dysplasia (see p. 196-8). Because the joint surfaces are not gliding properly over one another, they wear irregularly and eventually arthritis results. The age at which signs appear depends on how unstable the joint is. Dogs with severe instabilities may develop arthritis within a few months of the joint being damaged. In the case of dogs born with faulty joints, some develop severe problems within their first year, but others only show signs late in life.

Some breeds have inherently faulty form that render the dog far more prone to this form of arthritis. Examples of such breeds are the Dachshund** and Basset*** and Labradors*** with hip dysplasia.

Treatment of arthritis in dogs

Treatment depends on the cause and is aimed at reducing further damage and relieving pain.

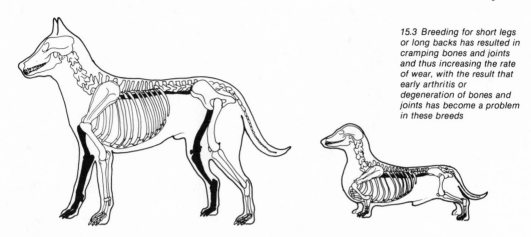

15.3 Breeding for short legs or long backs has resulted in cramping bones and joints and thus increasing the rate of wear, with the result that early arthritis or degeneration of bones and joints has become a problem in these breeds

In infectious arthritis antibiotics are used, but it is difficult to get antibiotics into the joint and to the site of infection. This is because there is no blood *within* the joint, but instead there is a filtered, purified and modified secretion called joint fluid (see p. 190). In the process of filtration, antibiotics (and other drugs) are often excluded. If thus "protected" from antibiotics, infections within a joint may flourish. (Sometimes the vet will inject the drug directly into an affected joint to overcome this problem.)

Treatment of auto-immune arthritis

Treatment is difficult, as any rheumatic sufferer knows. Relief of pain is usually the best we can do. Aspirin is effective, but should only be used for a short time and at the correct dosage or damage to stomach and kidneys may result. Dose is 10 mg/kg bodyweight (¼-2 tablets of 300 mgm aspirin, depending on size), every 12 hours. Consult your vet before you use aspirin for more than 3 days. A "buffered" aspirin is preferred (e.g., Bufferin). Other drugs, prescribed by your vet, can be used on a long-term basis.

Treatment of degenerative arthritis

If the instability of the joint can be corrected then repair of the loose or broken ligament is best. In many cases the damage to the joint is already done. Reduction of excess weight will help relief of pain and inflammation.

The use of replacement hips and other joints is possible but very expensive. Results are variable.

BROKEN BONES

Pain, swelling, and loss of use are the main signs of a broken bone. A broken leg usually hangs and the dog will not put *any* weight on it.

First aid

Be careful. A dog in pain may bite. If he shows any inclination at all to bite, first apply a muzzle (p. 276) before moving or examining your pet.

If you cannot immediately get the animal to a vet, to minimize further damage a temporary splint may be applied.

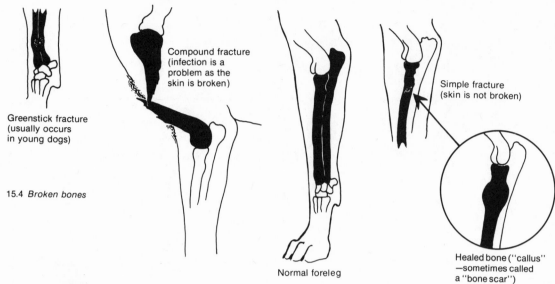

Greenstick fracture
(usually occurs
in young dogs)

Compound fracture
(infection is a
problem as the
skin is broken)

Simple fracture
(skin is not broken)

15.4 *Broken bones*

Normal foreleg

Healed bone ("callus"
—sometimes called
a "bone scar")

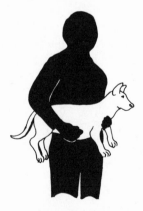

15.5 *Hind leg injury in a
large dog*

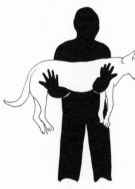

15.6 *Carrying a small dog
with a fractured foreleg:
support the dog's weight
with a hand under the chest
and the other hand spread
out to support the abdomen*

Transporting

Move the dog very slowly to minimize movement of the injured part.

For hind leg injuries
Pick the dog up under the chest and let the hind quarters hang very gently
(Fig. 15:5).

Front leg injuries
Put one arm under the chest and the other under his rump and let the
damaged leg hang free (Fig. 15:6).

If there is any suspicion that the spine has been damaged, *do not bend* the
dog's back. The best form of transport is on a firm board or door very carefully eased under the patient. (Note that a blanket sags too much.)

Treatment of broken bones

To mend, a bone must be set in the correct position and held rigidly in
that position for many weeks. While plaster casts are still used, many fractures are now immobilized by "internal fixation"; that is, using stainless steel
bone plates, pins, screws and wires. The increasing sophistication of veterinary surgery now allows us to successfully treat most fractures with minimum discomfort to the dog and rapid return to normal use.

SPRAINS

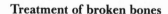

Sprains are injuries to the joints, usually due to overstretching or rupture
of the ligaments and joint capsule.

Pain and swelling are the main signs, and the dog will be very reluctant
to use the affected leg. X-rays may be necessary to distinguish between fractures and sprains.

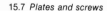

15.7 *Plates and screws*

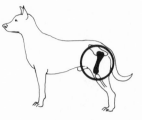

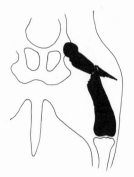

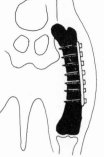

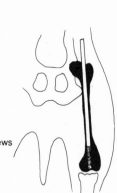

The femur, or thigh bone, is used for these examples

Fractured femur

Bone plate and screws

Bone pin

Treatment of sprains

Immediate application of cold will reduce the amount of swelling. This can be done with ice packs, ice wrapped in towels or cold water compresses. (Most dogs, however, will not keep still for long enough.) Cold hosing may help.

Do not apply liniments, ointments or preparations designed for human sprains—the dog's skin is very sensitive and is easily damaged by many of these preparations. Most dogs will also lick at the liniment or ointment and this can be most uncomfortable.

In most cases the dog will restrict himself. Pain is nature's way of telling him to slow down. Rest and time are needed for repair.

In the case of sprains, avoid painkillers such as aspirin and phenylbutazone in the first few days. Absence of pain may encourage the patient to move too much and possibly cause further damage.

How to avoid a sprain

Sprains usually occur when the dog slips and over-extends a joint. Keep him away from slippery floors, stairs, and loose rugs. Do not let your dog jump down on to linoleum or similar slippery flooring, or play with a ball on such floors.

When to call the vet if your dog has a suspected sprain

Mild sprains, especially in pups, may need only rest. If there is severe pain and swelling it is advisable to get expert attention.

You should also consult the vet:
• If swelling persists.
• If pain persists.
• If lameness persists without improvement over 48 hours.

THE KNEE (STIFLE JOINT)

There are three frequently seen conditions of dog's knees:
• Ruptured cruciate ligament.
• Slipping kneecap.
• Arthritis (see beginning of this chapter).

Ruptured cruciate ligament

The ligaments of the dog's knee are essential to stabilize the joint. Of these ligaments the most commonly damaged is the anterior (or front) cruciate ligament (see diagram). The posterior (hind) cruciate ligament is much stronger and less liable to damage.

When the anterior cruciate ligament breaks the dog experiences great pain. The knee becomes unstable and when weight is put on it, the thigh bone (femur) slides forward. This causes stretching of the joint capsule, wearing of joint surfaces and will lead to arthritis unless repaired.

Causes of ruptured cruciate ligament
The ligament may break as the result of a hard knock, or a violent twist to the knee. Some dogs have weak ligaments and are more prone to damage, e.g., Corgi and other short-legged dogs.

Treatment
Drugs give temporary relief only. Because the joint is unstable, arthritis develops after a few weeks or months. Broken cruciate ligaments do *not* heal by themselves. Surgical repair of the damaged joint will re-stabilize the joint and is the treatment of choice.

15.8 *Anterior cruciate ligament repair: this is one method of repair — by inserting an artificial tendon made of non-irritating and very strong synthetic material*

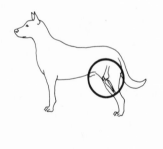

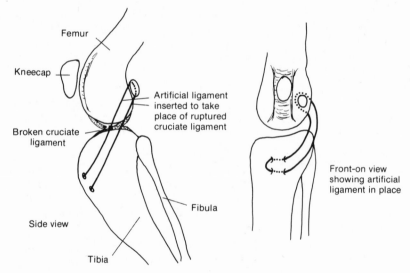

Femur

Kneecap

Artificial ligament inserted to take place of ruptured cruciate ligament

Broken cruciate ligament

Fibula

Side view

Tibia

Front-on view showing artificial ligament in place

Slipping kneecap (luxating or dislocating patella)

The dog's kneecap runs in a groove at the end of his femur (thigh bone).

In some dogs the kneecap occasionally slips out of its groove. It may then slip back spontaneously or it may stay out. This condition is hereditary in some breeds, especially Pomeranian**, Yorkshire Terrier*, Miniature* and Toy Poodle**, Chihuahua**, Boston Terrier.

Signs of a slipping kneecap
Some dogs appear to be only mildly discomforted, but others are acutely lame. The dog may suddenly yelp and hold the affected leg high. The kneecap sometimes slips back into place and the dog can use it again, but sometimes the dislocation persists and the owner (once trained) or a vet must put it back.

Veterinary treatment
Surgery may be advised to stabilize the kneecap and deepen the groove
in which the kneecap sits (Fig. 15:9). Dogs with slipping kneecaps should
not be used for breeding.

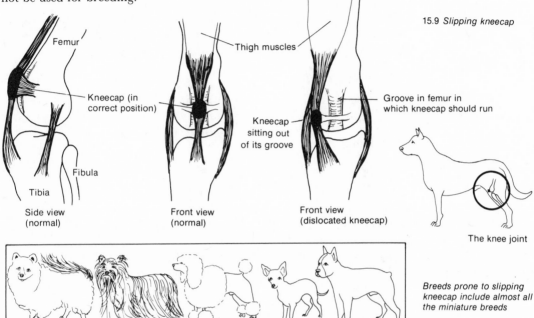

15.9 *Slipping kneecap*

Femur

Thigh muscles

Kneecap (in
correct position)

Groove in femur in
which kneecap should run

Kneecap
sitting out
of its groove

Fibula

Tibia

Side view
(normal)

Front view
(normal)

Front view
(dislocated kneecap)

The knee joint

Breeds prone to slipping
kneecap include almost all
the miniature breeds

The "all meat" syndrome (nutritional secondary hyperparathyroidism—rickets)

A diet based on meat alone is incorrect, and problems arise especially in
young, growing dogs. The mineral content of meat is too low in calcium.
The ratio of calcium to phosphate in meat is about 1:20. A correct ratio
should be about 1:1. Because calcium blood levels become low, calcium
is reabsorbed from the bones, resulting in weakening of the bones. Pain and
discomfort occur and the bones break easily—in some cases even collapsing
(termed a "folding fracture"). The pelvis may become narrowed resulting
in complications later in life, such as constipation or difficulty in giving
birth as pups cannot easily get through the narrow pelvis.

Treatment of the "all meat" syndrome
Correct the diet by supplementing with calcium carbonate at the rate of
one teaspoon per 400 g of meat fed until the pup is 6 months old (10 months
in large breeds).

How to prevent weak bones in pups
Feed balanced dog food, not all-meat diets, which caused the problems to
begin with.

BONE PROBLEMS OF LARGE DOGS

Young animals, especially of the large breeds*** such as Great Danes, St
Bernards, Newfoundlands, German Shepherds, Rottweilers, Retrievers and

Dobermans, are more susceptible to bone growth problems than the smaller breeds.

OCD (Osteochondritis dissecans)

OCD is a disease of the joint cartilage and is especially common in the shoulder joint, although other joints can be affected. It occurs primarily in young, fast-growing dogs, and more commonly in males.

What causes OCD?

The cause of OCD is not certain, although trauma, such as knocks or jolts, may be involved. The result is a flap of cartilage under which is an ulcer of raw bone (Fig. 15:10). OCD is a painful condition and can lead to chronic joint damage.

Signs of OCD

Dogs with OCD have a persistent and progressively more severe lameness of the affected leg—usually the foreleg. Although lameness often shows in only one leg, almost half of the dogs affected have bone ulcers in *both* legs. Diagnosis can only be confirmed by X-ray examination.

> Suspect OCD if you have a young, fast-growing dog of a large breed that has a persistent lameness, especially of the foreleg.

Treatment of OCD

Surgical treatment may be necessary to remove the loose flap of cartilage; curette the bone ulcer; and so allow healing to commence.

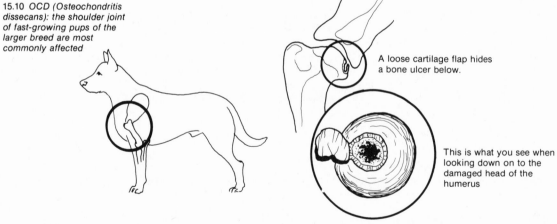

15.10 *OCD (Osteochondritis dissecans): the shoulder joint of fast-growing pups of the larger breed are most commonly affected*

A loose cartilage flap hides a bone ulcer below.

This is what you see when looking down on to the damaged head of the humerus

HIP DYSPLASIA

Hip dysplasia (HD) is a condition of the hind leg in which the hip joint is badly formed. A loose joint leads to abnormal wear and in some dogs to arthritis.

Hip dysplasia is the most common disorder of the hip in large-breed dogs.***

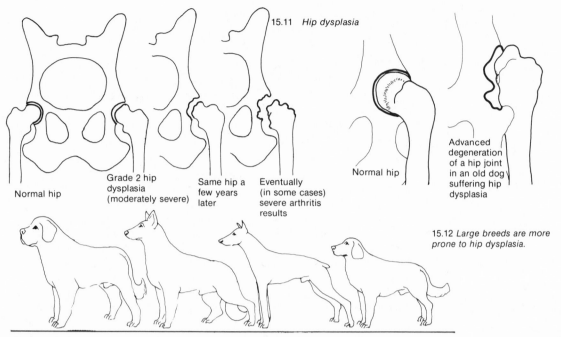

15.11 *Hip dysplasia*

Normal hip

Grade 2 hip dysplasia (moderately severe)

Same hip a few years later

Eventually (in some cases) severe arthritis results

Normal hip

Advanced degeneration of a hip joint in an old dog suffering hip dysplasia

15.12 *Large breeds are more prone to hip dysplasia.*

Signs of HD

The signs vary, and there is no way of being *absolutely* sure your dog has HD unless X-rays are taken. There are signs, however, that should make you suspicious.

The young dog with HD may walk with a swaying gait, and when running may "bunny hop," moving both hind legs together. He may sit with both legs on one side and have difficulty rising.

Although signs of discomfort may reduce or disappear as the dog gets older, the seeds are sown for arthritis to develop. In severe cases this arthritis can be crippling.

Genetics: Preventing hip dysplasia

Hip dysplasia is not caused by one gene, but by many. A dog may carry only some of the faulty genes that produce a poor hip joint. As a result, there are many "degrees" of hip dysplasia, from a mild case with no apparent signs, through to the "sloppy" joint and very flat hip socket (where the joint is virtually absent).

If good hip joints were the *only* factor considered when selecting dogs for breeding, hip dysplasia would rapidly be eliminated.

Breeders must decide what they want in their dogs: is it sensible to select for fashion (color and coat length) at the expense of good hips? Dogs known to be hip dysplastic should be eliminated from breeding programs.

Show ring entrants should be certified free of hip dysplasia by a vet before achieving "Champion" status.

> Hip dysplasia is largely an inherited defect appearing first during the time of rapid growth (4-9 months).

197

Treatment of hip dysplasia

Feeding

Feeding of the young growing dog is a strong influence on whether a potentially dysplastic hip joint matures into a normal or abnormal joint. The pup that is on a high calorie diet and is rapidly increasing in size and weight is far more likely to develop dysplasia than his littermate (of the same breeding) who is brought up more slowly and who does not carry excess weight during development.

Surgery

Once hip dysplasia is evident and is causing pain or lack of use of the legs there are several surgical procedures which may help. These are:

• Removing the pectineus muscle (Fig. 15:13). In some cases this seems to allow the ball of the femur to sit better in the socket of the pelvis.

• Removal of the ball of the femur. By removing the part of the femur which fits into the hip socket, the leg is left without a bony connection to the trunk. This immediately relieves pain. What then holds the leg? Hip muscles contract to firmly hold the leg in position, and a "false" joint is formed.

Dogs that have had the hip joint removed usually recover to walk normally. The results are better in small breeds but good results have been obtained in dogs as large as Great Danes.

• Remodelling the pelvis (technically, a difficult operation) by changing the architecture of the pelvis to give better seating of the joint.

• Artificial hips: In human medicine, total hip replacement with an artificial hip (or "prosthesis") has become a standard and highly successful procedure. Although possible in dogs, the results are variable. It is also an expensive undertaking.

15.13 *Hip dysplasia surgery*

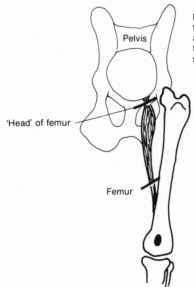

Pelvis

'Head' of femur

Femur

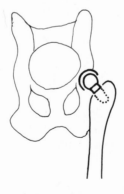

Pectineus removal. Remove the pectineus muscle to allow the head of the femur to sit deeper in the hip socket

Artificial hip. An artificial hip joint is a technique used frequently in man. It is feasible in dogs, but expensive.

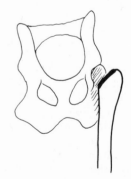

Removal of the ball of the femur. A "salvage" operation is to remove the ball-shaped head of the femur. The dog forms a false joint and usually copes well with good function in the leg

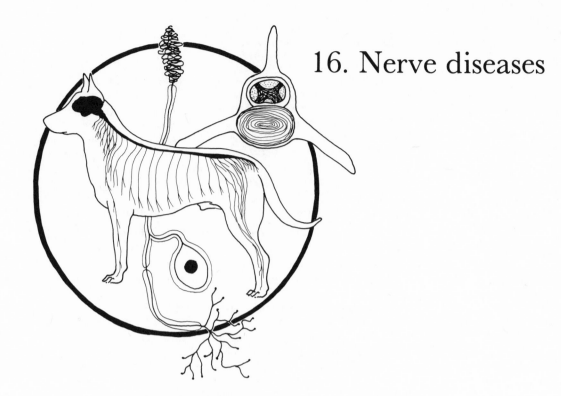

16. Nerve diseases

SPINAL INJURY

Nerve cells are highly specialized units; but the costs of specialization are high and one of the penalties that nerve cells have paid is that they lack the ability to heal: once injured beyond a certain degree, damage is permanent.

When spinal cord damage is suspected take great care to avoid further damage, such as could occur if the patient is handled roughly.

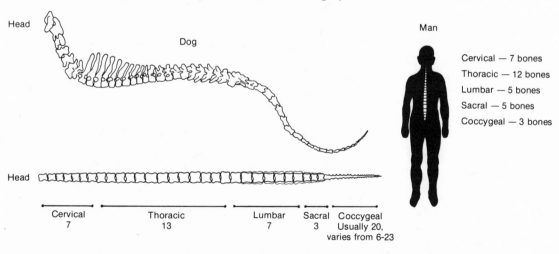

Head

Dog

Man

Cervical — 7 bones
Thoracic — 12 bones
Lumbar — 5 bones
Sacral — 5 bones
Coccygeal — 3 bones

Head

| Cervical 7 | Thoracic 13 | Lumbar 7 | Sacral 3 | Coccygeal Usually 20, varies from 6-23 |

*, **, *** indicate increasing likelihood of a particular trait or problem occurring.

16.2 *The spine*

199

Why spinal injury is so severe

The brain is the central control "computer" of the body and is linked to all parts by an intricate communications network of nerves. The main "cable" of nerves is called the spinal cord and all the nerve pathways in the body, except the nerves of the head, run for some part of their journey through the spinal cord. Any damage to the spinal cord can affect large sections of the body, as, once the spinal cord is cut, messages no longer get through. In this way, the dog can lose control, not only of the limbs, but of other organs such as the bladder and the gut and even the ability to breathe, depending on where the cord is injured.

Signs of spinal injury may include some of the following:

- If mild to moderate—pain or altered (usually increased) sensitivity to pain (hyperesthesia).
- Paralysis of limbs or weakness (paresis) of same.
- Loss of sensation (seen as no response to painful stimulus such as pinching the toes).
- Excessive arching backwards of the neck.
- Stiff forelegs.
- Loss of control of the bladder (urine flows out constantly in some cases or is involuntarily retained in others).
- Loss of control of the anus (feces run out) or the opposite (constipation).
- Lack of response (e.g., to being called by name).
- If the neck is damaged there is extreme pain on moving the head.

Causes of spinal damage

- Usually injury (e.g., car accident), kick (e.g., by horse), or a fall from a high place (e.g., roof).
- Disc disease (see later).
- Cancer of the spine.
- Some infectious diseases.

The bony spine (or vertebral column) contains a tunnel through which the spinal cord (which is made up of billions upon billions of nerve pathways) runs (Fig. 16:3).

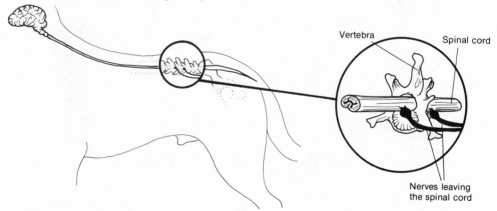

Vertebra

Spinal cord

Nerves leaving the spinal cord

16.3 *The Spinal Cord*

If pressure is put on the spinal cord, for example, when a diseased disc bursts, or due to a tumor, or if the spine is broken, then the delicate nerves that comprise the cord may be crushed against the hard and unyielding roof of this bone tunnel.

If the pressure is great enough damage is permanent. If the dog's spine is broken, the spinal cord may be severed, and this may be fatal especially if the cord is severed in the neck.

Treatment of spinal cord damage

Urgent treatment is essential and is aimed at reducing the pressure on the spinal cord. The outlook is poor if the neck or middle of the back is injured.

What to do if you suspect your dog has a spinal injury

• Muzzle him if he is attempting to bite, otherwise you may drop him as you try to avoid being bitten.

• Find a hard, firm surface to carry him on. A door or pet stretcher are ideal. A blanket has too much sag but will do in an emergency.

> Any dog with suspected spinal injury must be moved with extreme care to avoid further damage.

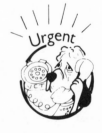

In the absence of such aids, your aim is to move the spine as little as you can. Carry the dog stretched out and do not bend his back or neck.

Get to a vet as soon as possible without bouncing the injured dog around—do not drive at breakneck speed or more damage may be done.

Treatment commenced less than 4 hours after the injury gives the best chance of recovery. Treatment commenced more than 24 hours after serious injury has very much less chance of success.

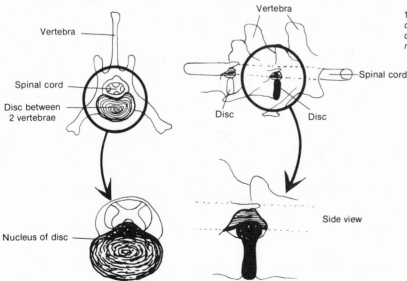

Vertebra

Vertebra

Spinal cord

Spinal cord

Disc between 2 vertebrae

Disc

Disc

Nucleus of disc

Side view

16.4 *Disc rupture: when the disc ruptures the spinal cord is compressed hard against the roof of the spinal cord*

DISC DISEASE

Between each of the vertebrae is a shock absorber called a "disc" (Fig. 16.4). This shock absorber absorbs the pressures when the dog bends, runs or jumps, and allows movement of what would otherwise be a rigid spinal column.

Breeds susceptible

The breeds more susceptible to disc disease include Dachshunds***, Pekingese*, Cocker Spaniels*, Miniature* and Toy* Poodles, Beagles* and Corgis**.

Causes of disc disease

The discs between the vertebrae degenerate with age. In some breeds the degeneration starts very early—even from a few months of age.

The central part (or nucleus) of a diseased disc can suddenly rupture and put pressure on the spinal cord, thus jamming the nerves against the roof of the bone tunnel through which the spinal cord runs (Fig. 16:4). The ruptured nucleus causes extreme irritation and marked inflammation occurs where disc material has extruded. Inflammation greatly increases the pressure on the spinal cord. Depending on the amount of pressure, the dog experiences pain, weakness, loss of sensation and in severe cases, paralysis.

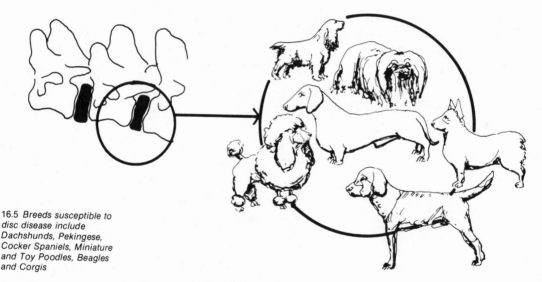

16.5 *Breeds susceptible to disc disease include Dachshunds, Pekingese, Cocker Spaniels, Miniature and Toy Poodles, Beagles and Corgis*

Treatment of disc rupture

The idea that a "slipped disc" can be pushed back into place is not true. The disc has burst and cannot be manipulated back.

Things the vet can do:

● Relieve the pressure that results from the inflammatory reaction that follows rupture of the disc. This is achieved usually by resting the dog, plus using cortisone and other drugs such as mannitol to reduce pressure within the spinal canal.

• Surgery (called disc fenestration) to remove the disc material.

• Surgery to remove the roof of the spinal canal, therefore releasing the pressure on the spinal cord. This surgery must be undertaken within 24 hours of disc rupture for the best chances of success.

> Confine your dog if you suspect a bad back.
> Do not let him jump!

RADIAL PARALYSIS

Paralysis of the radial nerve of the front leg results from hard knocks, such as occurs in car accidents or falls. The dog will drag the affected limb along the ground and if not protected, sores and ulcers will develop which lead to infection.

If the nerve is severely damaged, the paralysis may be permanent; and in this case, owners must consider having the now useless leg amputated.

In many cases, the nerve is only bruised and function slowly returns after a few days, although it may take up to six weeks.

FITS, SEIZURES, CONVULSIONS, EPILEPSY

The most frequent signs of a fit, seizure or convulsion are:
- Loss of consciousness.
- Stiffness of the body or rigidity, then intermittent stiffness.
- Slobbering (salivation).
- "Paddling" with the legs.

Most seizures take from ½ to 5 minutes from start to finish. Recovery may occur a few seconds to many minutes from the first onset of signs. The dog is usually "not quite with it" (disorientated) for a few minutes after recovery.

Causes of fits and seizures

The brain controls the entire body via electrical impulses transmitted through the nerves. A seizure is caused by a "burst" of electrical energy within the brain, similar to the violent discharge of energy seen as lightning during thunderstorms.

This electrical "storm" occurs within the brain when an irritation such as a blood clot, an old scar, or an acute inflammation due to poison or infection causes a build-up of electrical charge or potential. The electrical potential builds up to a peak, then violently discharges itself and this is expressed as a "seizure." The actual pattern of the seizure depends on which part of the brain is involved and on how big an area is affected.

The irritations which could lead to seizures include:
- Blow to the head.
- Scars forming following injury.
- Inflammation within the brain (encephalitis).
- Tumors.
- Malformation (e.g., hydrocephalus in Chihuahuas).

• Poisoning (e.g. strychnine, lead, organophosphates).
• "Worm fits"—associated with heavy worm infestation in puppies.
• Epilepsy.
• Milk fever (hypocalcemia in nursing bitches).
• Low blood glucose, e.g., in diabetes.
• Constipation.

The treatment of seizures

First eliminate the cause if possible, for example, give calcium in milk fever.

Drugs are available which reduce the build-up of the electrical "storms" within the brain. The most commonly used are phenytoin sodium (Dilantin), phenobarbital (phenobarb) and primidone (Mysoline).

Epilepsy is defined as a state in which *repeated* seizures occur. The interval between seizures may be only minutes, but is usually hours or days and may be several months. Epileptic attacks may start to occur some weeks or (usually) months after a blow to the head, such as might occur in a car accident. This is due to scar tissue contracting and producing a source of irritation within the brain.

Many epileptic attacks are classified as idiopathic epilepsy, which means the condition is of unknown cause.

Treatment of epileptic dogs is frequently very rewarding, but you will need a close liaison with your vet to find the correct drugs and most suitable dose rate.

> Once seizures are controlled with regular medication an epileptic dog can usually live a normal life.

Scottie cramp

Scottie cramp is a recessively inherited condition (see p.47). Signs include rigidity of legs, back and tail in Scottish Terriers. These episodes are due to nerve disease, not muscle disease, and are usually of short duration. The signs usually first appear when the pup is 6 months old or when exercise on the leash is begun. The dog may hop on one leg then the other in trying to relieve the spasm. Drug therapy usually relieves Scottie cramp and the dog enjoys a normal life expectancy.

Coon Hound paralysis (seen in the USA.)

The cause is unknown, but is probably due to a virus. It is contracted by some dogs which hunt raccoons.

Signs start with weakness of the hind legs, but gradually all four limbs are affected and the dog is unable to stand. The peak of the disease is usually around the tenth day. While there is no specific treatment, many dogs will recover.

Tick paralysis

In some areas ticks affect dogs by causing paralysis, or by transmitting diseases such as Rocky Mountain Fever. The female tick swells up to the size of a large pea after feeding (see p.24).

Cause
Some species of tick contain a poison within their salivary glands that causes paralysis. When the tick bites the dog some of this poison is injected into the dog.

Signs of tick paralysis
You usually see a weakness in the hind quarters gradually becoming a paralysis which spreads up to the forelegs. A change in bark may also be noticed. Death can occur due to breathing failure if treatment is not commenced in time.

> If you are entering a tick-infested area, examine your dog daily and use a tick wash regularly.

Treatment of tick paralysis
First kill the tick by applying alcohol or gin, or finger nail polish remover directly on the tick with the tip of a pencil. After a few minutes grasp the dead tick as close to the skin as possible and pull until the tick lets go. *Do not squeeze* the tick as you may inject more poison into the dog. You may lever the tick out with scissors like using a claw hammer to remove a nail. Tick anti-serum is available if paralysis has commenced, and is very effective in neutralising the poison. Get your dog to a vet quickly if he cannot stand properly.

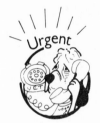

> Ticks must be removed carefully to avoid squeezing more poison from the ticks' salivary glands into the dog's system.

Prevention of tick paralysis
Examine your dog daily for ticks. Look under the ears, collar, tail and between the toes. Ticks like cover.

Ticks can attach themselves to all other animals and also humans, so check all children carefully.

> When travelling with your dog, find out whether you will enter tick-infested country. If so, use protective washes, powders or collars and check the dog daily.

Insecticides
Flea washes such as 4% Malathion and 1 per cent Ectoral can be used. Powders are also effective and flea collars assist control of ticks, but there is no substitute for a thorough daily check.

WOBBLERS

"Wobblers" is the name given to dogs suffering from a disorder of the neck vertebrae. An instability of these vertebrae results in compression of the spinal cord of the neck.

The most usual sign is inco-ordination of the hind quarters: the dog will appear to stumble or walk crabwise for a few steps. In more severe cases all four limbs may be affected.

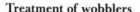

The large breeds are more commonly affected, especially Dobermans** and Great Danes**. Young, fast-growing dogs are at a greater risk than a pup raised at a slower rate of growth.

The cause of the looseness of the vertebrae is not certain, but overfeeding, injury and hereditary factors have been implicated.

Treatment of wobblers

Surgery is necessary in severe cases to reduce the laxity between the neck vertebrae. Surgery is sophisticated and can be expensive.

"WEAK MUSCLE" DISEASE—myasthenia gravis

Signs of this disease are a generalized weakness that is aggravated by exercise. This condition is not common in dogs, although it is now being recognized more often. It is well known in man.

SOME OTHER INHERITED NERVOUS DISEASES OF DOGS

German Short-haired Pointers* may inherit a nervous disease which causes an inability to learn at 6 months of age and later progresses to weakness, blindness, deafness and convulsions.

Cairn Terriers* and West Highland White Terriers* may inherit an enzyme deficiency which causes paralysis and loss of vision at a few weeks to a few months of age.

English Setters* may inherit a disease which shows up at about 12-15 months of age in which reduced vision, dullness, aggression, weakness and muscle spasms and fits may develop.

Irish Setters* are affected by a different disease causing an inability to stand or walk in young puppies, uncontrolled movement, seizures and blindness.

Swedish Laphund* puppies at 5-7 weeks of age can be affected by a progressive weakness which is inherited as an autosomal recessive (see p. 48).

Miniature Poodles* at the age of 9 weeks to 5 months can be affected by a disease of the brain in which not enough nerve covering or myelin is produced.

German Shepherds at about 9 or 10 years can be affected by a degeneration of the spine. Hind leg weakness is noted. Cortisone and other pain-relieving drugs may assist to relieve the condition but do not cure.

> If you breed a litter in which some pups grow weak, become dull, then beware: it may be an inherited condition.

17. Fashion and disease

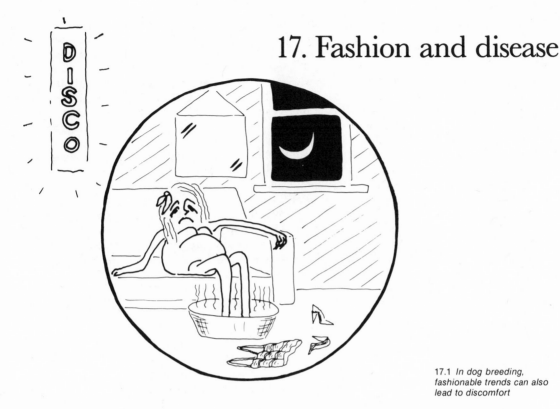

17.1 *In dog breeding, fashionable trends can also lead to discomfort*

The Bulldog was developed when man incorrectly thought that if a dog had a short snout he could hang on grimly to his quarry and still be able to breathe. There was a price to pay for this adaptation—the Bulldog could not smell as well and his teeth were crowded together, leaving him prone to gum disease, tooth infections and skin disease in the folds of his face. Some Bulldogs developed overlong soft palates and as a result simply could not breathe properly at all.

The Bulldog is only one casualty of man's capacity to breed dogs according to his whims. Sometimes the aim was to produce a breed for a specific

17.2 *Breeding away from origins: fashionable breeding* **programs have** *accentuated features such as short noses, excessive facial folds and short, crooked legs*

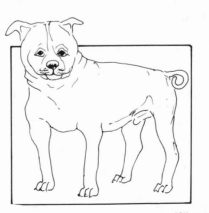

Short nose

Folds

20th century Bulldog

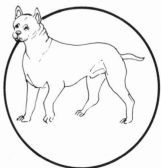

18th century Bulldog

objective but usually it was merely to suit the fashions of the time. Frequently these fashionable whims have cost the dog dearly in other ways. Breeders, in their quest for less important qualities such as coat color, have lost sight of an overall good, healthy dog.

In contrast, over the centuries, nature has selectively eliminated any traits in dogs that interfered with their vigor and ability to survive. Man has not followed nature's example. In only a few hundred years, and especially in the last fifty years, we have managed not only to reverse nature's selection, but in some breeds we now have some inherited defects accepted as normal for the breed. We have reached the stage where a dog with faulty conformation is thought to be desirable!

Breeding for fashion can cause discomfort. When the shape of the head is altered, the setting of the eyes is affected and eyes set poorly in the eye sockets become diseased. When the length of the back is altered, increased strain and stresses are put on the spine and limbs.

When the ears are long and floppy, the ears are adversely affected. All these fashionable changes have resulted in increased discomfort to the dog.

The influence of fashion is shown in this chart:

Dog and bitch are mated
▼
When female egg is fertilized a spontaneous change
in the genetic make-up of progeny may occur
▼   ▼

Because the puppies have an appealing color or appearance, they are line bred or inbred to perpetuate this change	To avoid undesirable consequences, any change from the original type should be culled and not used for breeding
▼	▼
Inadequate culling allows undesirable traits and risky conformation to appear, e.g : • Nose is too short • Face is wrinkled • Teeth do not meet • Eyelids are loose • Legs are crooked • Joints are diseased	Select progeny to retain or return to the original conformation and type
▼	▼
Continued line-breeding/ inbreeding for fashionable traits breeds many dogs with risky conformation	The original type of dog, free from disease, is maintained
▼	
These traits become so common that they are accepted as "normal" for the breed and the original type has been lost due to influence of fashion	

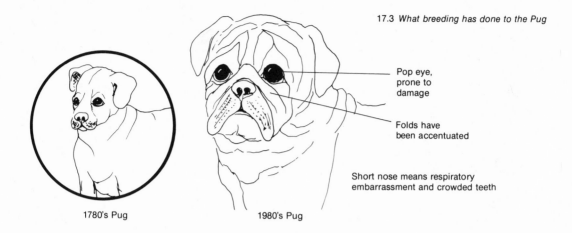

17.3 *What breeding has done to the Pug*

Pop eye, prone to damage

Folds have been accentuated

Short nose means respiratory embarrassment and crowded teeth

1780's Pug

1980's Pug

Below is a list of some of the risky conformations which occur in dogs called "normal" by today's standards, i.e., they comply with current breed standards for the show ring.

> Any breed standard which leads to disease or discomfort should be modified.

In this breed	this conformation	leads to:
Afghans	Unpigmented third eyelid.	Inflammation from the sun.
Australian Silky Terriers	Long hair on forehead (topknot); long hair on the skin of the eyelids; hair over the eyes.	Loose hair on the eyeball, eye irritation.
Basset	Long floppy ears.	Ear canal blocked off, poor ventilation leads to infection.
	Folds of skin on forehead/face.	Excess skin folds allow eyelids to irritate the eye. Excessive forehead skin allows upper lids to droop over eye and obstruct vision.
	Sagging lower eyelids.	Eye inflammation.
	Short legs.	Arthritis and nail conditions.
Bloodhound	Folds of skin on forehead/face.	Eyelids irritate the eye. Excessive forehead skin allows upper lids to droop over eye and obstruct vision.
	Sagging lower eyelids.	Eye inflammation.
	Long floppy ears.	Ear canal blocked off, poor ventilation leads to infection.

17.4 *What breeding has done to the Bloodhound: excessive folds of facial skin are far more apparent with the head lowered*

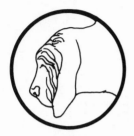

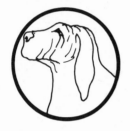

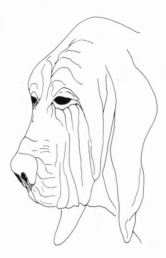

20th century Bloodhound

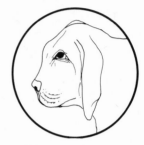

17th century Bloodhound did not have many folds in facial skin

In this breed	this conformation	leads to:
Border Collies	Unpigmented third eyelid.	Inflammation from the sun.
Boston Terrier	Prominent (pop) eye. Poor bony protection of the eye.	Eyes more prone to disease. Eye is easily dislocated out of its socket.
Boxer	Short nose.	Difficult breathing. Upper jaw too short for lower jaw, crowded mouth. Dental disease.
Bull Terriers	Unpigmented third eyelid. Deep set eyes.	Inflammation from the sun. Eyes collect matter, become irritated.
Chihuahua	No bony protection of eyeball; pop eyes.	Eye injury; eyes more prone to disease.
Cocker Spaniel	Fold below lower lip. Long hair on the ears.	Skin infection. Grass seeds collect in long hair. Ungroomed ears are heavy and block off the ear canal; poor ventilation causes ear infection.
	Extra long eyelashes. Folds of skin on forehead.	Eye irritation. Excess folds allow eyelids to irritate the eye. Excessive forehead skin allows upper lids to droop over eye and obstruct vision.

In this breed	this conformation	leads to:
Corgis	Unpigmented third eyelid. Long back.	Inflammation from the sun. Disc disease of the spine.
Doberman	Deep-set eyes.	Eyes collect matter, become irritated.
English (British) Bulldog	Short nose.	Difficult breathing; crowded mouth; upper jaw too short for lower jaw; dental disease; eye irritation.
	Screw tail.	Skin infection under tail.
German Shepherds	Unpigmented third eyelid.	Inflammation from the sun.
Greyhounds	Unpigmented third eyelid.	Inflammation from the sun.
Lhaso Apso	Prominent (pop) eye. Poor bony protection of the eye. Short nose.	Eyes more prone to disease. Eye is easily dislocated out of its socket. Difficult breathing.
Maltese	Long hair on forehead (topknot); long hair on the skin of the eyelids; hair over the eyes.	Loose hair on the eyeball, eye irritation.
Miniature, Toy Poodle	Hairy ear canal. Hairy eyelids (long hair on the skin of the eyelids*).	Poor ventilation of the ear leads to ear infection. Eye irritation, disease.
Old English Sheepdogs	Unpigmented third eyelid. Long hair on forehead (topknot); long hair on the skin of the eyelids; hair over the eyes.	Inflammation from the sun. Loose hair on the eyeball, less vision, eye irritation. (If topknot hair is allowed to cord, these effects are avoided.)
Pekingese	Prominent (pop) eye. Poor bony protection of the eye. Short nose.	Eyes more prone to disease. Eye is easily dislocated out of its socket. Difficult breathing. Upper jaw too short for lower jaw, crowded mouth. Dental disease, eye irritation.
Pug	Prominent (pop) eye. Poor bony protection of the eye. Short nose.	Eyes more prone to disease. Eye is easily dislocated out of its socket. Difficult breathing. Upper jaw too short for lower jaw, crowded mouth. Dental disease, eye irritation.

*We are not referring here to a disease in which extra eyelashes are present on the eyelid margin.

In this breed	this conformation	leads to:
Scotch (Rough) Collie	Deep-set eyes.	Eyes collect matter, become irritated.
Scottish Terrier Welsh Terrier	Hairy ear canal.	Poor ventilation of the ear leads to ear infection.
	Hairy eyelids (long hair on the skin of the eyelids*).	Eye irritation, disease.
Shar Pei	Wrinkled face.	Eyelids irritate the eye.
Shetland Sheepdog (Sheltie)	Small deep-set eyes.	Eyes collect matter, become irritated.
	Elongated upper jaw.	Poor "bite" leads to dental problems.

17.5 *What breeding has done to the Shetland Sheepdog: by elongating the upper jaw and nose, the seating of the eye has deteriorated*

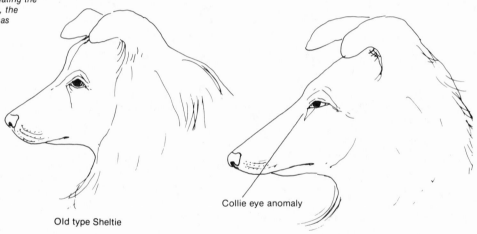

Old type Sheltie

Collie eye anomaly

1980's Sheltie

Shih Tzu	Prominent (pop) eye. Poor bony protection of the eye. Short nose.	Eyes more prone to disease. Eye is easily dislocated out of its socket. Difficult breathing. Upper jaw too short for lower jaw, crowded mouth. Dental disease.
St Bernard	Folds of skin on forehead/face.	Eyelids irritate the eye. Excessive forehead skin allows upper lids to droop over eye and obstruct vision.
	Sagging lower eyelids.	Eye inflammation.

*We are not referring here to a disease in which extra eyelashes are present on the eyelid margin.

In this breed	this conformation	leads to:
White-coated breeds	Decreased pigment in the coat, skin, ears.	Sun irritation, sunburn.
	Blue eyes	Poor tolerance of bright light, some parts inside the eyeball may be defective.

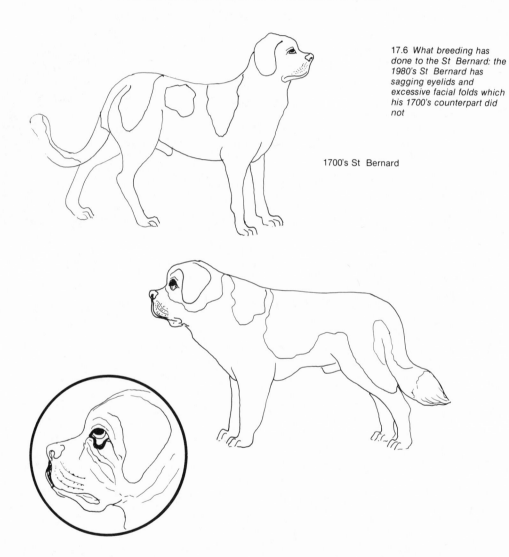

17.6 *What breeding has done to the St Bernard: the 1980's St Bernard has sagging eyelids and excessive facial folds which his 1700's counterpart did not*

1700's St Bernard

18. Mating, pregnancy and breeding

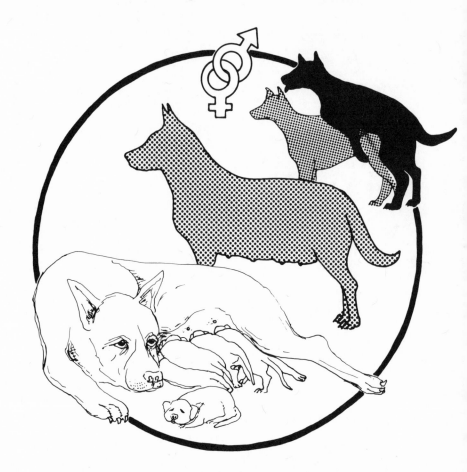

NEUTERING (DESEXING OR SPAYING)

What is meant by spaying?

Spaying is the term applied to the operation in which the ovaries and uterus are removed from the female dog (bitch). (Note the verb is spay and the operation is called a spay.) The spay operation is described later in this chapter.

The object of spaying is to stop the bitch from coming 'on heat' (see later) and from reproducing.

Should your female be spayed?

There are four main advantages in having your bitch spayed:

• Avoids bitch coming in to heat twice a year with the accompanying messy discharges and invasion by all the neighborhood dogs who can smell a bitch in season from literally miles away. Dogs are extremely persevering in their attempts to mate and to gain access to any bitch in heat ("in season").

persevering in their attempts to mate and to gain access to any bitch on heat ('in season').

• Avoids unwanted pups.

• Almost eliminates any chance of breast cancer (if spayed before 2 years of age).

• Helps keep the huge number of unwanted dogs down. Population control in our pets is a very real and serious problem.

Should my bitch have a litter before being spayed?

No. Well-meaning people may tell you that your bitch should have a litter of puppies or at least a "heat period" before she is spayed. There is no evidence to support this view.

At what age should she be spayed?

Your vet may have his own view but we believe 6 months is best.

The operation: what happens

The operation, termed a spay or an ovariohysterectomy (meaning the ovaries and part of the womb are removed) is performed while the dog is deeply asleep under a general anesthetic. She will feel nothing.

The surgeon sterilizes the instruments and prepares the skin before opening the abdomen, thereby minimizing the chance of bacteria entering. Some surgeons will open on the flank, others enter the abdomen near the belly button (Fig. 18:3).

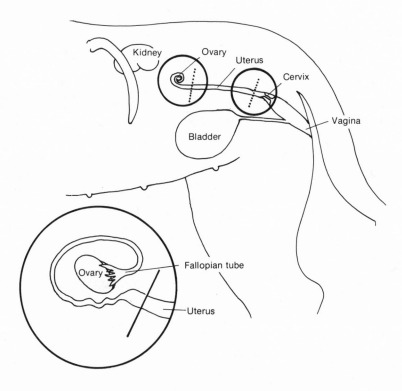

18.2 *Spaying (neutering) the bitch: in the "spay" operation, usually the entire genital tract, comprising the uterus and both ovaries, is removed*

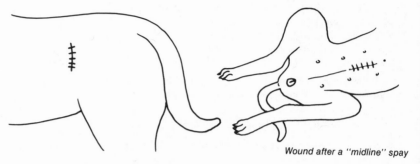

18.3 *Wound after a "flank" spay*

Wound after a "midline" spay

Both ovaries and the uterus are removed. The abdomen is closed using suture material that "dissolves" or is absorbed by the body in other ways.

The skin may be sutured with stitches that have to be removed (in 7-10 days) or dissolving sutures may be used.

How long after the operation before the patient is herself again?

It does not take long. After 3 days she is usually back to normal.

What precautions do I take after surgery?

Do not allow your bitch to jump or exercise vigorously until the stitches are removed. There should be no games or forced exercise for the first week.

Will she come on heat again?

No.

Will she become fat?

Not necessarily, although some bitches have a tendency to put on weight. Diet control will prevent excess weight gain.

Overweight after spaying is due to overfeeding and
lack of exercise.

MALE DOGS: NEUTERING, CASTRATION OR DESEXING

In this operation, which is performed under general anesthetic, both testicles are removed, removing the source of sperm and male sex hormone (testosterone).

Why should I consider castrating my dog?

There are many advantages:
- Usually the dog becomes less aggressive and more placid.
- The dog is less likely to wander and chase bitches on heat.
- Many councils charge more for entire (or not desexed) males.
- Neutering your dog helps the overall aim of reducing the number of unwanted pups.
- Desexing prevents tumors of the testicles.
- Desexing decreases problems occurring in the prostate gland, perineal hernias, hepatoid adenomas (tumours).

Disadvantages of castration

The dog can become overweight *if* the owner overfeeds him.

Will castration change my dog's nature?

There is no great character change, although the dog is quieter. A good watchdog will still be a good watchdog, barking at strangers. Ability to guard your territory is not altered.

Will it cure him of viciousness, biting, etc.?

Maybe. It depends on the dog and the nature of his aggression. If it is due to sex urges the chances are good that he will bite less after castration. If he is aggressive while "guarding" his territory then he will usually keep on doing so. (Talk with your vet if you have this sort of a problem.)

Note that the dog's libido remains the same for up to two months after the operation. The change is not immediate and he will still wander about and mount bitches at first.

HEAT AND CONTRACEPTION

What is meant by a bitch "in heat"?

Twice a year most bitches become fertile. Their ovaries produce a crop of eggs which may be fertilized and pups conceived if she is mated at the correct time. Accompanying this egg production is a distinct change in the bitch's behavior due to hormones produced by her ovaries and she becomes extremely attractive to the male dog.

The period during which she remains attractive to the male dog is termed "heat" or "season."

When do bitches first come into heat?

Usually between 6 and 12 months of age, and most commonly around 8 months. Some of the larger breeds do not come into heat until 12-14 months. Other factors can influence first heats—for example, many greyhound bitches do not start to come into heat until after they have finished their racing career.

How often do bitches come into heat?

Most bitches come into season every six months. Heat lasts for about 18-21 days but there is wide variation, ranging from 14-28 days. Some breeds, such as the Basenji and Samoyed, cycle only once a year.

Will the bitch in season mate with more than one dog?

Yes—several males can each sire part of the same litter by mating with the bitch during the one heat period.

How do I prevent unwanted matings?

When your female is in heat you should keep her confined for the entire three weeks or so. If your yard is not dog proof and you cannot keep her inside the house, it may be necessary to send her to a kennel for the duration. Any exercise should be done on a leash or in isolation. Do not let her urinate on your front garden.

217

MATING, PREGNANCY AND BIRTH

Breeding

Should my bitch have pups?

The female does *not* need to have a litter to become physically or psychologically fulfilled. The choice to breed your female should be taken only after due consideration of the time, effort and expense. The world already may have too many dogs. Haphazard and irresponsible breeding is to be discouraged.

In favor of breeding your bitch is the great enjoyment and pleasure you can gain from the experience, plus the educational value for children—not only in sex and reproduction but as a lesson in care and responsibility.

The sexual cycle of the bitch

"Heat" or "season" is the time during which the bitch's reproductive system becomes active. The ovaries produce hormones, with changes in the bitch's behavior.

The stages of heat and when to mate

	Estrus cycle of the bitch				
	Duration of Stage	**Proestrus**	**Estrus**	**Metestrus**	**Anestrus**
Average	9 days	9 days		30 days	4 months
Range	2-27 days	3-21 days		up to 90 days	2-8 months

18.4 *Sexual cycle (the figures are a guide only and vary from bitch to bitch)*

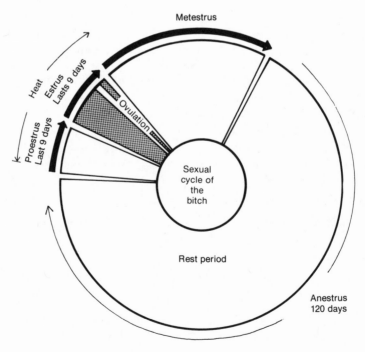

The first stage of heat *(Proestrus)*

The ovaries produce hormones (estrogens) that stimulate the womb (uterus), which swells and produces a lining ready for pregnancy. There is a noticeable discharge of a blood-stained fluid from the female passage (vulva), and the vulva swells, enlarges and becomes firm. It drops further down between the bitch's hind legs.

The bitch becomes attractive to males and more interested in their company, but will not yet accept the male for mating. If mating is attempted she will sit down and growl or snap at the male.

The second phase *(Estrus or "standing heat")*

At this stage the bitch is ready to mate. The eggs are ready for release from the ovary and fertilization. The bitch will accept the male and may actively seek out males. She will raise her tail to one side. The discharge from the vulva is straw colored and clear of blood spots.

It is only during this stage that conception and pregnancy can occur. Standing heat lasts from 6-12 days.

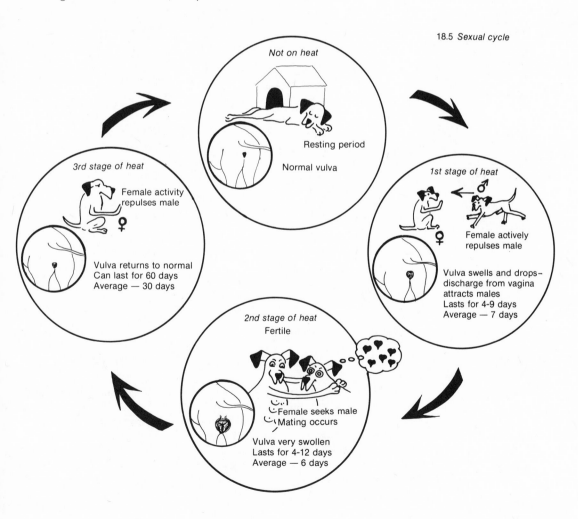

18.5 *Sexual cycle*

Not on heat

Resting period

Normal vulva

3rd stage of heat

Female activity repulses male

Vulva returns to normal
Can last for 60 days
Average — 30 days

1st stage of heat

Female actively repulses male

Vulva swells and drops–
discharge from vagina
attracts males
Lasts for 4-9 days
Average — 7 days

2nd stage of heat
Fertile

Female seeks male
Mating occurs

Vulva very swollen
Lasts for 4-12 days
Average — 6 days

219

The third phase *(Metestrus)*

There are now two states into which the bitch may enter. If mating has been successful, pregnancy commences. Otherwise she enters the phase of 'metoestrus'.

The start of metestrus is signalled when the bitch refuses to stand for the male. After a few days of metestrus she will no longer be attractive to males. The vulva gradually loses its swollen appearance and returns to its previous size. Note that the vulva of a bitch that has been on heat is always slightly larger than that of an immature bitch.

Metestrus lasts through the period of uterine shrinkage, and is followed by the period of sexual "rest."

The fourth phase *(Anestrus)*

This is the period of sexual rest or inactivity within the reproductive system. It lasts from 4-6 months in most cases.

18.6 Egg cycle: this chart shows how follicles develop in the ovary then burst to release the eggs. These eggs take about three more days to become ready for fertilization by sperm. Sperm from matings up to 8 days prior to this date can still be capable of fertilizing the eggs, although fresher sperm has a better chance.
The timing of fertilization is most accurately determined only by hindsight: 3 days before the vaginal discharge changes colour from a red color to a "straw" color. Determining the best time for breeding is a mixture of art and science, although if left to their own devices, dogs usually do pretty well

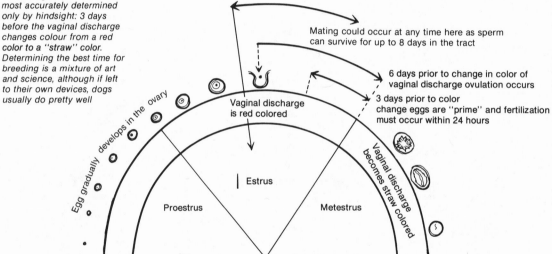

Mating could occur at any time here as sperm can survive for up to 8 days in the tract

6 days prior to change in color of vaginal discharge ovulation occurs

3 days prior to color change eggs are "prime" and fertilization must occur within 24 hours

Egg gradually develops in the ovary

Vaginal discharge is red colored

Vaginal discharge becomes straw colored

Estrus

Proestrus

Metestrus

When to mate

The actual time to mate varies with the individual bitch. Usually the tenth and twelfth days are chosen (but some may not be right until the fifteenth or even eighteenth day) and some are ready earlier, so the only way to be certain is to have a vaginal smear examined by the vet to determine precisely the stage of heat.

The behavior of the bitch tells us when to mate her: when she is showing great interest in the male, acting coyly, showing her vulva by lifting her tail to one side, and if the discharge from the vulva is a pale, straw color. The behavior of an experienced stud dog is often an accurate guide.

Because of the great variation in the day of highest fertility—some dogs have mated successfully as early as the fourth day, others as late as the nineteenth or twentieth day—it is advisable to get veterinary advice if you are having difficulty in finding the correct days for your bitch to mate.

SEXUAL INTERCOURSE

The act of sexual intercourse in the dog is different from human beings in several ways, the most remarkable being the "tie."

During intercourse, the dog mounts the bitch and inserts his penis into her vagina. After intromission, a gland at the base of the dog's penis swells to four or five times its original size, making the penis now much larger than the vulva's opening. The dog is unable to pull his penis out. Simultaneously, two muscles in the bitch's vagina constrict over the penis and hold the penis within the vagina so that the two animals are locked together in a union called the "tie." The tie may last only a few minutes but can last over 40 minutes.

Once the tie is formed, the male dog will usually throw one leg over the female and turn to face in the opposite direction—still locked together. It is thought that the stance evolved in the wild where dogs in a "tie" were more vulnerable to attack. Dangers were reduced by standing with a set of fangs facing in each direction.

Why do dogs form a tie?

The function of the tie is not certain. One theory is that it prevents loss of semen, and allows plenty of time for the seminal fluids to enter into the female genital tract. This theory seems reasonable, but why is such a method not important in other species?

What to do when dogs form a tie?

A tie is a natural and normal part of mating in the dog. Do nothing—simply leave the two alone and they will separate naturally, even if this takes 30-40 minutes. Watch that the bitch does not try to lie down or pull away if she is excitable or anxious.

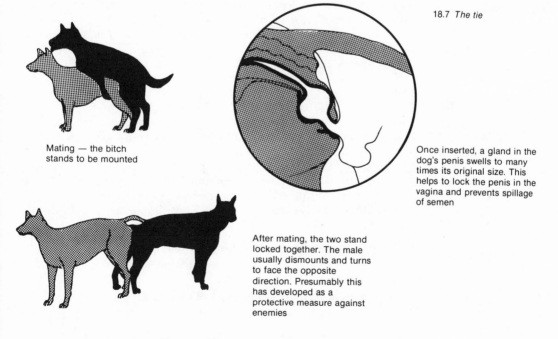

18.7 *The tie*

Mating — the bitch stands to be mounted

Once inserted, a gland in the dog's penis swells to many times its original size. This helps to lock the penis in the vagina and prevents spillage of semen

After mating, the two stand locked together. The male usually dismounts and turns to face the opposite direction. Presumably this has developed as a protective measure against enemies

RELUCTANCE TO MATE

Male reluctance

The male may be unsettled if he is brought to a strange area or another dog's "territory" and this may result in his refusal to mate. For this reason it is often the bitch that is taken to the stud male to mate.

Some males may have been discouraged by their owners from showing sexual advances towards other dogs or people, and associate attempted mounting with punishment and are therefore reluctant to mate.

Reluctant males can often be helped to overcome this initial reluctance if let run with an experienced bitch on heat known to be easy to mate with, who will not bite or snap at the male.

Female reluctance

The most common cause of sexual reluctance in the female is trying to breed at the wrong time of the heat cycle. Many bitches show signs during proestrus that can confuse some owners into thinking that their bitch is ready to mate. The bitch may even accept being mounted, but refuse any penetration. Patience is required—wait until the bitch comes fully into estrus (standing heat).

Some bitches have had little to do with other dogs and it may take some time to relieve their initial apprehension.

ARTIFICIAL INSEMINATION

Artificial insemination (AI) is the procedure in which semen is collected from the male and deposited into the genital tract of the female. AI may be necessary in some shy breeders, or where some anatomical problem exists, such as a constriction of the vulva (female passage).

Used correctly, artificial insemination should produce the same results as a natural mating. It does not spoil the bitch for future natural breeding nor does it produce any abnormalities in the pups.

AI is usually performed by a vet.

ACCIDENTAL PREGNANCY

Bitches on heat will usually mate with *any* male, and as males are often persistent and determined enough to get through, over or under all but the best security fences, accidental matings are common. If an accidental mating occurs, the pregnancy can be stopped by an injection of stilbestrol, or other drugs that prevent development of pregnancy, from your vet. It is preferable to give the injection within 24 or 48 hours of mating, although it can be successful up to a week after in some cases.

Will my bitch mate again after this injection?

Yes. She must be locked securely away from males.

A dog is mating with my bitch, can I untie them?

No. You cannot cause the dog to dismount as his penis swells inside the bitch and locks him in position. Until the swelling reduces (2 to 40 minutes), he cannot disengage.

Can a bitch become pregnant to more than one dog?

Yes. Each egg can be fertilized only once and therefore by only one father. However, as many eggs are shed in each season, those that are missed by one dog's sperm can still be fertilized by the next, so members of a litter may have different fathers.

If my pure-bred bitch is mated to a mongrel, is she spoiled for further breeding?

No. Previous matings have absolutely no effect on subsequent litters.

Can I postpone heat?

Yes. If holidays are coming up and so is your bitch's heat period, then tablets (Ovarid, Ovaban) are available to postpone the onset of heat for up to 45 days. Matenon or Cheque are drugs which, if given daily, allow heat to be postponed almost indefinitely.

CONTRACEPTION–THE AVAILABLE METHODS

The pill

Dosage is commenced on the first day of heat and continued for 8 days or so. This stops the development of heat and the bitch returns to her previous "neutral" state.

It is important to commence dosage immediately heat starts—on day one of heat; that is, at the first sign of bloody discharge or swelling of the vulva. A long acting hormone injection can also be used to prevent heat from starting. Lasts 5 to 6 months.

IUD

Intra-uterine devices, similar in action to those used in women, are available but have not found wide acceptance. They are awkward to fit and are liable to loosen and fall out.

The "morning after" injection

If mating has occurred, your vet can stop the pregnancy by an injection, for example, of the hormone stilbestrol, provided he sees the bitch within 48 hours—and preferably within 24 hours of the mating. After 48 hours it is difficult to abort a pregnant bitch.

How soon after having the pups can the bitch be spayed?

Most vets prefer to wait until the pups are weaned, which usually occurs 6 weeks after birth.

FALSE (PHANTOM) PREGNANCY

Some bitches exhibit signs of pregnancy even when they are not pregnant.

False pregnancy can occur after the bitch has been in season because a hormone called progesterone, which is produced by the ovaries, provokes many of the signs of pregnancy. The influence of the progesterone is vital in maintaining pregnancy and prepares the uterus for fertilized eggs. In cases of false pregnancy progesterone is produced by the ovaries even though its influence is *not* appropriate. In some cases, signs of false pregnancy may be confined merely to some enlargement of the breasts (mammary glands). But in other cases the signs are more dramatic. Some bitches become excitable, tremble, pant and even prepare a nest to receive the imaginary or phantom pups. She will often adopt toys or other objects and begin nursing them. If the signs are severe, false pregnancy can be treated with hormone shots or pills.

If the mammary glands become very enlarged and are causing the bitch pain or discomfort, you should try to reduce the pressure within the glands. Pressure may be relieved by milking a *small* amount of milk away from the swollen gland (do not take much or you will stimulate further milk production), or by applying a warm compress to the gland with gentle massage. If swelling or pain persists consult your vet.

FEEDING AND CARE OF THE PREGNANT BITCH

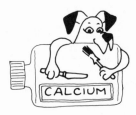

Vitamin supplements are probably not necessary but many breeders are convinced they help. A supplement of calcium is a good idea, as after the pups are born a lot of calcium is excreted in the milk. Give one teaspoon of calcium carbonate per 10 kg of body weight per day.

Many bitches lose their appetite in the last week or so of pregnancy. Don't worry unduly—although it is preferable for the bitch to eat well right up to delivery—as neither the bitch nor pups seem to suffer ill-effects from a pre-delivery fast.

Encourage moderate, regular exercise in the bitch right up to the birth of the pups. This improves muscle tone and reduces the chance of problems during birth. The lazy bitch is more liable to have difficulty delivering and may have weak or dead pups.

18.9 *Growth of pups from fertilized eggs — Cocker Spaniel*

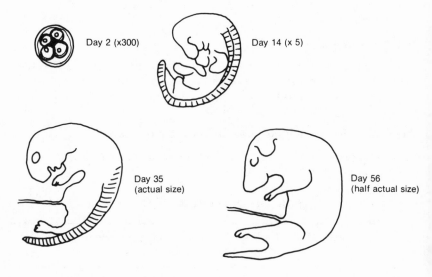

Day 2 (x300)

Day 14 (x 5)

Day 35
(actual size)

Day 56
(half actual size)

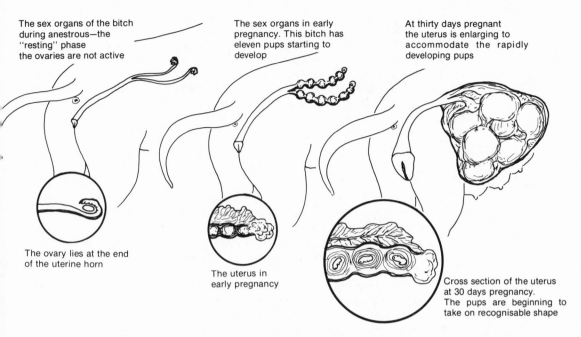

The sex organs of the bitch during anestrous—the "resting" phase the ovaries are not active

The sex organs in early pregnancy. This bitch has eleven pups starting to develop

At thirty days pregnant the uterus is enlarging to accommodate the rapidly developing pups

The ovary lies at the end of the uterine horn

The uterus in early pregnancy

Cross section of the uterus at 30 days pregnancy. The pups are beginning to take on recognisable shape

18.10 *Uterus horns*

PREPARING FOR THE BIRTH

The whelping area

Left to herself, the bitch will often find a quiet, dark, out-of-the-way area in which to have her litter. Try to get her to choose an area which is convenient for you and is dry and easily cleaned. Show her such an area well before the pups are due and supply plenty of newspaper and other bedding materials for her to make the nest.

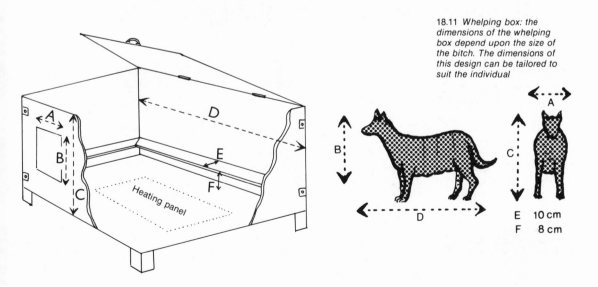

18.11 *Whelping box: the dimensions of the whelping box depend upon the size of the bitch. The dimensions of this design can be tailored to suit the individual*

Heating panel

E   10 cm
F   8 cm

Signs that birth is imminent

The bitch will usually refuse all food about 24 hours before delivery, and become restless. If she has not already done so, she will rummage in the bedding and tear up paper as she makes her nest.

The bitch's temperature usually drops about a degree centigrade (2°F) in the 12-24 hours before birth (from 38.5°-37.5°C or 101.5°-99°F).

She may start looking at her flanks; pacing; pawing at the ground and, if it is her first litter, become a bit nonplussed by it all. Sometimes she will vomit.

The birth

Most bitches are capable of giving birth with no help, although it is best if *one* person stays with her to ensure that if something goes wrong, the problem can be quickly dealt with. If the bitch is having her first litter, a little reassurance is a big help. Avoid having a crowd of people, although you may encourage children to watch after the first one or two pups are delivered.

The bitch usually lies on her side or front to give birth. Contractions of the uterus carry a pup from one of the horns of the uterus through the cervix which is now wide open and into the vagina. The water bag which surrounds the puppy bursts and fluid flows from the vulva. The membranes may appear as a dark, fluid bag bulging through the vulva but usually they break before they appear. The bag breaks (either spontaneously or due to the mother licking it) releasing a rush of straw-colored fluid. More commonly it is the head and legs of the pup that are first seen at the vulva and the pup should be delivered within a few minutes of these appearing by the bitch contracting her uterus and abdominal muscles.

Instinctively, the mother will now lick away the membranes surrounding

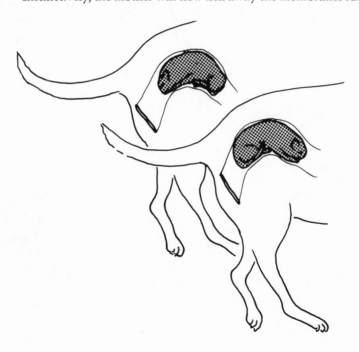

18.12 *Pups may be born head or tail first ('breech'). Both presentations are normal in the bitch*

the pup and bite the umbilical cord. She will lick the pup clean, stimulating it to breathe and sometimes to cry. Once cleaned, the pup gropes its way towards the warmth and softness of its mother's flank, nuzzles in and searches for a nipple.

The rest of the litter will appear head first and sometimes hind quarters first. Both presentations are considered normal in the dog.

There are two horns of the uterus and usually a pup is born alternately from one side and then the other.

The after-birth

Each pup has its own set of membranes (or placenta). After the birth of each pup, you should watch to see that the placenta comes either with the pup or soon after. A retained placenta can cause a serious infection within the uterus (metritis).

The bitch usually eats the placenta. This is natural and normal, although some breeders prefer to restrict the bitch to eating one or two placentas. Placenta eating can cause the bitch to vomit.

18.13 *Tying umbilical cord*

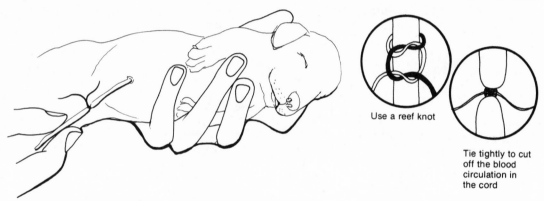

Use a reef knot

Tie tightly to cut off the blood circulation in the cord

COMPLICATIONS OF WHELPING

Bleeding umbilical cords

If the bitch cuts too cleanly instead of chewing the cord it may bleed. If so, tie the cord off with a sterile piece of thread about 6 cm from the pup's body (Fig. 18:13).

Membranes not removed by bitch

If the bitch does not lick the membranes off, or sever the umbilical cord, you must clear them from the pup's head as soon as possible to allow the pup to breathe. Then "present" the pup to the bitch to coax her into cleaning the pup. If she does not respond within a few minutes, you should:

• Tie off the cord with thread (that has been left to sterilize by soaking for 15 minutes in a disinfectant solution).

• Tie off the cord about 6 cm from the pup's body.

• Cut the cord between the membranes and the thread you have tied. Use scissors that have been sterilized (by boiling them for 20 minutes).

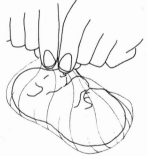

18.14 *If the bitch does not lick the membranes off then you must do it and coax the bitch into cleaning the pup*

227

Delays in pup emerging

> If the bitch has been straining for 60 minutes without any
> issue, telephone your vet.

If the pup is partly out but is not completely delivered within 2 minutes
of the head or legs emerging, you may need to help.

> When you assist delivery keep in mind that the pup is very
> delicate and easily damaged. Be gentle.

DELIVERING A PUP

• Push the lips of the vulva back and over the emerging pup. A little
pressure applied just below the bitch's anus (Fig. 18:15) will often stop the
pup from slipping back into the vagina.

18.15 *Assisted delivery: delays in pups emerging*

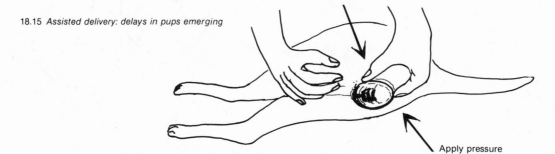

Apply pressure

• Grasp as much of the puppy as you can with a clean piece of rough
towelling and gently pull downwards and out (Fig. 18:16). Try to avoid
pulling one leg by itself as damage is easily done. Attempt to pull to
coincide with the bitch's expulsive efforts.

If the pup is stuck, gently rotate or "rock" him as you exert a firm but
gentle pull. Often the pup will come out more easily if rotated slightly
sideways.

18.16 *Assisted delivery:
gently pull downwards and
towards the bitch's back
paws while drawing the pup
out of the birth canal*

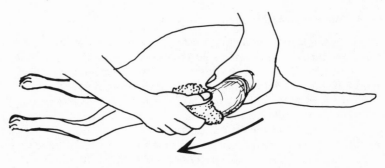

Pup not breathing

• Clear any membranes away from the mouth.

• Holding the puppy between both hands, swing him downwards in an arc towards your feet. Stop abruptly when his nose points directly to the ground (Fig. 18:17). In this way you may clear mucus obstructing his mouth or throat and help to clear the lungs of fluid.

• Rub the puppy briskly with a rough towel. This mimics the action of the mother's tongue and stimulates breathing.

• Mouth-to-mouth resuscitation may be necessary. Blow *gently* into the pup's nose and mouth until the chest starts to lift (Fig. 18:19). Do not blow hard or you risk rupturing the lungs.

• Persist with your efforts for 15 minutes before admitting defeat.

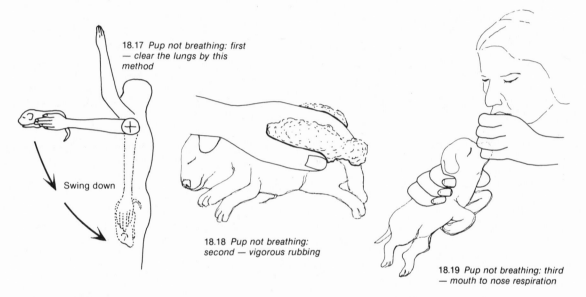

18.17 *Pup not breathing: first — clear the lungs by this method*

Swing down

18.18 *Pup not breathing: second — vigorous rubbing*

18.19 *Pup not breathing: third — mouth to nose respiration*

When to call the vet

• Bitch straining for 1 hour or more without any pup presented. (Some vets suggest waiting for 2 hours.)

• Membranes have ruptured but no puppy is presented within 30 minutes.

• There is over 3 hours between pups being born.

• Bitch is not straining ("uterine inertia").

• Bitch goes over 65 days.

• Bitch is lethargic.

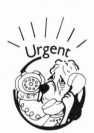

How long a time span should there be between pups?

Most bitches deliver a pup every 15-30 minutes, which gives them time to clean up each pup, but this time span varies and tends to get longer as labor continues. An interval of 2 hours between pups is not uncommon in larger litters as the muscles of the uterus become tired and contractions become less frequent and weaker.

If the interval between pups is over 3 hours or if the bitch is straining without producing a pup then telephone the vet.

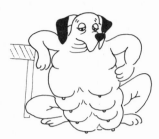

18.20 *Uterine inertia — lazy uterus: a cause can be excess weight*

UTERINE INERTIA—LAZY UTERUS

The uterus sometimes fails to contract to expel the pups. The most common causes are:

• Excess weight of bitch.

• Emotional upsets and anxiety may prevent normal labor. This may occur in a bitch with her first litter, especially in strange surroundings or in the company of an anxious, worried owner. A familiar atmosphere and calm reassurance from the owner can prevent this situation.

• Hormone deficiencies: there may be insufficient release of the hormone which stimulates contraction (oxytocin).

• After several pups have been delivered, the uterine muscles may become exhausted, especially after a very large puppy or a difficult delivery.

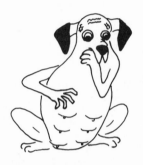

18.21 *Uterine inertia — lazy uterus: another cause can be emotional upset and anxiety*

CARE OF THE NEWBORN PUPS

The pup has no ability to control its temperature and can easily become chilled, which may be fatal. While the bitch is busy delivering further pups, those already born should be put into a draught-free box, which has been warmed to a temperature of 30°C (85°F) by a heating pad or a warm water-bottle. Do not overheat the pups or heat them too quickly.

Between deliveries, put the pups onto the bitch's nipples. Pups must suckle early as the first milk or "colostrum" is food which contains antibodies and will protect them against disease.

THE PUPS' EARLY DAYS

The newborn pup cannot see or hear, but will home into any source of warmth. The puppy will burrow its nose into anything soft and warm, its mouth automatically searching for a teat.

Newborn pups spend most of their first weeks asleep, waking only to eat. The mother will carefully monitor their temperature and keep them just right. She will also keep them clean, licking the anus to stimulate defecation and the belly to stimulate them to urinate.

Pups quickly burn up energy and must drink milk often, especially in the first 2 weeks of life. Pups that are not feeding well are liable to die. Pups should double their birth weight in 8-10 days.

Why newborn puppies die (see p. 234, 237).

The runt (see p. 237).

18.22 *New born pups*

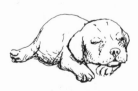

Newborn

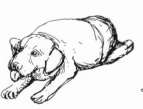

2-3 weeks

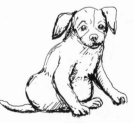

3 weeks

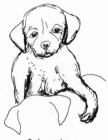

3-4 weeks

CARE OF THE BITCH AFTER WHELPING

Feeding

It is virtually impossible to overfeed the bitch after whelping while she is nursing pups. Give her several meals a day of high quality foods, including dry foods, meat, cooked eggs, cottage cheese, rice and cooked vegetables and a calcium supplement, such as calcium lactate, calcium gluconate or calcium carbonate. (See p. 80-83, 85.)

Vitamin supplements seem to help, especially the B group. Always allow free access to clean water.

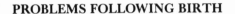

Veterinary check

About 12 hours after the birth your vet should check the bitch for any retained pups or membranes; to check pups for any deformities; and to make sure the bitch's milk supply is adequate and that there is no mastitis.

PROBLEMS FOLLOWING BIRTH

Mastitis

What is mastitis?

Mastitis is inflammation or an infection of one or more of the breasts, or mammary glands. It may be caused by infection, by physical damage (such as a knock) or by excessive build up of milk.

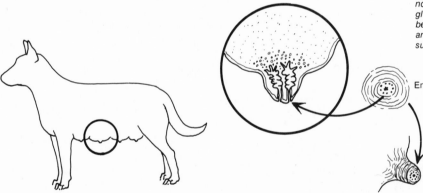

18.23 *The mammary glands: normally the mammary glands are firm, but if they become hot to the touch, and tight and swollen, suspect mastitis*

End of teat

Signs of mastitis
The breasts become swollen, hot and sometimes discolored. They are tender to touch. Often the bitch is uncomfortable and her appetite is poor. A fever is usually present.

The milk may be changed—sometimes straw-colored fluid only can be expressed or the milk may be blood-stained or thin and watery. In a few cases the milk appears normal.

Treatment
If infection is present, antibiotics are required. In some cases the gland may have to be opened and the affected area drained of the infected matter.

Will the pups be harmed?

The pups will not feed from the affected nipple. If mastitis affects several of the milk glands they will cry, due to hunger, and if these signs are not noticed and the pups are neglected, they will lose weight and may die.

How do you feed the pups?

The pups may be fed using an orphan pup formula (see p. 235 for orphan pup formula) or by a foster mother.

How can I reduce the chances of mastitis?

Keep the kennel area clean and free from abrasive surfaces. Avoid knocks or bumps to mammary glands.

If milk is building up in one or more glands and the pups are not drinking, gently express *a little* of the milk to take the tenseness from the gland. A warm salt water compress or warm soaks may help to reduce the swelling.

If too much milk is expressed, the gland will be stimulated to produce more milk and the tightness in the gland will quickly build up again.

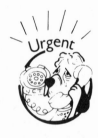

Metritis (infected uterus)

The infection can occur due to membranes or a dead pup being retained in the uterus, or from infection spreading upwards from the vulva into the uterus. Infection can follow use of dirty instruments or hands or a pre-existing vaginal infection.

> An infection of the uterus is a serious problem which
> may be fatal.

Signs
- Fever—temperature of (39.5 °C) or higher.
- Lack of appetite, excessive thirst, vomiting, diarrhea.
- Discharge from the womb, which is dark colored and often foul smelling. Color varies from deep red (like tomato soup) to a greenish or yellow color.

Note that it is normal for a bitch to discharge a dark greenish-black fluid for a few days after whelping. This becomes lighter and more watery. A straw-colored discharge for 2 or 3 weeks after whelping is normal.

Treatment
Veterinary treatment is essential to control the infection. The bitch's milk may be affected so that the pups refuse to drink and the milk may dry up. It is usually necessary to take the pups away and hand feed them.

Pyometra (pus in the womb)

Pyometra is a condition in which the uterus becomes filled with pus. It is a condition occurring usually in middle-aged or older, unspayed females. It is more common in bitches that have never had pups.

Is pyometra dangerous?

Untreated cases can certainly be fatal.

Signs of pyometra

Sometimes the pus discharges, so a vaginal discharge is seen. Sometimes there is no discharge and these cases are frequently the most severe, as toxic products build up in the body.

The bitch may show a variety of signs including:
- Increased thirst.
- Appetite loss.
- Depression.
- Vomiting.
- The vulva may enlarge.
- The abdomen may swell and feel "doughy" or tense

When does it start?

The onset of pyometra usually follows a heat period. Frequently this heat period is not as "strong" as normal and may last a shorter time than normal.

Veterinary diagnosis

Blood tests, X-rays and vaginal swabs may help diagnosis.

Treatment of pyometra

The most satisfactory treatment is surgical removal of the entire genital tract—ovaries and both uterine horns and body.

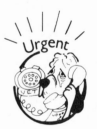

Milk fever (eclampsia)

Milk fever is due to a low level of calcium in the bloodstream. It is especially common in small breeds** and in bitches having their third or more litter**. Signs usually start about 3 weeks after whelping, but it may be much earlier, even before whelping.

Signs of milk fever

At first:
- Abnormal appetite (e.g., eating soil, etc.).
- Increased thirst.
- Rapid breathing.
- A stiff, unnatural gait progressing to loss of balance and paralysis, with stiffening of the legs.
- 'Glazed' expression.

> Rapid breathing of the bitch in milk can herald milk fever.
> Take the pups from the mother.

Treatment of milk fever

Treatment by a vet is required urgently. Intravenous injections of a calcium solution usually gives rapid relief, but *the bitch is liable to have further episodes if the pups are allowed to suckle* and thus drain more calcium from the mother's system. If the pups are old enough they should be weaned, but if still too young, then a replacement formula (see p. 235) should be fed for 24 hours. Then the pups should be started on a program of alternate feeds of hand feeding and nursing from the mother, so that the drain on the bitch's calcium is reduced.

Supplement the bitch with calcium: Calcium carbonate, calcium lactate or calcium gluconate should be used at a dose of 1-3 grams per day for one month. Do *not* use dicalcium phosphate (DCP).

19. The newborn pup

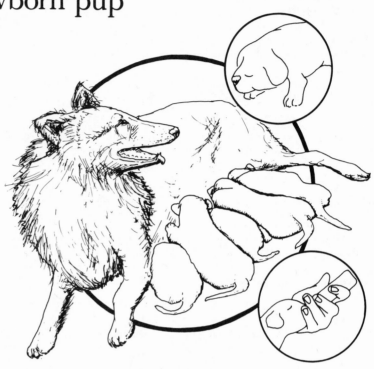

NEWBORN PUPS

> Newborn pups must be kept constantly warm and well fed.

Warmth

Pups have no ability to control their temperature for the first few weeks of life. It is essential to give them warm, draught-free accommodation. Pups will home in on any source of warmth, which usually means they snuggle into their mother or pile up amongst themselves. Chilling is the single greatest danger to the new pup and if pups are chilled they may die. But beware of overheating also. An overheated pup may become dehydrated and this can also be fatal. Aim for a temperature in the whelping box of 30°C for the first week of the pup's life. This temperature is gradually reduced over the next few weeks as the pup's ability to conserve heat improves—to 27°C by end of first week and 23°C by end of fourth week.

The importance of weight gain

A healthy pup spends most of his time asleep and the rest feeding. It is not normal for a pup to cry much unless he is cold or hungry, although

*, **, *** indicate increasing likelihood of a particular trait or problem occurring.

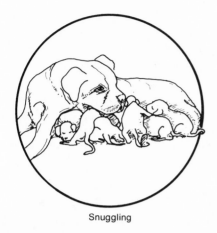

Snuggling

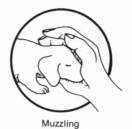

Muzzling

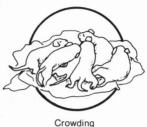

Crowding

19.2 *Pups seek warmth*

he may squeak as he struggles to get onto a nipple. The pup should be warm, and feel full and rounded and suck with enthusiasm on a finger placed in his mouth.

> Weigh pups daily in the first two weeks of life.

Pups may lose weight in the first two days of life, but this weight loss should not exceed 10 per cent of birth weight. The pups should start a weight gain by the time they are at least 48 hours old and if they do not then you should have the mother checked to make certain she is healthy and feeding the pups properly.

Hand feeding pups

If pups are not getting sufficient milk they need to have supplementary feeding. Ordinary cows' milk is *not* an adequate substitute. The easiest supplement is a commercial bitch's milk, which has been produced to conform closely to the composition of natural bitch's milk (e.g., Esbilac, Animilac).

You can make your own formula, as shown below. This should be fed warm.

4 oz (114 ml) evaporated milk (Carnation)
4 oz (114 ml) boiled water
1 teaspoon malt with cod liver oil
2 teaspoons Glucodin (medicinal glucose)
1 egg yolk
10 drops of Pentavite or some multi-vitamin mixture
(This formula provides 1½ calories per ml)

or

1 cup homogenised milk
3 egg yolks
1 tablespoon vegetable oil (e.g., corn oil)
10 drops Pentavite or some multi-vitamin mixture
(This formula provides 1¼ calories per ml)

For the 1st week of life, a pup needs 60 cals for every lb of his bodyweight divided into 6 feeds per day. (13 cals per 100 grams)

For the 2nd week of life, a pup needs 70 cals for every lb of his bodyweight divided into 3 or 4 feeds per day. (15 cals per 100 grams)

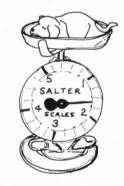

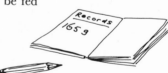

19.3 *The importance of weight gain: weigh the pups daily for the first 2 weeks and record the weight so that you can chart this progress*

For the 3rd week of life, a pup needs 80 cals for every lb of his bodyweight divided into 3 feeds per day. (18 cals per 100 grams)

For the 4th week of life, a pup needs 90 cals for every lb of his bodyweight divided into 3 feeds per day. (20 cals per 100 grams)

How to feed the orphan pup

A puppy nursing bottle, a doll's bottle or a small baby bottle can be used if the puppy is sucking well. Make the teat hole large enough for milk to drip out otherwise the puppy will find sucking too hard and may not feed properly.

19.4 *Feeding aids*

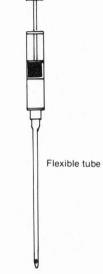

Flexible tube

Stomach tube feeder   Tube feeder   Eye dropper   Dolls bottle   Glass foster feeder

If the pup is not sucking well, you may use an eye dropper (Fig. 19:5) but be careful not to *squirt* milk down the mouth. Milk accidentally squirted into the pup's lungs will cause pneumonia.

Very sick pups may need to be fed by a tube inserted into the stomach. This must be done with great care.

19.5 *Hand feeding pups*

Eye dropper feeding: don't squirt — let the drops gently fall into the mouth

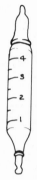

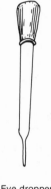

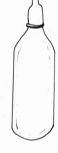

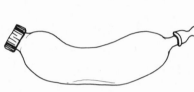

Tube feeding: measure the distance from the pup's nose to his last rib. Mark this distance on the rubber stomach tube and do not insert any more than that length of tube

Bottle feeding

After feeding of hand-reared pups
It is necessary to stimulate the pup to pass urine and feces. This is done by gently massaging around the anus and genitals with damp cotton wool. This mimics the action of the mother's tongue as she would normally perform this service for the pup.

DIARRHEA

Diarrhea in pups is a serious condition, quickly causing dehydration. Compared with older dogs newborn pups have little resistance and mild diarrhea can be fatal.

The most common cause of diarrhea is overfeeding, especially when a pup is being hand fed. If the pup develops diarrhea reduce the amount you are feeding him. Check your formula (see p. 235) and do not make it too rich.

One or two mls of Milk of Magnesia helps to slow gut movements and ease the diarrhea. It may be given three times daily.

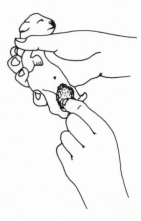

19.6 *After feeding stimulate urination and bowel motions by massaging gently around genitals with damp cotton wool or a flannel*

> If you cannot quickly control newborn puppy diarrhea,
> consult your vet at once.

UNDERFEEDING

The best way to avoid underfeeding is to keep a close check on weight gain. Weigh the pup *every* day so that if he fails to gain weight you can detect the problem early.

The underfed pup will usually cry and then become listless and feel cool to the touch. The suckling reflex is not strong in weak pups and the pup will need to be force fed (see p. 236) if he becomes weak.

SORE NIPPLES

In their enthusiasm to feed, 3 to 4 week old pups may damage the bitch's breasts with their sharp claws. This can make the bitch reluctant to allow the pups to suckle. The points of the pups' claws can be nipped off—but be careful only to take the very tips, or you may cause bleeding.

FADING PUPPIES

Fading pups fail to gain weight, become weak, feed poorly and eventually lose interest in feeding. They become listless and eventually die.

The fading puppy syndrome is not due to one single disease or condition, but may be caused by a number of factors. Often the cause is not known. An easy method of identifying a sick pup for ease of treatment and increased observation is to put a small streak of nail varnish on his toenails.

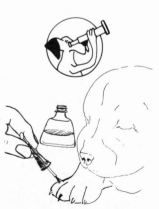

19.7 *Sick puppies: one puppy looks much like the next. To identify one, such as a sick puppy, paint one particular nail. This prevents treating the wrong pup*

Some of the causes implicated include:
- Herpes virus infection.
- Chilling.
- Inadequate feeding.
- Birth defects.
- Problems in the mother, for example, toxic milk.

HERPES VIRUS

The herpes virus may be an important factor. The newborn pups' temperature (about 36.5°C or 98°F) is ideal for the virus to thrive. The virus may be carried by the mother, where it causes no problem as her temperature is 38°C (101°F). When passed on to the pup, herpes virus may cause a severe illness and even death.

Signs of herpes virus infection

Most pups are 5-21 days of age when they contract the disease. Pups will stop nursing, cry, be unable to settle and show signs of abdominal pain. Sometimes the pup develops diarrhea, shows considerable pain and may die within 24 hours.

Treatment is not usually successful, although raising the environmental temperature to over 38°C (101°F) may sometimes help. There is no vaccine available yet.

Subsequent litters whelped by the same bitch do not necessarily become sick from herpes virus.

TOXIC (POISONOUS) MILK

Cause
If the mother's milk is affected by mastitis (see p. 231-3) or other infections, the pups may become ill due to toxins in the milk.

Signs
Pups are restless and distressed. They may have diarrhea and are often bloated with gas or "wind." The mother's breasts are hard and when they are squeezed produce abnormal milk (see p. 231).

Treatment
The pups must be hand reared until the mother's milk returns to normal.

NAVEL INFECTIONS

The umbilical or "birth" cord should be severed by the mother a few centimeters from the pup's body. This cord then shrinks and falls off, leaving a small scar or "navel."

If the cord becomes infected, a condition termed "navel ill" develops. The navel is swollen and red and there may be some pus discharging. The pup often looks sick.

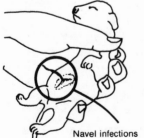

19.8 'Navel ill' in pups

Navel infections occur here

Where does the infection come from?

Infections can be picked up from droppings in the whelping box, from the mother's dirty teeth or from contamination during handling of the pups.

Treatment of navel infections
Clean the area of the navel with warm water and a *mild* soap. (Never use strong solutions or Phisohex on a young pup.) Treat the stump with an antiseptic such as iodine, mercurochrome or acriflavine.

> If the navel infection persists, consult your vet.
> Navel ill can be rapidly fatal.

WORMING THE PUP

The main worm parasite to be concerned about in the puppy is *Roundworm*. The pup may be born with an infestation and can pick up more worms immediately after birth. Although dog roundworms can not survive in humans, the eggs of these roundworms can cause a serious problem in children (see p. 109-10).

19.9 *Roundworm: it is essential to worm puppies for roundworm, not only for their own health, but because they can be a danger to young children*

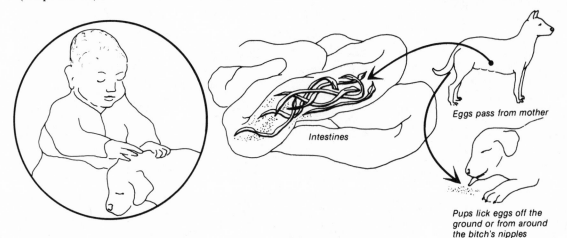

Intestines

Eggs pass from mother

Pups lick eggs off the ground or from around the bitch's nipples

For the sake of the puppy and also in view of the human health risk, pups should be treated after 28 days of age based on the results of a fecal sample. Drugs such as piperazine (e.g., Antoban) are used. The dose is 100-200 mg per kg bodyweight or pyrantel pamoate (Canex). 1 tablet per 7 kg bodyweight.

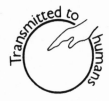

Hookworms can also kill pups.

Tapeworm is another worm parasite to be concerned about. If you see tapeworm segments in the pup droppings (see p.112-14) treat with praziquantel (e.g., Droncit). The dose is 1 tablet per 10 kg bodyweight, maximum dose 3 tablets.

WEANING THE PUP

Weaning means changing the pups' diet from the bitch's milk to other foods. Weaning can be achieved from 3-6 weeks of age, although 5 weeks is the most common age.

You can introduce most pups to solids as early as 3 weeks of age. Try a mixture of half evaporated milk and half baby cereal. Put a little on your finger and let the puppy suckle it, then gradually lower the sucking puppy's head down into a shallow dish full of the mixture. Eventually it will learn to take the mixture from the bowl.

Other foods that can be added to the mixture include glucose, egg yolk (raw or cooked), cottage cheese and eventually a little cooked, minced meat. Dry puppy foods can be fed so long as they are well moistened first.

As the pups take more of these foods, reduce the amount you feed the mother. This will reduce her milk supply and the pups will seek more and more food from elsewhere. Weaning should be quickly achieved from this point. The mother will help by starting to reject demands from the pups for food.

19.10 Weaning the pup: put a little food on your finger and let the pup suck it in, then gradually lower the sucking puppy's head down into the bowl of food

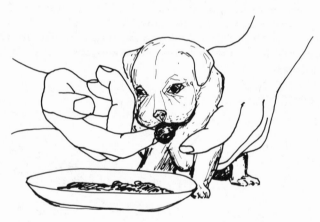

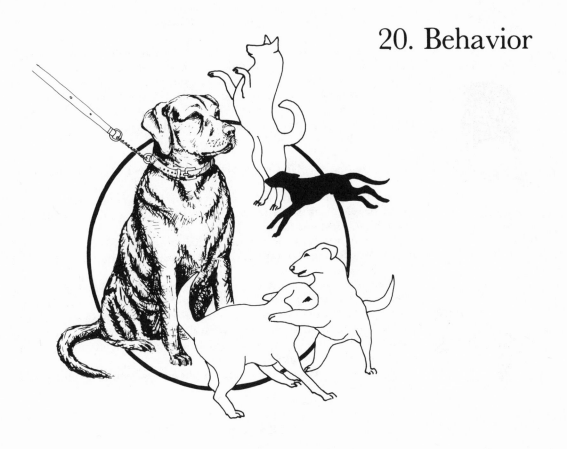

20. Behavior

The pup's relationship with you over the first weeks is vital for his future behavior. Establish from the start a proper understanding that you are the teacher and he is the pupil.

Much of the influence on a pup's future behavior occurs within the first 16 weeks of life. After purchase, at about 8 weeks of age, the owner has eight weeks to mold much of the dog's future attitude and character.

> Be consistent and calm and your new pup will adapt
> quickly and well to his new home.

THE AGE TO INTRODUCE A NEW PUP TO YOUR HOME

After the age of 5 weeks the pup looks for a substitute for his mother's affections. The ideal time to bring a new pup into your home is when the pup is from 6-16 weeks old, and preferably between 6 and 10 weeks old.

In the early days a pup is very impressionable, and your treatment of him at this time will form the basis of his future reactions and behavior.

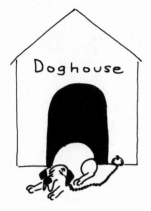

20.2 'How should punishment be used?'

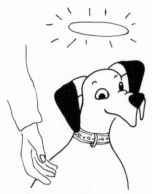

20.3 Praise is often reward enough. A food reward may be necessary in some cases

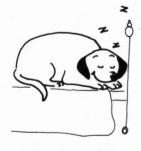

20.4 Pups grow up. Habits that are 'cute' in a pup can be a nuisance in older dogs

COMING HOME

Allow your new pup to investigate his new home freely. Supply him with some type of bedding where he can easily find it and establish his own little corner. A blanket in an upside-down carton box with a doorway cut out is a temporary bed favored by pups, as it has a cozy atmosphere. Do not isolate your pup on his first night, but put his bed inside. If you want the pup to sleep outside, start that from the second night.

CRIME AND PUNISHMENT

Never strike your puppy, as this can result in him becoming distrustful or shy of people. Fear is readily imprinted into a young pup, especially between 8-10 weeks of age.

It is enough to show displeasure by the tone of your voice: a firm tone makes your feelings crystal clear to the new arrival. Use the single word "no" when you can.

When he passes a motion in the correct spot, stops chewing your rug when reprimanded or eats up all his breakfast, then praise him. Do not allow bad habits to develop; what may seem amusing in a puppy can be a real problem in an adult, so allow no liberties as a pup that you do not intend to allow him as an adult, such as begging at the table, or sleeping at the foot of your children's bed.

Avoid rough handling at all times as physical or mental trauma can result.

TRAINING YOUR PUP

It is an advantage to begin teaching simple commands soon after weaning. Single words should be used and "sit," "stay," "drop," "come," and "heel" are commands to which your dog must respond. Have one or two 5-10 minute training periods daily.

Some Seeing Eye guide dogs that lead the blind eventually respond to 60 words of command and will learn to respond to words like "forward," "butcher," "hairdresser" and "delicatessen."

> Be patient when training your pup. Reward a dog or pup with praise. If you use food you will find it a hard habit to break.

My pup likes being cuddled, can this cause any problems?

Yes. Your pup is soon spoiled when petted too much for no reason. Praise and petting should be used as rewards when the pup does something *you* want him to do.

My pup mounts my leg, is this normal?

Pups learn sexual behavior at a young age and will mount littermates in early sex play. Your leg substitutes for a littermate.

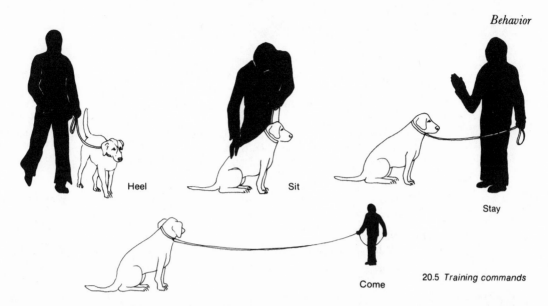

Heel

Sit

Stay

Come

20.5 *Training commands*

Do not let your pup learn to mount legs, but move your leg away immediately he starts or lift your knee and push him away—gently but firmly. Mounting can become imprinted and be a vice for the rest of his life if you allow it to go on too long.

My pup passes water when he greets me. What should I do?

Urinating is a normal act of submission when the pup greets you. It does not warrant punishment. Instead, to avoid this special greeting do not act excited when you return home. Pay attention to your puppy *only* after he has calmed down.

Always greet your dog in a calm and placid manner.

HOUSE TRAINING

House training should be simple and quickly achieved but, as in all training, you must be patient. Before you start, be sure the pup is healthy and has a good, balanced diet. (It is expecting too much to house train a pup with diarrhea.)

A toilet area must be decided on. This may be an area outside or paper on the floor inside.

Take your pup to the toilet area immediately he looks like passing urine or feces, after eating or playing and when he first wakes after a snooze.

When the pup uses his toilet area you should immediately praise and pet him. Let him know how pleased you are and how clever you think he is.

Do's and don'ts of house training

Accidents
When accidents are discovered some time after the event, don't make a fuss. Clean them up, but don't let your pup see you doing it. Do *not* rub his nose

in the mess. This only confuses the pup. He really has no idea what you are trying to teach him. If scolding is to be effective you must catch him in the act. Physical punishment only confuses the pup and will often prolong the house training program. It also makes the pup "sneaky" about house soiling.

If you notice the pup is about to pass a motion, take him immediately to his toilet area. If he then passes a motion, praise him liberally. Learning to use his proper toilet area usually takes only a few days.

Water
It is not advisable to have water available at night or when the pup is left alone until after he is house trained. This should only take about a week.

Older dogs
Older dogs can be house trained by the same methods, but it can take longer—especially with nervous dogs.

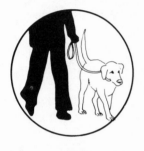

Always lead dogs on left

PULLING ON A LEAD

To stop a dog pulling on a lead, a choker chain is very useful. The choker is only a tool and should be used as such—you will get nowhere by simply pulling on the choker as this often leads to a tug of war.

The choker is designed to be jerked on and not pulled. At the same time that you jerk, tell your dog to "heel," always remembering to praise your dog for a job well done.

Your aim is to have your dog walk level with you and dog trainers consistently insist on the dog walking on the left side.

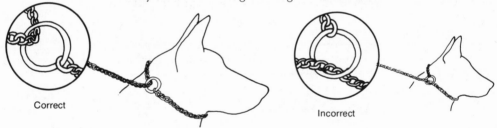

Correct

Incorrect

20.6 *Correct use of choker chain*

DIGGING

Why does my dog dig holes?

Some dogs dig holes and lie in them as a way to keep cool. Such dogs should be given access to cooler areas such as shade trees. Close clipping of the hair during summer will help the long-haired breeds.

The majority of "problem" diggers are bored or frustrated. Digging is a tension outlet in much the same way as children relieve tension by sucking their thumbs, or the Greeks do by playing with their "worry beads."

Stopping destructive digging

If possible, remove the cause of the problem by alleviating the boredom and underlying frustration. This might be achieved by allowing your dog inside, providing regular and vigorous exercise, or even getting a companion dog.

If you give your dog a lot of attention when he behaves badly, he will actually accept this as a reward and continue his bad behavior.

Create his own "area." Have a corner of a room with your dog's blanket or rug in it, where he will go on command. When you are out, he will have his own corner to go to and is less likely to feel the frustrations of isolation.

Favorite sites for digging

Some dogs will dig in a certain area of the garden whether they are isolated or not. In some cases, these dogs can be stopped by applying a repellent (available in pellet or aerosol form at some veterinary surgeries and plant nurseries) to the digging areas. These repellents may need renewing after heavy rain.

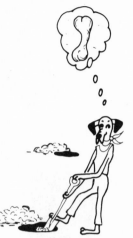

This method does not seem to work if the underlying problem is boredom. Another method that may work is to place a handful of marbles in a tin can. When you catch your dog in the act of digging, throw the tin near him. This will startle him. It should not take long for the dog to associate the act of digging with something unpleasant—in this case, a sudden noise and fright.

How can I stop my dog from digging out?

This can be an awkward problem. The only certain way is to have a dog-proof enclosure with high fences that lean in at the top, or have an overhang projecting into the compound, plus either a concrete surround to prevent the dog digging under or have the fence project down at least half a metre below the surface of the soil.

This sort of compound is beyond many owner's budget, but sometimes the *reason* for the dog digging out can be discovered and perhaps the answer lies therein.

Why do dogs dig out?

Breed and temperament: Some breeds such as the Border Collie, German Shorthair Pointer and the Kelpie are bred for an active working life. If these dogs are constricted in a suburban area they may rebel against their limited range and try to escape. The answer here is don't select the wrong breed if you have only limited space.

Loneliness: Frequently this is the problem. Dogs that are in the company of their owners or children may be perfectly content, but when left alone become anxious or lonely and many dig out to find companionship. Such a dog may benefit from another dog or company, or arrange to leave him with other people or dogs when you are out. If neither of these solutions is possible then the problem is hard to overcome. Tranquillizers and sedatives can be effective if this occurs only infrequently, but cannot be used as an everyday solution.

Sex: A male dog will do almost anything to get to a bitch in heat. This is a powerful basic drive. A neutered male is a far better pet for suburbia. In the case of a bitch, when she is in the fertile phase of heat she, too, will try to find a male and fences become only a frail barrier. Read the section on heat and contraception (p. 218-23).

Neutering your pet, especially in the case of a male, usually results in a quieter dog that is less inclined to wander and cause mischief, but it is not 100 per cent effective and does not solve the problem in all cases, but is often well worth a try.

Some other causes: Some dogs are well behaved most days but are attracted to garbage on collection days. These dogs should be routinely chained up or locked in on garbage days. Other dogs join in with children on their way to or from school: again you must pay special attention to confining these dogs when children are about.

To conclude: Dogs that dig out or escape in some other way can be a nuisance to other people and are liable to be injured on the road or picked up by the dog catcher. If you can deduce why the dog is trying to escape and rectify the cause then you are fortunate. If not, then sound dog-proofing may be the only solution.

BARKING

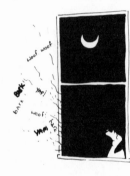

Barking can be a sign not only of protecting your property but of boredom, frustration or loneliness. Eliminating these stresses can be achieved by the same method that was discussed under "Destructive digging." Give your dog plenty of exercise and play and regular periods of your time.

A dog will often bark at people or cars passing his gate or window. Boarding up gates so that the dog can no longer see out or preventing access to a window will usually stop these barkers.

Chaining a dog up often creates the sort of stress that produces a barker. It is estimated that in a suburb of medium density a dog's bark can be heard by 200 surrounding houses (about 1000 people).

CHASING CARS

Chasing cars and people on bicycles is a serious anti-social habit which can lead to injury or death. A severe reprimand at the first offence is needed. If you cannot teach your dog to stop this habit you must confine him to the backyard. If this is not feasible an obedience school is advisable.

Road sense

You can teach your dog road sense, but this teaching can never be relied upon to save your dog from serious injury. Attendance at an obedience school will teach instant response to your command when your dog's life is in danger.

Use a choker as gentle restraint to train your dog to pause at the curb—and stay in the "down" or "drop" position on command before crossing the road. Remember praise and pats follow a good performance.

Perhaps one of the more important disciplines is to teach your dog not to cross the busy road to join you on the far side. Puppies in their exuberance may rush across the road and this has caused many dogs to die young.

> Do not let your dog run free in the city—he is a hazard
> to himself and others.

CHEWING

Why does my dog chew everything?

As with digging, the underlying reason for destructive chewing is usually the monotony of isolation or similar stress situations. It is normal for pups to chew when teething (p. 89) and over-pampered pets tend to be chewers.

The "aerosol spray technique" works in many cases: hold an aerosol container of *unscented* underarm deodorant at 90° to the dog's face and your face. Crouch down facing your pet at about 2 yards away and say, "What's this?" When the dog approaches to sniff the can and is about 1 foot from it then give one short spray and jab the can abruptly at your dog's nose. Then stand, saying "Good dog!", thereby ending the session. Put the can away out of sight. When the dog is not around, *lightly* spray objects that have been chewed or are likely to be chewed. Do not saturate the atmosphere with the spray. Your dog will associate the smell of the spray on the objects with that nasty experience with the can. This procedure *may* need daily repetition for several days.

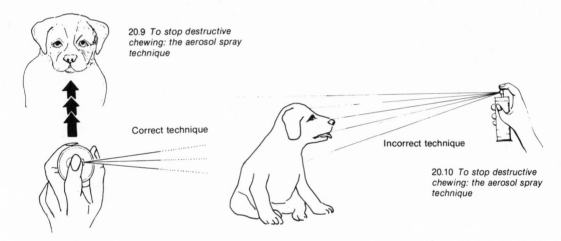

20.9 *To stop destructive chewing: the aerosol spray technique*

Correct technique

Incorrect technique

20.10 *To stop destructive chewing: the aerosol spray technique*

SIT-STAY TRAINING

Spend a week practicing sit-stays. Always reward the dog with praise. After he has learned the task and is performing well, put him on an intermittent schedule of food rewards.

After the dog has learned to sit quietly while you walk away, place an object in which the dog has absolutely no interest—perhaps a glass ash tray—on the floor at a distance of 3 yards from the dog and then pick it up again. If the dog sits quietly and does not object, walk back and give him a food reward. Then put an object down and pick it up at a distance of 2½ yards from the dog, then at 2 yards until the game is played right in front of the dog.

Perform with a variety of objects in which your dog has no or little interest. The dog must sit quietly until the object is removed before he receives a reward. These sessions *should be fun* for the dog. Stop before he tires of the game.

Gradually, items which are progressively more appealing are used. If the

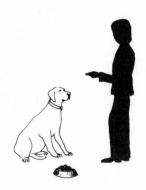

20.11 *Sit-stay training*

dog should get up or try to take the object, firmly say *"no"* and *"sit"* and give no reward. You may have to repeat the exercise several times at either a distance that is farther away or with an item that the dog is less interested in. (Food which the dog prefers to the reward should not initially be used as an object to be placed in front of the dog.)

Take opportunities to give the dog the command "sit-stay" whenever you think the dog is naturally motivated enough to obey. Have him sit before he is petted, let outside or inside, before the car door is opened or he is fed his regular meal. If he gets up and takes the object, return him to the original position and start again.

My dog growls at me when I try to remove his bone. What should I do?

You need to regain your dog's trust. Start by teaching him to "sit-stay" for delicious food rewards. A dog that is confident of his master will not be protective of his food and will trust you.

AGGRESSIVE BEHAVIOR IN DOGS

Aggressive behavior accounts for about half of all behavior problems brought to vets. Many people think of aggressive behavior as a sinister disease—but most cases of aggression are within normal behavior patterns for the dog. People ask for advice because their dog worries them, but this aggression may be a normal way to act according to the canine code of behavior.

Aggression within a group of dogs

In the wild, a definite social order will form within any group of dogs like the "pecking order" of chickens. The dominant dog wins first choice of food, mate or whatever else is up for grabs. To become top dog of a group of dogs, violence or aggression is necessary. After establishing his place, threats of aggression or play-fighting are usually sufficient to maintain his place until a real challenge is given by an up-and-comer, at which time another fight will take place, the victor becoming the dominant dog. In this way the fittest dogs survive to continue the line while the old, weak or unhealthy dog goes under, especially in times when resources are limited. Compare this with modern breeding selection, when a dog may be selected to breed simply because his coat is a pretty color or his muzzle is just the right fashionable length.

Crowding will increase aggression within the group; so will a scarcity of food. When groups of dogs are fed you can reduce aggression by either feeding each dog separately, or having only dry food available, or feeding a bulky meal food which is less appetising than meat. Less palatable food may mean fewer fights, whereas a hunk of juicy meat tends to provoke fighting.

Aggression towards humans

If you own a large breed dog it is essential to establish your dominance early while the dog is still a pup. Many problems of a dog's aggressive behaviour towards his owner occur when the dog thinks he is dominant or if there is doubt as to who is dominant. *One way to establish dominance is simply to pick the puppy up when he starts to misbehave,* in the same way as the mother would pick up the errant pup.

If you are frightened of big dogs, do not get one.

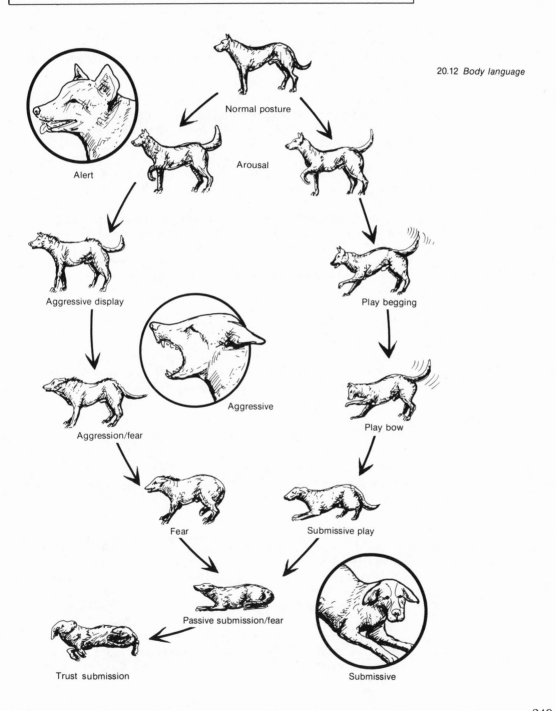

20.12 *Body language*

Normal posture

Alert

Arousal

Aggressive display

Play begging

Aggressive

Aggression/fear

Play bow

Fear

Submissive play

Passive submission/fear

Trust submission

Submissive

Breeding and aggression

Breeding programs strongly influence the temperament of a breed. In Britain and the USA a "rage syndrome" has become common in at least three of the four most popular breeds and many of these dogs have had to be destroyed. In these cases vicious attacks started suddenly, usually when the dog was 6-18 months old. On investigation, evidence clearly showed a genetic defect that could be traced back to a tiny handful of "champion" ancestors.

Because it has been the fashion to breed for looks and not temperament it has become increasingly difficult to recommend *any* breed with confidence that their temperament is sound.

The temperament of many breeds is deteriorating and owners must start to demand excellence in more than just looks if this trend is to be reversed.

With large dogs, avoid play-fights. Not only can they get out of control, but the needle-sharp teeth of pups can give painful nips. Discourage immediately and firmly any characteristic you do not want to develop, such as aggression towards strangers or other pets. Obviously if the dog has been acquired for protection this may be a desirable characteristic.

Once an aggression problem has been established, there are several avenues of treatment. A dog will always show aggression for a reason. Mistrust of or insecurity towards humans can be an important factor. Take your puppy for walks in shopping centers or busy streets so that he becomes used to people. Where possible let the people pat the pup. Your relaxed and confident manner with people will give the pup more confidence and hopefully overcome any distrust.

Protection training

If you want your dog to serve you specifically in a protection role it is advisable to find a reputable obedience and protection training school. Here you will find experienced handlers who can usually train your dog safely and efficiently. Trying to train the dog yourself, even with the help of a book, is not advisable.

Can aggression be cured?

Tranquillizers
Tranquillizers have a temporary effect only. The most common tranquillizers used are chlorpromazine derivative, e.g., acetyl promazine. Valium (diazepan) is also widely used. Tranquillizers can be useful as a short-term control of a problem.

Hormones
The male sex hormone testosterone stimulates aggression. Removal of the source of testosterone by castration is very effective in many (but not all) cases of aggression in males. It is more effective when performed while the dog is young.

Some hormones can be used to "chemically castrate" the dog. These hormones exert a temporary effect only and the unwanted behavior may return once the hormones are withdrawn. Hormones can be a useful tool in changing the dog's behavior pattern—you train the dog while he is on drug treatment, then when his behavior is modified, the drug is gradually withdrawn.

Euthanasia

There is no treatment that is guaranteed to stop aggressive and harmful behavior in dogs. The problem is a complicated one, and while some dogs may be completely controlled by treatment, many are never completely trustworthy. Where there is danger to the family, and especially where children are at risk, you must consider having the dog destroyed. Do not let your heart rule your head—much as you may deplore having your dog destroyed, in some circumstances it is the best solution.

Some aggressive dogs may be trained out of their aggressiveness, provided the temperament of the dog is sound. But you must be prepared to spend a considerable amount of time and effort training the dog and often the aid of a professional dog handler is advisable.

OTHER BEHAVIOR QUESTIONS

How can I avoid my pup disliking the vet?

Pups visit the vet at 6-8 weeks of age for their temporary vaccinations. The injection will not hurt the pup so make this trip pleasurable, as fear can be imprinted at this stage unless you are calm and handle the pup calmly. Once the pup has associated a visit to the vet with fear and apprehension, it is difficult to alter his feelings, so try to create an atmosphere of fun and relaxation. Subsequent visits will be much easier as a result.

My dog scratches to get inside. How do I overcome this?

You must ignore your dog. He may scratch dozens, even hundreds, of times before he gives up, but do not reward your dog by letting him in unless you want him to come in whenever he scratches.

My dog is frightened by thunderstorms. How do I overcome this?

Ignore your dog's fear if you want him to improve. Speak words of reassurance, but avoid petting and too much attention during a storm or his behaviour will be worse in later storms. Tranquillizers or other drugs may be given when thunder is in the air to help teach your dog to forget his fear.

Should I take my dog to obedience class?

This is an excellent idea—you will both learn a lot and you will get more joy from dog ownership. You will learn to command and your dog will be taught to obey. Using an obedience school does not mean you want a servile, brow-beaten dog, but instead it establishes a healthy rapport and the dog will trust and obey you.

What effect does castration have?

When a dog is castrated, his testicles are removed. This removes the source of the male sex hormone, testosterone, and as a result there can be marked changes in the dog's behavior. Aggression toward other males, urine marking of territory and mounting of other animals (or of people's legs) are reduced in castrated males. Roaming is decreased in most and aggressiveness is reduced or stopped in many dogs.

My dog is unruly. What can I do?

This problem needs your self-control to allow your dog to develop his. Ignore your dog when he is excited, for example when you first arrive home. Greet him in a calm and restrained manner. Praise and pet him when he is quiet.

Can drugs help problems of behavior?

Drugs should be used only as tools to help modify behavior. It is not sufficient to tranquillize a dog to a state of lethargy and believe that you have controlled or solved the problem. Tranquillizers and other drugs such as the hormone progestin can be used as aids to change behavior. Your patient and firm teaching is more important than drugs.

How should punishment be used?

You can change your dog's ways if you punish immediately after bad behavior and every time he does something wrong. Punishment even a few minutes after a misdemeanour is too late as the dog will not understand why you are annoyed. Punishment should not be used in an attempt to control fears and phobias such as fear of thunderstorms.

> Misused or excessive punishment is harmful and useless. It can break a dog and he will become frightened and unpredictable.

My dog tends to be jealous. How can I avoid him harming our new baby?

A dog showing signs of jealousy must be kept away from young children. If you are expecting a new baby, give a jealous dog away to someone else before the baby arrives. Never leave a jealous dog alone with a new baby.

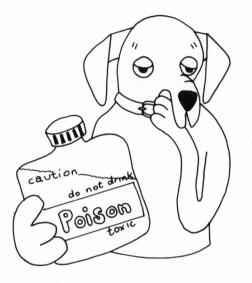

21. Poisoning

WHAT TO DO IF YOU THINK YOUR DOG HAS BEEN POISONED

• *Don't panic!* Consult the chart in this chapter to determine the immediate home treatment while you telephone the vet.

• If an emetic is suggested, this means getting the dog to vomit. This can be done by giving a nauseating solution, such as 1 teaspoon salt in a cup of warm water placed down the side of the mouth or using syrup of ipecac (available from pharmacists). The dose of ipecac is 1-2 ml per kg of the dog's weight. Your vet can also give an injection to cause vomiting. Do *not* try to induce vomiting if petroleum distillates, acids or alkalis have been consumed or if the dog is depressed and not fully alert and conscious.

• Collect any suspected source material, such as any empty packets, or any loose pills, or any chemicals, solvents, pest control products, medicines, cleaners or sprays that the dog may have come in contact with. Take these with you to the vet.

• A sample of vomit may be useful for diagnosis.

• Do not give anything by mouth if the patient is convulsing, depressed or unconscious.

• Allow the dog to drink as much water as he wants.

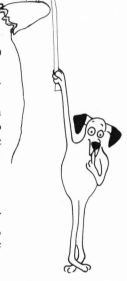

21.2 *Don't panic!*

Why are dogs easily poisoned?

Dogs are actually attracted to some poisons, for example, some rat poisons and snail baits.

RULES FOR THE HOME (FOR DOG AND CHILD SAFETY)

• Keep your medicines out of reach and in a *locked* cabinet.

• Pay attention to *all* poisons such as garden chemicals, petroleum products, insecticides, detergents, scourers. Make certain they are out of reach, and cannot be knocked down.

• Never use old food or drink containers for poisons—confusion and accidental poisoning can occur very easily.

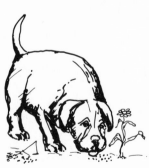

21.3 *Dogs are actually attracted to some poisons — for example, snail and rat poisons*

Name	Source	Signs	Immediate home treatment	Comments
Acids	Battery acids, some solvents.	Abdominal pain. May be blood-stained vomiting. Shock. Possibly mouth burns or ulcers.	*Do not induce vomiting.* Give sodium bicarbonate if possible (5%). Give milk of magnesia, alum. If nothing else is available, give lots of water. See a vet as soon as possible. Acid on skin: flush with lots of water.	
Adhesives	Glues and pastes.	Discomfort in mouth: drooling saliva, smacking lips.	Give milk (preferably) or water.	Not very attractive to dogs, but are potentially quite toxic.
Alcohol, methylated spirits	Alcoholic drinks. Industrial alcohol.	Depression, vomiting, collapse.	Bicarbonate of soda in large quantities. Warmth. See your vet.	Dogs may be induced to take large quantities of alcohol for "fun." Such "fun" can be fatal.
Alkali (strong bases)	Fluid cleaners, solvents, etc.	Abdominal pain. May be blood-stained vomiting. Shock. Maybe mouth burns or ulcers.	*Do not induce vomiting.* Try to neutralize by giving copious amounts of water or, preferably, dilute vinegar, lemon juice, etc. On skin: flush with vinegar. See vet as soon as possible.	
Ammonia	Household cleaner.	Irritates nose and throat: sneezing, salivating and drooling. Maybe vomiting.	Fresh air.	Rarely a problem as dogs are repelled by smell.
Antibiotics	Dispensed tablets for human or animal infections.	Penicillin: Large numbers can cause vomiting and diarrhea 6-12 hours later. If dog is allergic reaction can occur. Tetracycline: Vomiting and diarrhea.	If large numbers are taken induce vomiting. Induce vomiting.	
Anti-depressants	Valium.	Depression. Loss of consciousness. Coma—depends on dose.	Vomiting—induce if still conscious.	Take animal to vet as soon as possible.
Anti-freeze (ethylene glycol)	Some anti-freeze preparations.	There are two types of signs: If a lot has been drunk, "acute" poisoning occurs. Otherwise, "chronic" occurs—the signs of which are due to kidney damage.	Immediate treatment may save dogs with potentially fatal doses. If the dose is greater than 10 ml per kg bodyweight there is no effective treatment. *Intensive veterinary treatment is essential.*	Cats like the sweet taste, as do some dogs.

When poisoning of any sort is suspected see your vet as soon as possible.

Name	Source	Signs	Immediate home treatment	Comments
Anti-freeze (*cont'd*)		*Acute:* Initially apprehension (worried look), then the dog sits about, staggering and vomiting. Wobbling becomes worse and the dog collapses. His back legs are paralysed and coma and death follow. *Chronic:* (If dog survives for up to 24 hours.) Signs vary but may include vomiting, thirst and depression. Progresses to kidney failure and death.		
Ant killers	See "Arsenic" if it contains arsenic. If it contains Chlordecone there are usually no signs.			
ANTU	Rat poison (odorless white powder).	Restlessness, leading to lethargy. Cherry red gums. Difficulty breathing.	*Immediate* emetic. Preferably injection given by vet.	Treatment is usually not successful.
Arsenic	Some rodent poisons, paints, herbicides, ant poisons, insecticides. (**Note:** The uses of arsenic in these compounds is decreasing. Poisoning by arsenic is uncommon).	Depending on dose, signs occur from hours to weeks after eating arsenic. Death may occur within hours or may take weeks, or the animal may survive. **Signs:** initially vomiting, severe abdominal pain. Watery diarrhea, often with blood flecks. Shock and collapse precede death.	Purge immediately to induce vomiting. Treatment by vet as soon as possible.	Samples of urine, bowel motion, vomit and any suspected source material should be kept and submitted to vet for analysis.
Aspirin (Acetylsalicylic acid) Disprin, Aspro	A common widely used household drug.	*Can be very toxic if large numbers eaten.* Appetite loss. Depression and vomiting which may be blood stained. Convulsions—maybe death if a very large overdose is taken.	Give an emetic if large numbers have been eaten. See a vet.	Cats are especially sensitive. This drug is very toxic if large quantities are taken or if overdosed over some days.
Baby oil	Baby oil.	Nil. Maybe diarrhea about 12 hours later.	Nil.	
Barbiturates	Some tranquillizers, some sleeping tablets.	Depression, sleepiness. Loss of consciousness. Coma.	If the dog is conscious, induce vomiting. *Keep animal moving.* Take to vet as soon as possible.	
Carbon monoxide	Car exhausts—when dogs are locked in garage with exhaust fumes building up.	Cherry red gums.	Place in fresh air. Artificial respiration (firmly depress chest with flat of hand, then release. Repeat about 15 times a minute.) Smelling salts.	

255

Name	Source	Signs	Immediate home treatment	Comments
Carbon tetra-chloride	Some worming preparations (rarely used today).	Fumes are poisonous. Breathing problems and respiratory failure.	Artificial respiration.	
Caustic soda	See "Alkalis, strong bases."			
Chlorinated hydro-carbons	Flea rinses, Benzene hydro-chloride, Dieldrin, BHC, DDT, Gammexane, malathion, lindane, toxophene, chlordane, methoxy-chlor. *These are absorbed through intact skin.*	Initially excitement. Twitching, then muscle tremors, starting at face. Convulsions or seizures may develop—these are fairly short but recur and may be stimulated by handling.	There is no specific antidote. Treatment is aimed at reducing amount of poison absorbed. • *If dog has tremors or convulsions,* take to vet as soon as possible, with minimal handling and preferably in a *darkened* vehicle. • *If not yet convulsing,* wash off as much from the body as possible—soap and water will suffice. (This only applies in cases of skin absorption. If dog has swallowed the poison, take to vet as soon as possible.) An emetic should only be used if muscle tremors are not present.	Samples of vomit or bowel motions should be collected if malicious poisoning is suspected.
Chlorine	Water sterilizers. Swimming pool water contains too low a concentration of chlorine to cause acute poisoning.	Reddened eyes and sometimes mouth if strong solutions contacted.	If in eye wash out well. If much is swallowed, a little milk may ease discomfort.	
Cosmetics		Most are fairly non-toxic. After shave lotion and perfume may contain a lot of alcohol but their powerful smell is unattractive to dogs.		
Detergents		Vomiting and frothing or foaming at mouth. Diarrhea.		Dogs are not attracted much. Low toxicity.
Disinfectants				Dogs are not attracted much. Low toxicity.
Drain cleaner	See "Alkali."			Very dangerous and corrosive.
Felt pens		Non-toxic.		

Name	Source	Signs	Immediate home treatment	Comments
Flea collars		Allergic reaction (reddening) of the skin of neck, eyes.		Do not use a flea collar unless fleas are a problem.
Glass		Ground glass and/or small glass chips do not seem to cause any damage. Large pieces could cut the intestine and even perforate the gut, but the authors have never known a dog to eat any.	If large amount or large piece swallowed do not induce vomiting. Surgery may be necessary.	Ground glass is not established to be fatal.
Golf ball centres	Golf balls.	Nil. Non-toxic.	Phone your vet if you suspect a golf ball has been swallowed.	Main danger is as a "foreign body" causing bowel blockage (see p. 105).
Hexachloro-phene	Skin creams etc. e.g., Phisohex.	In very young pups can cause brain damage. The signs are dullness and listlessness. In theory the damage is temporary, but permanent damage has been known to occur.		Do not use Phisohex on very young dogs (up to 6 weeks of age).
Kerosene (paraffin)	Heating and lighting fuel, cleaning fluids.	Abdominal pain.	Give milk and vegetable oil. *Then* purgative such as sodium sulphate, (glauber salts 10-25 g). Take to vet.	
Lead (Note "Lead" pencils do not contain lead.)	Lead-based paints—primers. (These are less common now but *were* very common, therefore be very suspicious of old painted objects.) Linoleum, batteries, putty, some lubricants, lead weights (sinkers, curtain weights, etc.), solder, some pipes.	First the dog gets gut signs, then nervous signs. *Gut signs:* (in about 9 out of 10 dogs poisoned by lead) Abdominal pain ("colic"). Vomiting. Appetite loss. *Nervous signs:* These signs follow the gut signs. They vary from dog to dog, so do not expect all of them—dog looks worried, even hysterical. Nervousness, whining. Dislike of light (photophobia). Inco-ordination and staggering. Eventual paralysis.	Lead poisoning can be fatal if untreated. Treatment is usually effective if started early enough. Your vet will probably need to do blood tests to confirm the diagnosis as the signs are not specific for lead poisoning. Induce vomiting if substances containing lead have been eaten within previous half hour.	Usually happens to young dogs due partly to their youthful appetite and curiosity. Chronic, slow build up of poisonous levels can occur.
Match heads (NB: Striking surface contains red phosphorus which is non-toxic.)	Matches.	Contains potassium chlorate. Causes stomach irritation and vomiting if enough are eaten. Pups usually chew the wood rather than eat the ends.		

Name	Source	Signs	Immediate home treatment	Comments
Metaldehyde (snail poisoning)	Slug and snail poisoning.	Inco-ordination and muscle tremors, twitching convulsions, continuous salivation.	Get to a vet. Induce vomiting as soon as possible. If treatment is commenced soon enough, the outlook is reasonable.	Snail poisons may be attractive to dogs. Lock the packets away and do not heap the poison, but scatter it over the garden.
Methylated spirits		Refer "Alcohol" (methylated spirits is 95 per cent alcohol). Poisoning is rare due to unattractive smell and terrible taste.		
Organo-phosphate carbamate	Insecti-cides—via skin, mouth or lungs. Some worming preparations.	Muscle tremors and twitching. Profuse drooling. Often dog will urinate, pass motions. Difficulty in breathing—eventually paralysis of the breathing muscles and death. Sometimes paralysis of the hind legs.	None. Take to vet. Wash off any excess poison with cold water or soap and cold water.	Common.
Paracetamol	Type of pain killer.	After few days liver damage may occur and signs include yellow membranes, vomiting, diarrhea, restlessness, depression, abdominal pain.		
Phenol (carbolic acid)	Some disinfectants, fungicides, wood preservatives, some photographic developers (can be absorbed through the skin).	Staggering, twitching. Depression, leading to a coma. Muscle twitching can be very severe.	Give milk, egg and/or oil. *Then* purge. Wash off any excess phenol (use methylated spirit).	Never use disinfectants on dogs unless the label specifically allows use on dogs. If so, follow the instructions strictly.
Strychnine	Pesticides.	Apprehension, tenseness and stiffness, progressing to violent seizures or convulsions, stiffness of the limbs. These seizures last from a few seconds to minutes. Convulsions become more frequent and death occurs in 1-2 hours.	None. Induce vomiting and get to a vet as soon as possible.	Get to vet as soon as possible. Any suspected source matter should be collected. Strychnine is one of the most common agents used by malicious poisoners.
Tobacco	Cigarettes.	Vomiting due to irritation.	Charcoal tablets.	If vomiting is severe, consult your vet.

Name	Source	Signs	Immediate home treatment	Comments
Warfarin (Ratsac)	Rat and mice poisoning.	Is a blood anticoagulant (stops blood clotting) therefore signs are related to bleeding, and vary according to site of bleeding. Sometimes the dog has difficulty breathing and there may be blood in the vomit or bowel motions. The heart rate is fast and weak, and there may be small hemorrhages or blood spots on the gums. Weakness progresses to staggering, collapse and death.	Treat gently. Do not knock, bump or handle roughly, as bleeding may be increased. Keep warm. Get to a vet as soon as possible as antidote is highly successful if given early.	These poisons can be attractive to dogs. Keep Warfarin in a closed cupboard. When using rat poison make sure the dog has no access.
1080 (sodium fluoroacetate)	Vermin poison for rats, rabbits, foxes, etc.	Signs occur half to 2 hours after eating. Intermittent excitement and depression. Convulsions. Vomiting, urinating and repeated bowel motion. Death in 2-12 hours.	Nil. Induce vomiting but get to vet immediately.	Cats are less susceptible than dogs. Treatment may be successful in mild cases.

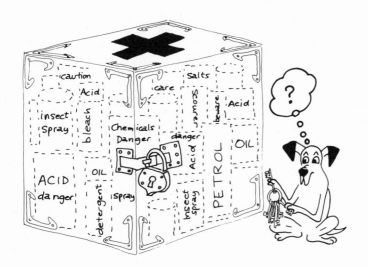

22. Cancer

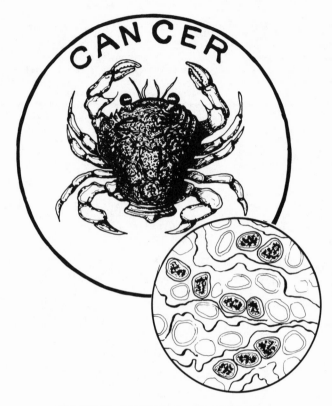

CANCER (TUMORS, GROWTHS)

A cancer is a growth which is beyond the body's control. Few words evoke such fear as cancer. We should bear in mind many cancers are treatable and some do not even require treatment. Although cancer can be a serious or fatal condition it is *not* an inevitable death sentence.

To understand this chapter, a few terms must be explained:

Neoplasm (noun):   Any new growth or growths usually referring
Neoplasia: to tumors.
Neoplastic (adjective):

Cancer: Any malignant neoplasm tumor.
Tumor = swelling/lump: A new growth of cells or tissues characterized by lack of control by the host's body. "Tumor" can refer to a *harmless* lump or a *harmful* cancer.

BENIGN TUMOR

One that grows by expanding or swelling from within somewhat like a balloon being blown up. A benign tumor is usually surrounded by a capsule.

*, **, *** indicate increasing likelihood of a particular trait or problem occurring.

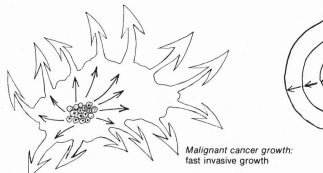

Malignant cancer growth:
fast invasive growth

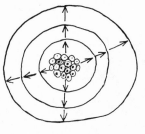

Benign tumor growth:
slow growth. The tumor
expands like a balloon being
blown up

*22.2 Malignant tumors are
invasive and destructive,
while benign tumors grow
to passively occupy space*

If my dog has a benign tumor, should it be removed?

The vet will decide each case on its own merits. The position of the tumor must be considered. A growth on an elbow or eyelid could worry a dog even though it is not life threatening. Benign tumors may be knocked, or ulcerate, bleed or otherwise cause inconvenience and the vet may recommend removal for these reasons.

LIPOMA (FAT TUMOR)

Lipomas are very common, especially in older dogs and in Labradors*, Terriers* and overweight dogs. They are composed of fat tissue and grow very slowly. They are usually found just under the skin.

They feel soft, have smooth borders and, as they are not very firmly attached, can usually be moved around under the skin. Lipomas are usually small, varying from a tiny size to a few cms in diameter. Occasionally lipomas become very large and "melon" sized.

> Lipomas are almost invariably benign.

BREAST TUMORS (mammary tumors)

Breast tumors account for over half the total number of tumors in bitches. Mammary tumors are much more common in bitches over 6 years of age, especially if they have not had any litters, and are rare in bitches that have been spayed *before* they are 2 years of age. After 2 years, spaying appears to make little difference to the incidence of breast cancer. Males are rarely affected.

These tumors are felt first as irregularly shaped, firm masses within the mammary glands (Fig. 22:3). An observant owner may discover them when they are only pea-sized and smaller. If neglected, they can become very large and some types spread to involve many or all of the bitch's 5 sets of mammary glands.

Early detection of breast cancer means that if surgery is needed, it is less extensive and more likely to be successful.

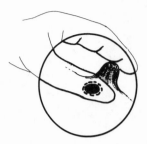

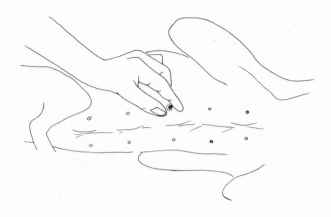

22.3 *Early detection of breast cancer: regularly feel both rows of mammary glands for swelling or lumps. These are easier to feel in bitches than in human females, as there is very little breast tissue present in the non-lactating bitch. Growths larger than ½ cm should be discussed with your vet*

> Feel your bitch's mammary glands regularly for
> any lumps or nodules.

MALIGNANT TUMOR (cancer)

A cancer grows out from its borders, invading and destroying surrounding tissues. Cancerous cells may break away from the parent tumor and take root some distance away. Such tumors are termed "secondaries" (the parent tumor being called the "primary").

> Malignant tumors are progressive and can spread, rapidly.

The treatment of malignant growths

If a malignant tumor is suspected it should be removed at the earliest opportunity. This is not always possible: the tumor may already have spread, either branching out locally or by seeding tumor cells to other parts of the body ("secondaries").

As an alternative to surgery, new treatment methods are being developed. The use of X-rays to destroy malignant cells is very effective in some cases but in veterinary medicine this form is not always available. Sometimes radioactive needles are inserted into a tumor. The radioactivity emitted is capable of destroying some tumors without affecting surrounding healthy tissues. Drug treatment (or "chemotherapy") is still in its infancy, but effective safe drugs to control cancers may soon be developed.

How can we tell the difference between a benign growth and the much more dangerous malignant tumor?

Some types of tumors are fairly easily recognized and the vet can give you a confident assessment of their usual course and likely dangers. But no matter how "typical" a tumor appears to be, the final diagnosis can only be

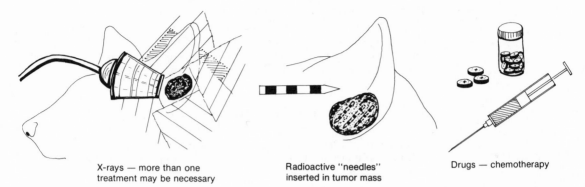

X-rays — more than one
treatment may be necessary

Radioactive "needles"
inserted in tumor mass

Drugs — chemotherapy

22.4 Treatment of malignant cancer: various methods may be employed, depending on the site of the tumour, its size and other factors, which are discussed in the text

made by a pathologist. By studying the microscopic structure of a tumor, pathologists determine how it will behave and whether it is likely to recur after removal. Many tumors are not easily classified as benign or malignant but lie somewhere between.

Common characteristics of benign vs malignant skin tumors

This chart is a guide only. Tumors can be deceptive and do not always follow the rules.

	Benign	**Malignant**
Rate of growth:	Slow	Usually fast
Shape:	Regularly shaped, often rounded or oval with well-defined borders.	Irregular in shape, often hard to determine where the growth finishes.
Pain:	Often does not worry the dog at all—but it depends on the position of the tumor.	Often inflamed—area may be swollen, painful. Varies with the stage of growth of the tumor.
Other features:	Often can be moved slightly.	Held firm to surrounding tissues.

What are some of the difficulties in offering a firm prognosis?

Although we speak of "benign" and "malignant" tumors it is not really as clear cut as that as there are degrees of malignancy. Some malignant tumors rarely spread, or perhaps only after a very long period of growth. On the other hand, we can never be to confident. A tumor which has been termed benign may change its nature and become malignant, although this is not particularly common.

If my dog has a malignant tumor, what should I do?

If a malignant tumor is suspected, the situation is serious.
Some malignant tumors spread very quickly. If the tumor has already spread, for example, to the lungs or liver, it is pointless to operate.

Euthanasia offers a comfortable release from a cancer which has spread.

A malignant tumor may be so large or extensive that it is impossible or extremely difficult to remove, e.g., tumors of bone, liver, lung or pancreas, however malignant tumors involving the skin can often be completely removed, so the prognosis for a successful outcome can be good.

THE OLD DOG AND CANCER

Cancer tends to be more common in old dogs. If a very old dog is suffering from a malignancy, surgery is not always the kindest thing to do. Euthanasia is considered before suffering starts.

Do dogs get leukemia?

Leukemia in the dog is usually called lymphosarcoma or malignant lymphoma. It is a different disease to that of man and resists treatment. Leukemia may show in a variety of ways—from a general slowing down of the body, lumps appearing under the skin to uncomfortable red eyes. Diagnosis is by examination of a blood sample or tissue section (lymph node biopsy) from the dog.

22.5 *Dogs over five years of age seem more susceptible to many forms of cancer*

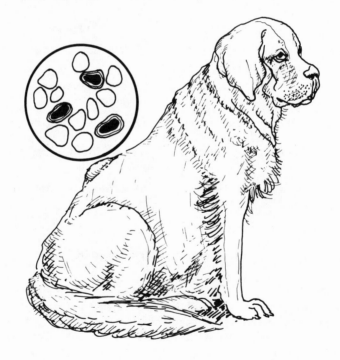

23. The old dog

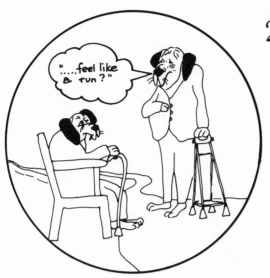

As your dog ages he needs extra care and attention as there is a greater likelihood of him developing chronic problems, such as heart or kidney disease. Aging is inevitable and irreversible, but early recognition of warning signs allows you to protect him from unnecessary discomfort.

> Some conditions attributed to old age are diseases that are treatable and may be cured.

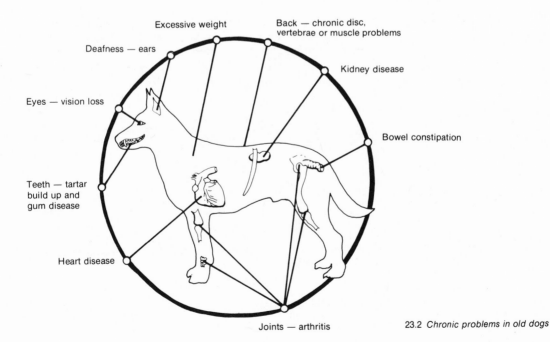

23.2 *Chronic problems in old dogs*

For how long do dogs live?

Few dogs live past 16 years of age and for some breeds the expected life span is much shorter. Large breeds such as the Great Dane and Scottish Deerhound have a life expectancy of only 8 or 9 years, while others, such as the terrier breeds, can be expected to live for 12-15 years. The greatest age reliably recorded for a dog is 27¼ years for "Adjutant," a black Labrador who died in England in 1963.

23.3 One year of a dog's life does not equal seven of a man's. See the chart to find out the equivalent human age of your dog

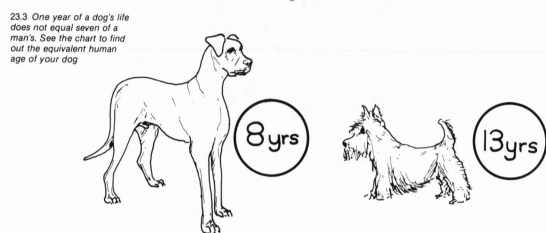

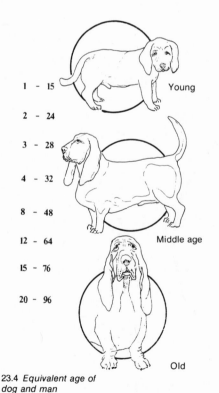

1 - 15   Young

2 - 24

3 - 28

4 - 32

8 - 48

12 - 64   Middle age

15 - 76

20 - 96

Old

23.4 Equivalent age of dog and man

It is often said that one year of a dog's life equals seven of a man, but this is inaccurate. A pup develops very rapidly in his early months and by a year has far outstripped the relative development of a 7-year-old child. As early as 8 months a bitch is sexually active and capable of becoming pregnant—somewhat more advanced than a 5-year-old child.

A French vet called Dr Lebeau has worked out a realistic guide to the equivalent ages of dog and man:

Age of dog	Equivalent age of man
1 year	15 years
2 years	24 years
3 years	28 years
4 years	32 years
8 years	48 years
12 years	64 years
15 years	76 years
20 years	96 years

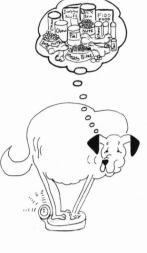

WEIGHT AND DIET

Overweight dogs do not live for as long as they otherwise would. Obesity puts an extra strain not only on the heart, lungs and joints, but, indirectly, on all vital organs.

> With age, dogs become less active. They need less food for their daily needs as they burn less energy.

Avoid rich and starchy foods such as bread, biscuits, all sweet foods and "treats." Reduce the amount of milk, cereals or dry food.

If your dog is already overweight, read the section on obesity (see pp. 86-7). Dieting a dog is usually more successful if the daily intake is decreased over a 3 week period. Also weigh the dog weekly and note his weight and chart your progress. Bear in mind that weight loss should be gradual and slow; a few hundred grams lost each week is good enough.

The average-sized elderly dog (weighing about 20 kg or 44 lbs) needs about 60 calories per kg of bodyweight daily. This figure can vary greatly from dog to dog and according to exercise.

A good canned dog food supplies about one calorie per gram. The semi-moist foods supply 3 calories per gram and the dry food 4 calories per gram. (These figures are a guide only as there is great variation between individual products.)

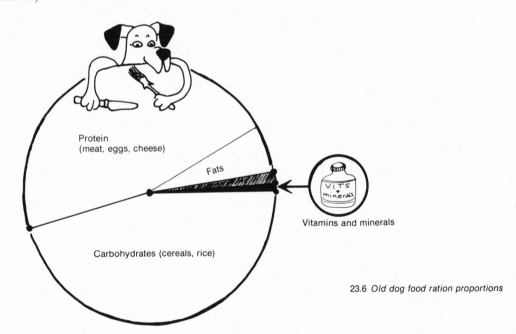

23.6 *Old dog food ration proportions*

Although the older dog is fed less, the ration must supply all essential nutrients, and should contain:

Protein
(e.g., meat, egg, cheese)

Should account for no more than 50 per cent of the dog's total intake.

Carbohydrates (e.g., cereals, rice, pasta)	Should be cooked to make them more digestible.
Fats	The diet should contain *some* fat, but fat is high in calories and can be difficult to digest, therefore only give a small amount.
	Commercial dog foods contain sufficient fats, so it is *not* necessary to add any fat.
Vitamins and minerals	Old dogs usually benefit from a vitamin and mineral supplement.

CONSTIPATION

The old dog's bowel loses muscle "tone" and this could lead to constipation or diarrhea. Constipation could also be caused by prostate enlargement in males or conditions such as a rectal diverticulum. The bowel motions can be made regular by adding bran cereals, Normacol or Isogel granules to the diet. Foods that are known to cause constipation, such as bones, should be avoided.

Passing wind

A common complaint from owners is that their beloved pet is putting a strain on the relationship by passing a lot of foul wind (flatus/farting).

Foods that increase the amount of gas or wind passed include beans, cabbage, root vegetables, soybeans, onions and cauliflower. Large quantities of milk may also cause a lot of gas to be passed. (To avoid the passing of wind see p. 103 on the gastro-intestinal system.)

KIDNEY PROBLEMS

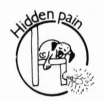

The kidneys are the first organs to fail in many old dogs. The warning signs include excessive thirst and passing of greater amounts of urine than normal; increased hunger (this happens at first, later there may be a *lack* of appetite); weight loss; foul breath; dark bowel motions; listlessness; vomiting and loss of skin tone.

A urine sample can be quickly analysed by the vet and, if necessary, further tests taken to determine how efficiently the kidneys are working.

23.7 *Excessive thirst may be a sign of kidney disease*

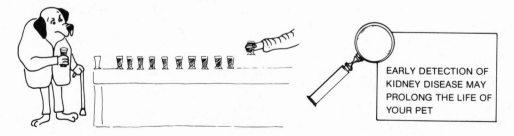

EARLY DETECTION OF KIDNEY DISEASE MAY PROLONG THE LIFE OF YOUR PET

URINE DRIBBLING IN OLDER FEMALE DOGS

A common problem in spayed bitches is urinary incontinence—they start to dribble urine, usually continuously. Owners often report that their old pet is apparently surprised to find she has wet the floor or her bed. Fortunately, in most cases, this condition is easily remedied by giving a small supplement of the female sex hormone, estrogen. This results in an improvement in the muscle tone of the bladder, especially the bladder sphincter muscle.

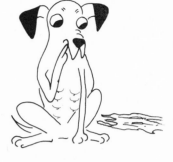

23.8 *Urinary incontinence*

HEART

Heart disease is the major killer of humans. This is not so in dogs, but heart disease is still a very important condition and if recognized early enough allows more effective treatment to minimize your pet's distress.

Warning signs include a cough, especially at night or on first waking in the morning, decreased exercise tolerance, fluid build-up in the abdomen (seen as a "pot" belly), panting and listlessness (see p. 127-8).

THE JOINTS

Arthritis and rheumatics: see p. 189-90.

THE SENSES CHANGE WITH AGE

Ears

Unhappily many older dogs go deaf and there is little that can be done. Fortunately, the deaf dog copes well at home. Clearing the ear canal of wax with an ear wax solvent may help, e.g., Waxsol, Ceramol.

23.9 *The joints: arthritis is quite common in older dogs, especially those of large breeds or in dogs with poorly formed legs, such as Bassets*

> Beware of hearing loss in the old dog. A road accident can result
> if he wanders on the streets or even around driveways.

Eyes

Generally speaking old age alone does not cause vision loss. Blindness is caused by *disease* of the eye.

One common condition of the eye that is associated with age is a characteristic "blue" look. This is because the protein that forms the lens of the eye gradually hardens to become slightly cloudy. The lens, which is normally invisible, becomes more obvious. In spite of aging, light penetrates through an old lens and the dog can still see well.

> A blue lens from old age should not be confused with a
> white lens or cataract. Cataracts can cause blindness—
> a blue lens does not.

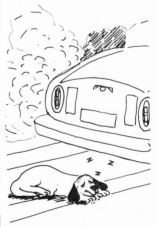

23.10 *Always be very careful when backing out of your driveway if your old dog has a hearing problem*

23.11 *The senses*

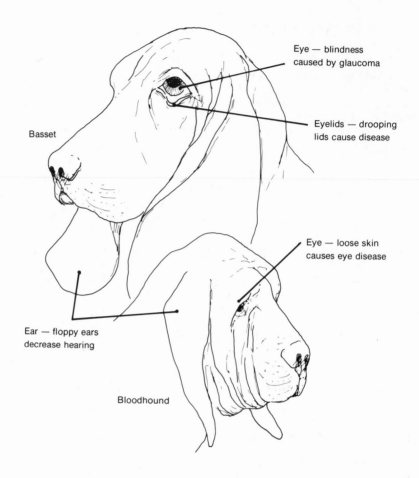

Basset

Eye — blindness
caused by glaucoma

Eyelids — drooping
lids cause disease

Eye — loose skin
causes eye disease

Ear — floppy ears
decrease hearing

Bloodhound

EUTHANASIA

Most of us hope that when the time comes our beloved pet will quietly pass away one night. If not, then a difficult decision will have to be faced: should you have your dog's life painlessly ended or should you persevere with treatment to ease discomfort and prolong life? The decision is never easy, but for your dog's sake you must weigh up the future carefully. Is there any joy left for him? Is treatment available which will give a reasonable chance of recovery to a near normal life? If the answer is no, then you owe it to your pet to be brave enough to make the decision for euthanasia. Euthanasia means he can die quietly and with dignity and without unnecessary pain.

Euthanasia is painlessly performed by a vet who will simply inject your dog with an anesthetic overdose. It is a gentle, swift and humane exit that will cause the dog no distress.

HOW TO TELL IF YOUR DOG IS DEAD

If your dog is found lying apparently dead after an accident, poisoning or due to old age the following will help you decide if the dog is dead:

• **Breathing stops:** This may be checked by holding a mirror next to the nose. Any breath will cause a fogging on the mirror's surface.

• **Heart stops:** Heartbeat is normally felt on the left side of the chest just behind and below the point of the elbow (see below).

• **Eyes—no reflex:** Touch corners of the eyelids or the surface of the eyeball with the tip of your finger. If the dog is dead there will be no blink. The position of the eye may help you. When the dog is asleep or not conscious the lids are closed and the third eyelid moves across the eye hiding the eyeball from sight. Following sudden death the eyelids are open and the eyeball is easily seen. The eye also feels softer.

• **Wide pupil:** The pupil is widely dilated in the dead dog.
Later on the dead dog will go stiff from rigor mortis.

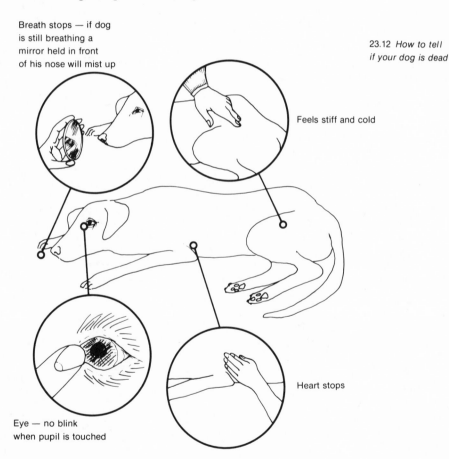

Breath stops — if dog is still breathing a mirror held in front of his nose will mist up

23.12 *How to tell if your dog is dead*

Feels stiff and cold

Heart stops

Eye — no blink when pupil is touched

Appendix

TEMPERATURE

The normal temperature of the dog is approximately
101.3°F (± 1.0°F) or 38.3°C (± 0.5°C)

Why the body temperature varies

The dog's temperature rises and falls a little every day, being slightly higher, for example, in the evening than in the early morning. The temperature

rises after exercise	*falls* in cold weather (by 1° or 2°F)
when the dog is excited	during sleep
in hot weather	

Young dogs experience greater ranges of body temperature than older dogs, and react more to various stresses. For example, a young dog with an infection may run a high fever of 104° or 105°F, while an old dog with the same infection may have little or no temperature rise.

In general, a temperature of over 103°F (30.5°C) in a dog (assuming normal conditions, that is, no hot weather) indicates a focus of inflammation in the body—perhaps due to bacterial or viral infection.

HOW TO TAKE A DOG'S TEMPERATURE

A dog's temperature is taken by inserting a thermometer into the rectum. A thermometer with a short, stubby bulb should be used. (Thermometers with long, thin bulbs are designed for use in human mouths. They are more liable to break than stubby bulb thermometers.)

Temperature taking

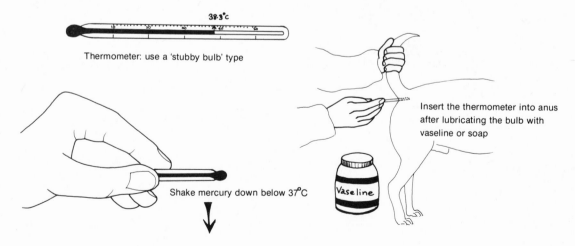

38.3°C

Thermometer: use a 'stubby bulb' type

Shake mercury down below 37°C

Insert the thermometer into anus after lubricating the bulb with vaseline or soap

Vaseline

1. Shake the thermometer until the silver column of mercury reads less than 37°C (98.5°F). Hold the thermometer by its top end, and with a flicking action of the wrist, force the column of mercury back into the bulb.

2. Lubricate the bulb with vaseline or soap.

3. Lift the dog's tail, insert the thermometer into the anus and gently push it in to about one-third of the thermometer length. *Never* force it. If there is resistance, maintain a gentle pressure and rotate the thermometer clockwise and anticlockwise and it will slip in eventually.

4. Leave the thermometer in for 15-20 seconds. Discourage the dog from sitting while the thermometer is in place.

5. Remove, and wipe with cotton wool, then read to the top of the mercury column.

NOTE: • *Never* clean a thermometer with warm water. It may shatter.

        • *If* the thermometer breaks while in the dog's rectum, do not try to fish it out. The dog will usually pass it in his next motion; the mercury in the thermometer is not toxic.

PULSE

With each heart beat, a pulse of blood can be felt coursing through the major arteries. This pulse is most readily felt where an artery runs near the surface and over a bone—such as in your wrist.

The easiest place to find your dog's pulse is the inside of the hind leg, about midway between knee and hip. The femoral artery runs along the thigh bone here.

Feel for the pulse with the balls of your fingers (don't use your thumb—sometimes you can be confused by your own pulse which can be quite strong in the thumb).

Feel for a distinct groove between the muscles and you will detect the hardness of the thigh bone beneath. The femoral artery runs over this bone and by using gentle pressure you should be able to detect the pulse. Be patient and don't press too hard.

Count the number of pulses through the artery over 15 seconds. Multiply by 4, and you have the rate per minute.

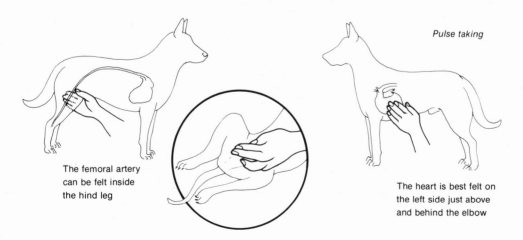

Pulse taking

The femoral artery can be felt inside the hind leg

The heart is best felt on the left side just above and behind the elbow

Normal resting pulse rate:

		Range
Small dogs	130	(110-140)
Medium dogs	100	(90-115)
Large dogs	80	(60-90)

Variations in the pulse rate can be normal. The pulse rate rises:
- After exercise,
- When frightened,
- When hot,
- With age (as the heart becomes less efficient);

The pulse rate falls:
- When asleep
- If very fit (e.g., Greyhound in training),
- In some specific heart diseases.

RATE OF BREATHING (respiration rate)

Normal 18, (range 12-35) breaths per minute.
Large breeds tend to have lower respiration rates than small or toy breeds.

GESTATION PERIOD (length of pregnancy)

63 days (range 59-66 days)

COMMON MEASURES

1 teaspoon	=	5 mls
1 dessertspoon	=	8 mls
1 tablespoon	=	15 mls
1 cup	=	240 mls
1 pint	=	480 mls
1 fluid ounce	=	30 mls

Note: One ml occupies a volume of one cc and measurements of mls and cc are interchangeable.

TEMPERATURES

°C	°F
37	98.6 (normal for human)
38	100.5
38.5	101.3 (normal for dog)
39	102.2
39.5	103.1
40	104
40.5	105

USEFUL HOUSEHOLD DRUGS

Drug	Use	Dose
Aspirin	Pain relief (also decreases inflam-mation in the eye)	10 mg per kg—one-third of a tablet per 22 lbs (10 kg) every 12 hours (one tablet contains 300 mg). Note: Cats are dosed no more than every 52 hours.
Charcoal	Diarrhea, flatulence	1 tablespoon in 4 ozs. water per 30 lbs (13½ kg). 2-6 tablets 3 or 4 times daily.
Dramamine	Travel sickness	25-50 mg 1 hour before travel.
Glauber's Salts (Sodium Sulphate)	Constipation	1 teaspoon per 10 lbs (5kg).
Hydrogen Peroxide	As emetic	2 teaspoons per 30 lbs (13½ kg) every 10 minutes for 3 doses, or until dog vomits.
	As antiseptic	3% solution.
Kaopectate	Diarrhea	1 teaspoon per 5 lbs (2¼ kg) every 4 hours.
Milk of Magnesia	Gastritis, diarrhea	1 teaspoon per 5-10 lbs (2¼-4½ kg) every 6 hours.
Mineral Oil (liquid paraffin)	Constipation	1 teaspoon per 5 lbs (2¼ kg).
Phenylbutazone (Butazolidine)	Pain (also decreases eye inflammation)	100 mg 2 or 3 times daily. Do not persist for more than 24 hours without veterinary advice.
Senokot granules	Constipation	1 teaspoon to 1 dessertspoon daily.
Salt (sodium chloride)	Emetic	2 teaspoons in a cup of warm water.
Syrup of Ipecac	Emetic	1-2 mls per kg.

These drugs may be used if veterinary attention is not readily available. If signs of disease persist or are severe, call your vet at once.

THE MEDICAL CUPBOARD

Antiseptic, e.g., Liquid Savlon/Cetavlon
Cotton buds
Cotton wool
Flea powder

Flea rinse, e.g., Nuvanol/Malathion

Gauze bandages. A two-inch bandage is also used to muzzle the injured dog, p. 15.

Insecticidal cream for fly-bitten ears

Nail clippers and/or file

Roundworm remedy, e.g., Antoban (routine for pups)

Salicylic acid 5 per cent, tannic 5 per cent in alcohol for moist spots on the skin (STA solution)

Scissors

Sebum dissolving shampoo, e.g., Seleen, to remove excess oil or scales on skin

Stubby bulb thermometer

10 ml syringe/or rubber bulb for flushing out pus, foreign body from the eye or for cleaning wounds

Tweezers

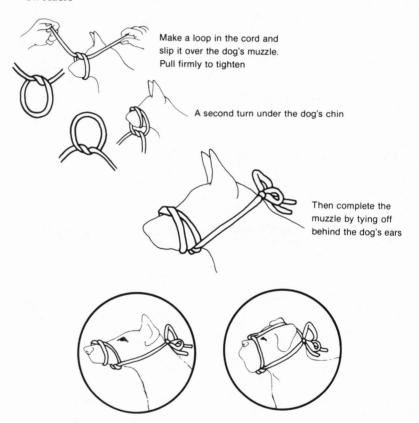

Applying a muzzle use a pyjama cord or a tie, a bandage or a piece of broad cordage. (Narrow rope or string may cut into the skin)

Make a loop in the cord and slip it over the dog's muzzle. Pull firmly to tighten

A second turn under the dog's chin

Then complete the muzzle by tying off behind the dog's ears

Veterinary drugs

- Make sure all retain their labels.
- Discard *all* old medications.
- Do not home dose with veterinary treatments.
- Keep drugs out of reach of children.
- Cortisone is described by many names. It can be dangerous if e.g., incorrectly used in the eye.

SIZE OF DOGS

Toy Dogs Less than 5 kg	Small Dogs 5-10 kg	Medium Dogs 10-25 kg	Large Dogs More than 25 kg	(kg x 2.2 = lb)
Affenpinscher	Australian	Australian Cattle	Afghan Hound	
Australian Silky	Terrier	Dog	Airedale Terrier	
Terrier	Border Terrier	Australian Kelpie	Bloodhound	
Chihuahua	Boston Terrier	Basenji	Borzoi	
Chinese Crested	Bull Terrier	Basset Hound	Boxer	
Dog	(Miniature)	Beagle	British Bulldog	
Dachshund	Cairn Terrier	Bedlington	Bull Mastiff	
(Miniature)	Cavalier King	Bull Terrier	Chow Chow	
English Toy	Charles	Elkhound	Collie	
Terrier	Spaniel	Finnish Spitz	Dalmatian	
Griffon	Dachshund	French Bulldog	Deerhound	
Bruxellois	(Standard)	Hungarian Puli	Doberman	
Italian	Dandie Dinmont	Irish Terrier	Foxhound	
Greyhound	Terrier	Keeshond	German	
Japanese Chin	Fox Terrier	Kerry Blue Terrier	Shorthaired	
Maltese	King Charles	Poodle (Standard)	Pointer	
Miniature	Spaniel	Schnauzer	German Shepherd	
Pinscher	Lakeland Terrier	Scottish Terrier	Dog	
Papillon	Manchester	Sealyham Terrier	Giant Schnauzer	
Pekingese	Terrier	Shetland	Great Dane	
Poodle (Toy)	Norfolk Terrier	Sheepdog	Greyhound	
Pomeranian	Norwich Terrier	Skye Terrier	Hungarian Vizsla	
Yorkshire	Poodle	Spaniel (Cocker)	Irish Wolfhound	
Terrier	(Miniature)	Spaniel (Cocker,	Mastiff	
	Pug	American)	Newfoundland	
	Schipperke	Spaniel (Field)	Old English	
	Schnauzer	Spaniel (Springer,	Sheepdog	
	(Miniature)	English)	Pharaoh Hound	
	Shih Tzu	Spaniel (Springer,	Pointer	
	Lhasa Apso	Welsh)	Pyrenean	
	Tibetan Spaniel	Spaniel (Sussex)	Mountain Dog	
	West Highland	Staffordshire Bull	Retriever	
	White Terrier	Terrier	(Golden,	
		Tibetan Terrier	Labrador)	
		Welsh Corgi	Rhodesian	
		Welsh Terrier	Ridgeback	
		Whippet	Rottweiler	
			St Bernard	
			Saluki	
			Samoyed	
			Setter (English,	
			Irish, Gordon)	
			Smooth Collie	
			Spaniel (Clumber,	
			Irish Water)	
			Weimaraner	

USUAL WEIGHT RANGE OF HOUND BREEDS

Breed	Dogs (kg)	Bitches (kg)
Afghan Hound	27-32	23-30
Basenji	11	10
Basset Hound	18-27	16-23
Beagle	13-16	11-13
Bloodhound	41-45	36-45
Borzoi	32-39	23-32
Dachshund (Long Haired)	8	8
Dachshund (Smooth Haired)	11	10
Dachshund (Wire Haired)	9-10	8-9
Dachshund Miniature (Long Haired)	5	5
Dachshund Miniature (Smooth Haired)	5	5
Dachshund Miniature (Wire Haired)	5	5
Deer Hound	39-45	30-36
Elkhound	23	20
Finnish Spitz	11-16	11-13
Foxhound	32	32
Greyhound	30-32	27-30
Irish Wolfhound	55	41
Pharaoh Hound	23	20
Rhodesian Ridgeback	34-39	30-34
Saluki	20-27	16-23
Whippet	10-13	8-11

USUAL WEIGHT RANGE OF GUNDOGS

Breed	Dogs (kg)	Bitches (kg)
German Shorthaired Pointer	25-32	20-27
Hungarian Vizsla	23-27	23-27
Retriever (Curly Coated)	32-36	32-36
Retriever (Flat Coated)	27-32	27-32
Retriever (Golden)	30-32	25-27
Retriever (Labrador)	27	25
Setter (English)	27-30	25-28
Setter (Gordon)	30	25
Setter (Irish)	27-30	25-27
Spaniel (Clumber)	25-32	20-27
Spaniel (Cocker)	11-13	11-13
Spaniel (Cocker, American)	11-13	11-13
Spaniel (Field)	16-23	16-23
Spaniel (Irish Water)	27	27
Spaniel (Springer, English)	23	23
Spaniel (Springer, Welsh)	16-18	16-18
Spaniel (Sussex)	20	18
Pointer	23-25	23-25
Weimaraner	25-30	20-25

Reproduced with permission from *Feeding the Dog and Cat,* Uncle Ben's of Australia.

USUAL WEIGHT RANGE OF THE TERRIER BREEDS

Breed	Dogs (kg)	Bitches (kg)
Airedale Terrier	20-23	20-23
Australian Terrier	4.5-5	4.5-5
Bedlington Terrier	8-10.5	8.10.5
Border Terrier	6-7	5-6
Bull Terrier	18-23	18-23
Bull Terrier (Miniature)	9	9
Cairn Terrier	6	6
Dandie Dinmont Terrier	8	8
Fox Terrier (Smooth)	7-8	7-8
Fox Terrier (Wire)	8-8.5	7-8
Irish Terrier	12	11
Kerry Blue Terrier	15-17	16
Lakeland Terrier	8	7
Manchester Terrier	8	8
Norfolk Terrier	6	6
Norwich Terrier	6	6
Scottish Terrier	8.5-10.5	8.5-10.5
Sealyham Terrier	9	8
Skye Terrier	11	10.5
Staffordshire Bull Terrier	13-17	11-13
Welsh Terrier	9.5	9
West Highland White Terrier	8-9	7-8

USUAL WEIGHT RANGE OF WORKING DOGS

Breed	Dogs (kg)	Bitches (kg)
Australian Cattle Dog	20-22	20-22
Australian Kelpie	20.5-25	18-27
Bearded Collie	20.5-25	18-27
Belgian Shepherd Dog (Groenendael)	24-25	22-24
Border Collie	19-24	18-22
Briard	36-41	32-36
Collie (Rough)	20.5-29.5	18-25
Collie (Smooth)	20.5-29.5	18-25
German Shepherd Dog	34-38.5	27-32
Hungarian Puli	13-15	10-13
Norwegian Buhund	15	14
Old English Sheepdog	27-41	23-27
Shetland Sheepdog	8-10	8-10
Stumpy Tail Cattle Dog	20-22	20-22
Welsh Corgi (Cardigan)	10-12	9-11
Welsh Corgi (Pembroke)	9-11	8-10

Reproduced with permission from *Feeding the Dog and Cat,* Uncle Ben's of Australia.

USUAL WEIGHT RANGE OF THE TOY BREEDS

Breed	Dogs (kg)	Bitches (kg)
Affenpinscher	3.0-3.5	3.0-3.5
Australian Silky Terrier	3.5-4.5	3.5-4.5
Cavalier King Charles Spaniel	4.5-8	4.5-8
Chihuahua (Long Coat)	1-3	1-3
Chihuahua (Smooth Coat)	1-3	1-3
Chinese Crested Dog	5-5.5	5-5.5
English Toy Terrier (Black & Tan)	3-3.5	3-3.5
Griffon Bruxellois	2-4.5	2-5
Italian Greyhound	3-3.5	3-3.5
Japanese Chin	2-4	2-4
King Charles Spaniel	3.5-6	3.5-6
Maltese	2-4	2-4
Miniature Pinscher	3-4	3-4
Papillon	1.5-2	2-3
Pekingese	3-5	3.5-5.5
Pomeranian	2	2-2.5
Pug	6-8	6-8
Yorkshire Terrier	3	3
	(max)	(max)

Reproduced with permission from *Feeding the Dog and Cat,* Uncle Ben's of Australia.

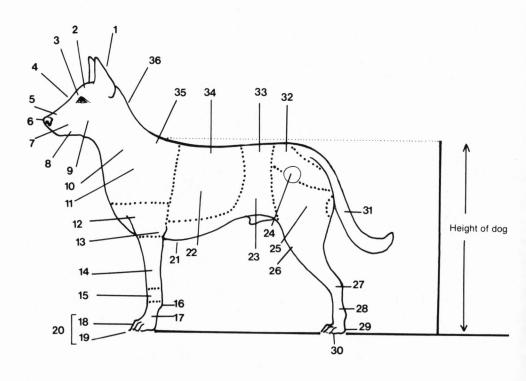

USUAL WEIGHT RANGE OF NON-SPORTING BREEDS

Breed	Dogs (kg)	Bitches (kg)
Boston Terrier	4.5-11	4.5-11
Boxer	30	28
British Bulldog	25	23
Bullmastiff	50-59	41-50
Chow Chow	23-32	18-32
Dalmatian	27	25
Doberman	34-41	29.5-36
French Bulldog	13	11
Great Dane	54.5	45.5
Keeshond	16-23	16-20.5
Lhasa Apso	7	6-7
Mastiff	57-89	57-89
Newfoundland	63.5-68	50-54.5
Poodle (Standard)	9-13.5	9-13.5
Poodle (Miniature)	5.5-7	5.5-7
Poodle (Toy)	3.5-5.5	3.5-5.5
Pyrenean Mountain Dog	45.5-54.5	41-52
Rottweiler	45.5-54.5	36-41
St. Bernard	73-78	63.5-73.5
Samoyed	20.5-25	16-20.5
Schipperke	5.5-7	5.5-7
Schnauzer (Giant)	41-50	41-50
Schnauzer	16-20.5	16-20.5
Schnauzer (Miniature)	7-8	7-8
Shih Tzu	4.5-7	5.5-6
Tibetan Spaniel	4.5-7	4-7
Tibetan Terrier	11-13.5	11-13.5

Reproduced with permission from *Feeding the Dog and Cat,* Uncle Ben's of Australia.

1. Ear
2. Skull
3. Eye
4. Stop
5. Foreface. The foreface, nose and jaws make up the muzzle
6. Nose
7. Jaws. The fleshy parts of the lips and jaws make up the jowls
8. Lips. Pendulous upper lips are called flews
9. Cheek
10. Neck
11. Shoulder
12. Upper arm
13. Elbow
14. Forearm
15. Wrist
16. Stopper pad
17. Pastern (metacarpals)
18. Toes
19. Nails
20. Forefoot
21. Sternum (breastbone)
22. Chest
23. Flank
24. Hip
25. Thigh
26. Stifle (knee)
27. Hock (heel)
28. Rear pastern (metatarsals)
29. Hind foot
30. Pads
31. Tail
32. Croup
33. Loin
34. Back
35. Withers (top of the shoulders)
36. Crest of neck

Glossary

Based on:
  The *A-Z of Australian Family Medicines*, Rosalind Spencer, Butterworths, 1980.
  Black's *Veterinary Dictionary*, edited by Geoffrey West, 13th ed., Adam & Charles Black, London, 1979.
  The Eye in Veterinary Practice, J. R. Blogg, Saunders, Philadelphia, 1980.

Purpose of this glossary:
To assist all your reading and help you understand your vet.

Abdomen: the portion of the body that lies between the chest and the pelvis
Abiotrophy: hereditary degenerative disease of late onset
Abnormality: an irregularity in any organ or system
Abortion: premature expulsion of the fetus
Abrasion: removal of surface layers of skin or eyeball
Abscess: a localized collection of pus, usually enclosed in a wall of fibrous tissue
Accommodation: the adjustment of vision for seeing at different distances. Produced by change in shape of lens
Acetylsalicylic acid: aspirin
Achondroplasia: a hereditary congenital disturbance of growth causing deformed limbs
Acidosis: chemical imbalance due to excess acid
Acquired immunity: immunity resulting from either vaccination or a previous attack of the disease which makes the body resistant to further infection
Action: the way in which a dog walks, trots or runs
Acuity: visual ability to distinguish shapes; applies to central vision
Acute disease: a disease which is rapid in onset
Adhesion: the joining of two structures by fibrous (scar) tissue
Adipose tissue: fat
Adrenal glands: two small organs found next to the kidneys; they secrete various hormones
Adrenalin: a hormone produced in the adrenal gland which has various functions including constriction of blood vessels and stimulation of the heart
Aetiology: the study of causes of a disease
Afterbirth: the tissue delivered after the newborn pup. It comprises the membranes that surround and nourish the pup in the uterus
Agenesis: absence of an organ
Albino: an animal lacking in the pigment melanin, so it is white
Albumin: one of the proteins found in blood
Alimentary canal: digestive system
Allele: one of two or more contrasting
    1. genes (on the same locus in homologous chromosomes)
    2. characters transmitted by alternative genes
Allergen: a compound (usually a protein) that can cause an allergic reaction in susceptible individuals
Allergy: a specific sensitivity which results from exposure to a particular allergen
Alopecia: absence of hair from an area normally covered with hair

Alveoli: the small air sacs within the lung

Amaurosis: blindness, especially blindness without apparent reason—from disease of the retina, optic nerve or brain

Amino acids: the building blocks which form proteins

Anabolic: tissue building; growth

Anemia: a deficiency of red blood cells

Anesthetic: a compound that produces contracted insensibility or unconsciousness

Anal: referring to the anus

Analgesic: a drug which causes loss of pain without loss of consciousness

Anaphylactic: possessing anaphylaxis

Anaphylaxis: an unusual or exaggerated reaction of the animal to a substance, e.g., a severe allergic reaction to a bee sting, or an acute allergic reaction to penicillin

Androgen: male sex hormone

Aneurysm: abnormal localized widening of a blood vessel following weakening of its walls

Ankylosing spondylitis: inflammation of the joints in the backbone which leads to loss of mobility

Anestrus: the state in the femal dog when it is not "in season"

Anomaly: marked deviation from the normal

Anorexia: loss of appetite

Anoxia: lack of oxygen

Antacid: substances which decrease the acidity of the stomach

Anterior: towards the head (a term used in anatomical descriptions)

Anterior chamber: the space filled with fluid (aqueous) in the front part of the eye, behind the cornea

Anthelmintic: a substance used to kill parasitic worms

Antibiotic: a substance derived from a living organism which is capable of killing or inhibiting growth of another organism, especially bacteria

Antibody: a substance found in the blood or other body fluids which has a specific restrictive or destructive action on a foreign protein, i.e., fights against infection

Anticoagulant: substances which prevent blood clotting

Antidote: a compound which neutralizes a poison

Antiemetic: substances which prevent vomiting

Antigen: a protein which enters the body from outside which leads to the formation of antibodies by the white blood cells

Antihistamine: a drug which neutralizes the effect of excess histamine release which can be caused by an allergic reaction

Antipruritic: substances which prevent itching

Antipyretic: substances which lower body temperature in fever

Antiseptic: a compound which kills bacteria and/or virus, used to prevent the harmful results of infection in living tissue

Antitussive: substances which relieve coughing

Anus: the posterior opening of the digestive system

Aorta: the main artery of the body

Aplasia: lack of development of an organ

Aqueous humor; aqueous: clear, watery fluid which fills the front chamber of the eye

Arrhythmia: irregular beating of the heart

Arteriosclerosis: hardening of the arteries

Artery: a blood vessel which carries blood away from the heart. This blood is rich in oxygen

Arthritis: inflammation of a joint

Ascites: swelling of the abdomen with fluid

Ascorbic acid: Vitamin C

Asphyxia: suffocation, due to lack of oxygen in the blood

Aspirin: a pain relieving, fever reducing anti-inflammatory drug

Astigmatism: faulty vision due to rays of light not sharply focused on the retina

Astringent: substances which shrink the outer layers of the skin in order to slow discharges from below the skin

Ataxia: loss of the power of movement, so a staggering step results

Atopic dermatitis: skin inflammation due to hereditary allergy

Atopy: a form of allergy which is hereditary, e.g., asthma, eczema

Atria: the two chambers at the top of the heart. These receive blood from large veins

Atrial septal defect: defect between two of the chambers or atria of the heart

Atrophy
1. a defect or failure of nutrition seen as a wasting away
2. decrease in size of the cell, tissue, organ or part

Atropine: potent drug used to enlarge pupil and reduce eye pain. Bottle of these eye drops can be fatal to children

Aural: relating to the ear

Auricles: another name for atria

Ausculation: a method of diagnosis by which internal organs are examined by listening to the sound they produce, usually with a stethoscope

Auto-immune disease: disease caused by the body producing antibodies against its own cells

Auto-immunity: a disease whereby the body's defence mechanisms act on normal tissues

Auto-immunization: reaction to its own tissues

Autolysis: self digestion

Autopsy: examination of the internal organs of the body after death

Autosomal: attached to an ordinary paired chromosome as distinct from a sex chromosome

Avitaminosis: the condition caused by lack of a vitamin in the diet

Bacteremia: bacteria in the blood stream

Bacteria: a type of micro-organism. Some bacteria cause disease

Bacteriocidal: an agent that kills bacteria

Bacteriostatic: an agent that stops bacteria from growing without actively killing the bacteria

Back-cross: the offspring resulting from mating an animal to one of its parents

Ball & socket: a type of joint where a sphere of bone moves within a cup, e.g., hip

Barbiturates: a family of drugs which can cause sedation or anesthesia

Benign: mild or not serious; not malignant

Beta blockers: drugs used in various heart and circulatory disturbances

Bilateral: on both sides

Bile: a fluid formed in the liver and stored in the gall bladder which aids in digestion

Binocular vision: the ability to use the two eyes simultaneously to focus on the same object and to fuse the two images into a single image

Biopsy: the examination of a specimen from live tissue, usually with a microscope

Bitch: a female dog

Bladder: a sac used for storing fluids, e.g., urinary bladder

Blepharitis: inflammation of the eyelids

Blind spot: blind area where light rays focus on the optic nerve head in the eye

Blindness: lack or loss of ability to see due to disorder of the eye, the pathways from the eye to the brain or in the brain

Bloat: a distended stomach, usually in cattle or sheep

Blood group: a red blood cell type

Blood poisoning: septicemia

Blood pressure: the pressure in the arteries

Blue merle: a color term—blue and grey mixed with black

Bone pinning: a method of treating fractures whereby a pointed, stainless steel pin is driven down the centre of the bone to hold the broken ends in place

Booster inoculations: injections given after the first vaccination to help increase immunity

Boracic acid: a mild antiseptic, now replaced by better drugs

Bowels: intestine

Bow-legs: the long limb bones bend outwards

Boxer ulcer: corneal epithelial erosion—ulcer on the eyeball

Brachycephalic: a skull where the forehead is high and the face is short, e.g., Boxer, Pug

Bradycardia: slow heart beat

Breech birth: a birth where the puppy's hind feet appear first (rather than the head)

Brindle: a color term for black hairs mixed with a lighter color

Brisket (sternum): the bone in the center of the chest joining the ribs

Broad spectrum antibiotic: an antibiotic which acts against a wide range of micro-organisms

Bronchi: the main tubes into which the windpipe divides

Bronchioles: small conducting tubes within the lung

Bronchitis: inflammation of the lining of the tubes in the lung

Bruise: an injury caused by a blow which leads to discoloration of the skin due to a localized collection of blood

Burn: an injury caused by dry heat

Bursa: a small fluid-filled cavity found where unusual pressure occurs, e.g., elbow

Bursitis: inflammation of a bursa

Buttocks: the rump or hips

Caecum: a blind ending sac found at the junction of the small and large intestine

Caesarean section: removal of unborn young from the mother by surgical incision into the uterus

Calamine: a substance used as an astringent and protective agent

Calcification: deposition of calcium salts in a tissue where it is not normally found

Calculi: stones composed of mineral salts found in various parts of the body, e.g., urinary or gall bladder

Calculus: a "stone" formed by the crystallization of certan salts

Callus: a piece of new bone laid down around the ends of a broken bone during the first few weeks after fracture

Calorie: a unit of heat used to give an indication as to the amount of energy in a food

Canaliculus: a small tear drainage tube at the inner corner of the upper and lower eyelids leading from the tear duct opening to the tear sac

Cancer: a malignant tumor, i.e., a tumor which continues to grow and spread at a rapid rate eventually leading to death of the animal, if corrective measures are not undertaken. See also Neoplasm

Candida: a type of fungus

Canine teeth: also called eye teeth. They are the large curved teeth seen towards the front of the mouth

Canker: an old term used to describe inflammation of the external ear

Canthus: the angle at either end of the eyelid opening

Capsule:
1. a soluble case made of gelatin which contains small doses of medicine
2. a protective envelope of fibrous tissue which surrounds certain organs such as the kidney, liver or lens

Carbohydrates: a group of chemical substances including sugars and starches used as an energy source for the body

Carbolic acid: a disinfectant

Carcinoma: a malignant growth which is derived from epithelial tissue, for instance skin or lung tissue

Cardiac: referring to the heart

Cardiac arrhythmia: an irregularity in the heartbeat

Cardiac output: the volume of blood pumped through the heart per minute

Cardiography: the recording of the phases of the heartbeat

Caries: a process of decay of teeth or bones

Carpal subluxation: dislocation above the front paw

Carrier: an animal which has a genetic defect without showing it; or an animal which possesses disease-causing organisms without being affected

Cartilage: a hard but flexible tissue found in certain parts of the skeleton, such as nose, ear or windpipe

Caruncle: small prominence at the corner of the eye near the nose

Castration: the removal of the testicles of male animals

Cataract: clouding of the lens or its capsule

Cataract, immature: a cataract where only part of the lens is involved

Cataract, juvenile: a cataract which develops during the first six years of a dog's life

Cataract, mature (or ripe): a cataract in which the whole lens is involved

Cataract, senile: lens cloudy due to old age. (Note that *all* old lenses become more "blue" with age and this is not disease)

Catarrh: inflammation of mucous membranes, especially the air passages, which leads to the secretion of mucus

Catheter: a soft, flexible tube which is passed into organs or blood vessels, e.g., into the bladder and used to remove urine when the animal is unable to urinate on its own

Caudal: towards the tail (a term used in anatomical descriptions)

Cecum: a blind ending sac found at the junction of the small and large intestine

Cell: the microscopic unit of which all plant and animal tissues are composed

Cellulitis: a rapidly spreading infection found just under the skin

Central nervous system (CNS): the brain and spinal cord

Central retinal atrophy (CRA, CPRA): an inherited disease which leads to degeneration of the retina. Found in some sporting dogs, e.g., Labrador Retriever, Border Collie

Cerebellar hypoplasia: underdeveloped part of the brain called the cerebellum

Cerebral: referring to that part of the brain containing its higher functions, e.g., thought

Cerebrospinal fluid: the fluid bathing the brain and spinal cord

Cervical: referring to the neck

Cervix: opening of the uterus

Cesarean section: removal of unborn young from the mother by surgical incision into the uterus

Chemotherapy: the treatment of disease with chemical substances, especially in relation to cancer

Cherry eye: prolapsed gland of the third eyelid

China eye: a light blue eye

Chlorhexidine: an antiseptic

Choking: obstruction to breathing

Cholecystitis: inflammation of the gall bladder

Cholesterol: a type of fat present in the blood

Chondrodysplasia: faulty cartilage and bone development

Choroid: the middle of the three coats of the eye. It possesses blood vessels which are responsible for nutrition of the retina

Chromosomes: minute bodies found within the cell nucleus which store genetic information

Chronic disease: a disease which lasts for a long time (weeks/months)

Chronic superficial keratitis (CSK): inflamed red mass on the cornea (and third eyelid may also be inflamed)

Ciliary body: a structure in the eye found between the iris and the choroid. It produces aqueous humor and contains the ciliary muscle

Cilium: eyelash

Cleft palate: a defect where the two halves of the roof of the mouth do not fuse

Clotting of blood: the process whereby the fluid portion of blood becomes jelly-like

Coagulation: another name for clotting

Cocaine: a local anesthetic

Cochlea: the region of the ear where sounds are converted to electrical impulses

Codeine: a pain killer

Cod liver oil: an oil rich in Vitamins A and D

Coitus: sexual intercourse

Coliform enteritis: gut infection

Colitis: inflammation of the first part of the large intestine

Collagen: the fibrillar substance of the connective tissue of the cornea and sclera

Collapsed trachea: deformed windpipe

Collie ectasia syndrome: collie eye anomaly

Collie eye anomaly: a common congenital hereditary defect in the back of the eye in Collies and Shetland Sheepdogs

Colobomas of the optic disc: pits in the head of the optic nerve in the eye

Colon: large intestine

Colostrum: the milk secreted by the mother, the first few days after birth. It is different from normal milk and provides the newborn with some defence against infection

Color dilute: possessing genes which dilute the coat color, e.g., merled dogs

Concussion: a temporary loss of consciousness due to an injury to the head

Cones: part of the layer of retina responsible for vision in bright light

Conformation: structure

Congenital: present at birth, not necessarily inherited

Congestion: excessive amount of fluid in a part of the body

Congestive heart failure: the heart is unable to maintain normal pumping of blood, resulting in fluid build-up in lungs and/or abdomen

Conjunctiva: the membrane which lines the eyelids and the front of the eyeball

Conjunctivitis: inflammation of the conjunctiva

Connective tissue: the structural elements of the body

Constipation: inability to defecate

Convulsions: powerful involuntary contractions of muscles

Cornea: transparent portion of the outer coat of the front of the eyeball forming the eye window

Corneal contact lenses: thin plastic lenses which fit directly on the cornea under the eyelids

Corneal graft (keratoplasty): operation to restore vision by replacing a section of opaque cornea with transparent cornea

Corticosteroid: drug used to reduce inflammation; harmful side-effects exist

Cortisone: one of the corticosteroids. It is also a hormone produced naturally in the adrenal gland

Costal: referring to the ribs

Cow-hocks: hocks pointing inwards

Craniomandibular osteopathy: deformity of the jaw

Crepitus: the grating of the broken ends of bones

Cruciate ligaments: a pair of ligaments in the stifle joint which prevent the joint from over-extending

Cryptorchid: a male with one or both undescended testes

CSF: cerebro-spinal fluid

CSK: chronic superficial keratitis—inflamed red mass, e.g., on the cornea and third eyelid

Cushing's disease: the result of production of excess corticosteroid by the adrenal gland

Cutaneous: pertaining to the skin

Cyanosis: lack of oxygen to the tissues which results in a bluish appearance of the lips, tongue, and mucous membranes

Cyclic neutropenia: a fatal blood disorder seen in silver grey Collies

Cyst: a swelling which contains fluid other than pus, whose walls are not inflamed

Cystine: Dicysteine, an amino acid produced by the digestion or acid hydrolysis of proteins. It is sometimes found in the urine and in the kidneys in the form of minute crystals, frequently forming cystine calculus in the bladder

Cystinuria: cystine crystals in urine

Cystitis: inflammation of the bladder

Dacryoadenitis: inflammation of the tear gland (tear-producing gland)

Dacryocystitis: inflammation of the tear sac (drains tears)

Dam: mother

Dapple: mottled marking of different colors due to genes for color dilution

Dark adaptation: ability of the eye to adjust to dim light

Day blindness: blindness during the day, due to faulty cones of the eye

Debridement: removal of damaged tissue from the surface of a wound

Defibrillator: a device which produces an electric shock used for restoring normal activity to the heart

Deformity: disfigurement

Degeneration: a deterioration. A change of a tissue from a higher to a lower or less active functional form

Degenerative pannus: an inflamed red mass, e.g., on the cornea

Dehydration: loss of water from the tissues

Demodex: a type of mite causing skin irritation

Depressed: decreased

Dermatitis: any inflammation of the skin

Dermatology: the branch of medicine concerned with disorders of the skin

Dermoid: a small tumor of skin present at birth on the eye

Dermoid cyst: cyst in the skin

Developmental abnormality: one which occurs between the time of fertilization and the adult stages of development

Dew claw: the first digit, found on the inside of the leg above the foot. It is often absent on the hind paw. It is functionless

Dextrose: a type of sugar

Diabetes insipidus: a disease due to disorder of the hypothalamus gland. The sufferer is unable to concentrate the urine and passes large volumes of very dilute urine

Diabetes mellitus: a condition where there is an excess of glucose in the blood stream and an ability of the body to utilize it

Dialysis: an artificial means of carrying out kidney function

Diamond eye: greatly oversized eyelid opening

Diaphragm: the structure which separates the chest from the abdomen

Diarrhea: increased amounts of and very fluid feces (stools)

Digestion: the preparation of food for absorption through the gut wall

Digitalis: a drug used for heart stimulation

Digits: toes

Dilation: to increase the size of a stricture

Diestrus: the last part of the estrus cycle. During this phase much progesterone is produced, a hormone which allows the maintenance of pregnancy

Diploid: the number of chromosomes found in most cells

Dislocation: movement of a bone from its normal position in relation to a joint

Distemper: a severe contagious viral disease of dogs

Distension: increase in size, usually of a hollow organ

Distichiasis: the presence of two rows of eyelashes on the one eyelid

Diuretic: a substance which promotes the production of urine

Diverticulum: a small outpouching of a hollow organ

DNA: a substance which makes up chromosomes

Docking: removal of part or all of the tail or other parts (ears)

Dolichocephalic: a skull which is long and narrow, e.g., Greyhound or Scotch Collie

Dominant inheritance: member of a gene pair which is capable of overriding the other member

Dropsy: see Edema

Duct: an enclosed channel used for conducting fluid

Duodenum: the first part of the small intestine

Dys-: a prefix meaning painful or difficult

Dysentery: a condition of the colon where blood is passed in the feces

Dyspepsia: disturbance to digestion

Dysphagia: difficulty in swallowing

Dysplasia: abnormal development of some part of the body

Dyspnoea: difficulty in breathing

Dystocia (or Dystokia): difficulty in giving birth

Dystrophy: inherited degeneration

Ear mange: ear irritation caused by a species of mite

Eclampsia: a disease occurring during late pregnancy or after whelping which causes muscle tremors, loss of consciousness, fits and can lead to sudden death. It is due to a deficiency of calcium

Ectasia: dilatation, distension

Ectropion: turning out of the eyelid

Eczema: a type of inflammatory disease of the skin which causes irritation and itching

Edema: the localized accumulation of fluid

Effusion: a collection of fluid in a space where it does not belong

Elbow dysplasia: faulty development of the elbow

Electro-cardiogram (ECG): a record of the different electrical phases of a heartbeat

Electro-encephalogram (EEG): recording of the electrical activity of the brain

Electrolyte: essential minerals present in body fluids

Elizabethan collar: a collar made of cardboard or plastic fitted over the dog's head, which prevents the animal interfering with wounds, dressings, etc.

Embolism: the plugging of a small blood vessel by a piece of material from another part of the blood stream. It can lead to a heart attack if the plugging occurs in the heart, or a stroke if it occurs in the brain

Embryo: an undeveloped fetus, i.e., the future individual soon after fertilization

Emesis: vomiting

Emetic: a substance which causes vomiting

Emollient: a substance which softens and soothes the skin

Emphysema: the abnormal presence of air in some part of the body. It usually refers to abnormally large air spaces being found in the lungs

Endocarditis: inflammation of the inner lining of the heart

Endocrine glands: glands which secrete hormones

Endothelium: the membrane lining certain vessels and cavities of the body

Endotracheal anesthesia: the anesthetic gas is passed down a rubber tube directly into the windpipe

Enema: introduction of fluid into the rectum usually to evacuate the bowels or loosen a constipated mass of faeces

Enteritis: inflammation of the intestines

Entire: not castrated or spayed

Entropion: a turning inward of the eyelid

Entropion medial: entropion at the corner of the eye

Enucleation: removal of the eyeball

Enzymes: substances formed within living cells which speed up biochemical reactions

Eosinophil: a type of white blood cell

Eosinophilia: the presence of abnormally large numbers of eosinophils in the blood

Epi-: a prefix meaning outside of

Epidermis: outer layer of skin

Epididymis: a structure associated with the testicle in which sperms mature

Epididymitis: inflammation of the epididymis

Epidural anesthesia: a local anesthetic is introduced into the spinal canal

Epiglottis: a structure in the throat which prevents material from passing into the larynx

Epilation: removal of hair

Epilepsy: a chronic nervous condition which leads to sudden fits

Epiphora: overflow of tears, a watery eye

Epiphysis: the end of a long bone

Epithelium: the layer or layers of cells of which skin and mucous membranes are composed

Epsom salts: used as a purgative

Epulis: a tumor-like growth on the gums

ERG: electroretinogram, records retinal function

Erosion: an eating or gnawing away, ulceration

Erythema: redness

Erythrocyte: a red blood cell

Esophageal achalasia: a malfunction of the gullet seen in Wire-haired Terriers

Esophagus: it is the tube which conveys food and drink down into the stomach; the gullet

Estrogens: female sex hormones

Estrus: season or heat in the bitch

Etiology: the study of causes of a disease

Euthanasia: humane killing

Everted third eyelid: turned out third eyelid

Excretion: disposal of waste materials

Expectorant: a substance used to clear phlegm

External parasites: organisms such as lice, ticks and mites which cause damage outside the body

Extremities: of the limbs

Exudate: a fluid, usually produced by disease, which escapes from the site of production

Eye shine: reflection from the eye seen at night

Eyelashes, extra: an additional row of eyelashes

Feces: solid excreta from the anus

Fallopian tubes: fine tubes which carry the egg from the ovary to the uterus

False pregnancy: a condition where all the signs of pregnancy are visible but the bitch is not in fact pregnant

Far-sighted (hyperopia): blurred close vision

Fascia: sheets or bands of fibrous tissue which surround muscles

Febrile: raised body temperature, fever

Femur: the thigh bone

Fetus: a fully developed individual within the uterus, i.e., one where all of the organs, limbs, etc., are similar in appearance to those of an adult

Fever: increased body temperature

Fibrin: a meshwork of fibers formed from blood which stops bleeding

Fibrosis: the formation of fibrous (scar) tissue

Fibrous tissue: one of the most abundant tissues of the body. It is composed of collagen (which when boiled gives gelatin), elastic fibers and fibroblasts surrounded by tissue fluid

Field of vision: the area which can be seen without moving the eyes
Filtration angle: See Iridocorneal angle
Fissure: a splitting or discontinuity of a surface, especially one that persists
Fistula: an abnormal passage often leading into an internal hollow organ
Fit: a seizure
Flank: the side of the body between the last rib and the hip
Flatulence/Flatus: passing wind
Flexor: a muscle that bends or flexes a limb or part of it
Foetus: a fully developed individual within the uterus, i.e., one where all of the organs, limbs, etc., are similar in appearance to those of an adult
Follicle: a tiny sac-like structure. Also refers to the structure which houses the hair
Follicular mange: another name for demodectic mange
Fracture: a break in a bone
Fundus: the back of the eyeball, includes retina
Fungal: caused by or relating to a fungus. Synonymous with the adjective fungous
Fungidical: an agent that kills fungi
Fungistatic: an agent that stops the growth of fungi
Fungus (pl. fungi): a primitive form of plant life
Floating rib: the last rib (which is not attached to the breastbone)

Gait: any of the co-ordinated leg actions of movement
Gall-bladder: a bag-like structure lying near the liver which stores bile
Gall-stones: hard masses formed in the gall-bladder
Gangrene: death of a part of the body accompanied by bacterial infection
Gastric: anything to do with the stomach
Gastritis: inflammation of the stomach
Gastro-enteritis: inflammation of the stomach and intestines
Gene: the unit of heredity found on a specific position on the chromosome
Genital organs: external reproductive organs
Genotype: the hereditary assortment of genes of an individual
Gestation: period of pregnancy
Gingival hyperplasia: overgrowth of the gums, epulis
Gingivitis: inflammation of the gums
Gland of the third eyelid: a gland surrounding the base of the third eyelid cartilage (formerly called Harder's or Harderian gland in the dog)
Glands: groups of cells which secrete substances which act on other organs
Glaucoma: increased pressure in the eye which harms vision
Globe: eyeball
Globoid cell leukodystrophy (also called Krabbe's disease): an inherited storage disease causing abnormal movements and vision loss
Glycogen storage disease: an inherited disease of the brain seen in toy breeds
Glycosuria: the presence of glucose in the urine
GM$_2$ gangliosidosis: storage disease due to enzyme deficiency
Goitre: enlargement of the thyroid gland due to iodine deficiency
Gonad: the ovary or testis
Goniolens: a lens placed on the cornea for gonioscopy
Gonioscopy: examination of the angle inside of the eyeball for the disease which causes glaucoma
Granuloma: a granular tumor
Growth: any formation of abnormal or new tissue

Haematemesis: the vomiting of blood
Haematocrit value: the percentage of whole blood which is composed of red blood cells
Haematology: the study of blood and blood producing tissues
Haematoma: an area of swelling that is filled with blood
Haematuria: blood in the urine

Haemoglobin: an iron-containing molecule found in red blood cells which transports oxygen

Haemolysis: the rupture of red blood cells

Haemoptysis: coughing up blood

Haemorrhage: bleeding

Haploid: half the number of chromosomes found in ordinary cells. The sperm and ova are 'haploid'

Hare lip: a malformation in the upper lip where the two halves do not fuse

Haws: protrusion of the third eyelids

Heart block: disturbance of electrical conductivity through the heart

Heat: popular term for a bitch in oestrus or in season

Heat-stroke: a condition caused by excess heat

Helminths: a class of parasitic worms

Hematemesis: the vomiting of blood

Hematocrit value: the percentage of whole blood which is composed of red blood cells

Hematology: the study of blood and blood producing tissues

Hematoma: an area of swelling that is filled with blood

Hematuria: blood in the urine

Hemeralopia: day blindness; defective vision in bright light

Hemiplegia: paralysis on one side of the body only

Hemoglobin: an iron-containing molecule found in red blood cells which transports oxygen

Hemolysis: the rupture of red blood cells

Hemoptysis: coughing up blood

Hemorrhage: bleeding

Hepatitis: inflammation of the liver

Hereditary: a condition passed on from generation to generation (not always evident at birth)

Heritable: a condition that can be inherited

Hernia: the pushing out through the abdominal walls or natural opening of any of the abdominal organs

Heterochromia: the eyes having a different color

Heterozygous: an individual with different alleles for a different character

Hexachlorophene: a powerful antiseptic

Hip dysplasia: an inherited condition affecting the hip joint

Histamine: a substance released by damaged tissues which causes part of the inflammatory response

Histology: the study of the microscopic structure of tissues

Homozygous: genetic term meaning possessing an identical pair of alleles for a character

Hordeolum: stye or inflammation of the sebaceous glands of the lids

Hormone: a substance produced in a particular region, which is carried by the blood and exerts its influence on another tissue away from the site of production

Horner's syndrome: damage to the sympathetic pathway which supplies sympathetic nerves to the eye. It is characterized by one sunken eye, prominent third eyelid, small pupil, drooping upper lid

Hot spot: an inflamed raw patch of skin that appears during hot weather

Humerus: the long bone found between the shoulder joint and elbow joint

Humor: any fluid of the body

Hybrid: a cross between two different breeds

Hydrocephalus: a condition where large amounts of fluid collect within the brain cavity

Hydronephrosis: blockage of the ureter leads to accumulation of urine within the kidney which causes it to expand and damages the kidney

Hygroma: a swelling occurring within a joint

Hyoid apparatus: the series of bones which support the tongue and larynx

Hyper-: a prefix meaning too much

Hyperemia: an excess amount of blood, still contained within blood vessels, in a part of the body

Hyperglycemia: an excess of glucose in the blood

Hyperopia (hypermetropia): farsightedness

Hyperplasia: an increase in the size of an organ or part due to an increase in the number of cells

Hypersensitivity: allergy. The body reacts to a foreign agent more strongly than normal

Hypertension: high blood pressure

Hyperthermia: increased body temperature

Hypertrophy: an increase in size of an organ or part due to an increase in the size of its cells

Hypervitaminosis: an excess of a particular vitamin

Hyphema: hemorrhage into the front chamber of the eye

Hypnotic: a drug which produces drowsiness

Hypo-: a prefix indicating too little

Hypocalcemia: a deficiency of calcium in the blood

Hypoglycemia: a deficiency of glucose in the blood

Hypomagnesemia: a deficiency of magnesium in the blood

Hypoplasia: malformation due to insufficient development

Hypopyon (Hi-*po*-pe-on): pus in the front chamber of the eye. The pus is usually sterile

Hypotension: low blood pressure

Hypothalamus: the part of the brain which regulates body temperature

Hypotony (Hi-*pot*-o-ny): a soft eye, reduced pressure in the eye

Hypoxia: decreased oxygen carriage in the blood

Hysterectomy: surgery involving removal of the uterus. (The ovaries are usually removed at the same time)

Ichthyosis: dry scaly skin

Idiopathic: a disease with unknown cause

Ileum: the last part of the small intestine

Ileus: distended intestine

Ilium: one of the pelvic bones

Immune response: the body's reaction to infection

Immunization: the production of artificial resistance to an infection

Immunosuppressant: a substance which blocks the body's defence mechanism

Impaction: a condition where two things are firmly lodged together, e.g., feces

Impetigo: a skin disorder, characterized by blocked skin pores

Implantation: the burrowing of the fertilized egg into the wall of the uterus

Inbreeding: the mating of closely related animals

Incisors: the cutting teeth at the front of each jaw

Incompetence, cardiac: the inability of the heart valves to function properly due to disease

Incontinence: the inability to control urination or defecation

Incubation period: the time between exposure to a disease-causing agent and the development of symptoms

Infarction: changes which occur in a tissue after its blood supply has been cut off

Infection: exposure to potentially disease-causing organisms

Infectious: a disease caused by micro-organisms which may or may not be contagious

Infertility: the inability to breed successfully

Inflammation: the series of changes which occur within a tissue after injury, providing that the injury has not caused death of the tissue. Inflammation is characterized by pain, swelling, redness, heat and loss of function

Inguinal hernia: a hernia usually made up of fat or intestines through the inguinal canal (between hind leg and the body wall)

Inguinal region: on either side of the groin

Inherited: due to genetic influences (not always evident at birth)

Injection:
  1. use of a hypodermic needle to give drugs
  2. congestion, e.g., injected blood vessel

Insulin: a hormone produced by the pancreas which causes a decrease in blood sugar levels. It is administered artificially to control diabetes mellitus

Interbreeding: the mating of the dogs of different varieties

Intercostal: between the ribs

Internal hemorrhage: bleeding into one of the body cavities

Internal parasites: worms

Intestine: a long hollow tube through which food passes and where most usable compounds are absorbed

Intervertebral disc: cartilage pads between the vertebrae

Intra-: a prefix meaning within

Intubation: the placement of a tube into the windpipe by way of the mouth, usually part of anesthetic procedure

Intussusception: a form of bowel obstruction in which part of the intestine folds in on itself; a telescoping of the bowels

In whelp: pregnant

Iridocorneal angle: the angle between the iris and cornea (deformed in some breeds causing glaucoma)

Iridocyclitis: inflammation of the iris and ciliary body

Iris: the colored circular membrane, the inner border of which forms the pupil behind the cornea and in front of the lens

Iris atrophy: a thin iris, loss of iris tissue

Iritis: inflammation of the iris

Irradiation: exposure to radiation, usually using X-rays

Irrigation: the washing out of wounds or body cavities with large amounts of warm water containing some antiseptic

Ischium: one of the pelvic bones

Ischemia: lack of adequate blood flow to a region or organ

-itis: a suffix meaning inflammation of that particular part

Jaundice: yellow coloration of the visible mucous membranes due to liver diseases, or due to blood conditions in the newborn

Jaws: the bones which carry the teeth

Jejunum: the central region of the small intestine

Jugular veins: the large veins running on either side of the neck

Juvenile amaurotic idiocy: storage disease due to enzyme deficiency causing blindness and death

Kaolin: a powder used to absorb toxins from the alimentary canal

Keratoconjunctivitis, proliferative: inflamed cornea and conjunctiva which grow in size from inflammation

Keratoconjunctivitis sicca (kcs): dry eye

Ketone bodies: abnormal intermediates in the breakdown of fatty acids, found during diabetes, starvation and other conditions

Ketosis: the presence of ketonbodies in body fluids and tissue

Knee: the lay name for joints in the foreleg of dogs between the elbow and paw which correspond to the wrists of humans

Laceration: cut

Lacrimal: relating to tears and the glands which secrete them

Lacrimal puncta: tear duct openings inside the upper and lower lids near the nose

Lacrimal sac: the dilated area at the start of the tear duct below the corner of the eye near the nose

Lacrimation: production of tears

Lactation: production of milk

Lactose: the main sugar found in milk

Lameness: abnormal movement of limbs

Laminectomy: a surgical procedure whereby the top or part of the backbone is removed to relieve pressure from the spinal cord

Lanolin: a grease used as the base for many skin preparations

Laparotomy: surgical opening of the abdomen

Larynx: the "voice box." It also prevents food from going down into the lungs

Lavage: washing out of the stomach or intestines

Laxative: a drug which promotes bowel evacuation

Lens: the structure in the eye which focuses light

Lens suture: a potential cleft inside the lens

Lesion: all changes to tissues produced by disease or injury; any abnormality

Leucocytes: white blood cells. These are involved in defence against invasion by micro-organisms

Leucopenia: a condition in which there are less than normal numbers of white blood cells

Leukemia: a condition where large numbers of abnormal white cells are released into the blood stream, a malignant disease

"Lick granuloma": a condition which arises due to the excessive licking of a wound, preventing healing. Large masses of scar tissue may form

Ligaments: strong bands of tissue which bind certain bones together

Limbus: a border in the eye, the edge of the cornea

Line breeding: the mating of dogs within a family to a common ancestor

Lipid: fatty material

Lipoma: a benign tumor of fat tissue

Lipoprotein: a complex molecule consisting of a lipid associated with a protein

Liver: a large organ lying in the abdomen whose functions are to aid in digestion of food, to break down harmful substances in the blood stream and to break down worn red blood cells

Local anesthetic: a substance which insensitizes one portion of the body leaving the rest of the animal fully conscious

Long-sighted: far-sighted

Lubricant: an oily substance used to reduce friction between opposing surfaces

Lumbar: the region of the back between the ribs and the pelvis

Lumen: the "hole" in a tubular organ

Lungs: the organs involved in oxygen and carbon dioxide exchange between the body and the atmosphere

Luxation: dislocation

Lymph: the excess fluid removed from body tissues

Lymph nodes, glands: structures distributed along lymphatic vessels which filter lymph

Lymphatics: the vessels which carry lymph

Lymphocyte: a type of white blood cell involved in defending the body from infection

Macule: a colored skin spot

Mastication: chewing

Mediastinum: the space in the chest between the two lungs. It contains the heart, major blood vessels, trachea, esophagus, nerves and other structures

-megaly: a suffix meaning an abnormal enlargement

Meibomian gland: a modified sebaceous gland of the upper or lower eyelid edge

Melanin: a dark pigment produced by cells called melanocytes which give rise to the color of skin, hair, eyes, etc.

Melanoma: a tumor of melanocytes

Membrana nictitans: third eyelid

Meninges: the protective membranes that surround the brain

Meningitis: inflammation of the meninges

Meniscus: a crescent-shaped piece of cartilage found in some joints which helps form a smooth surface for free joint

Merle: a color term. The coat color is diluted; usually blue grey with touches of black

Mesentery: the sheets of tissue which support the intestines

Metabolism: all the physical and chemical processes which occur in order to maintain the living body

Metacarpal: the bones between the wrist and the digits of the forelimb

Metaplasia: the abnormal change of one tissue type into another

Metastasis: the spread of a tumor to an area away from the original site of that tumor

Metatarsal: the bones between the hock and the digits in the hind limb

Micro-organism: a lower form of life so small it can only be seen under a microscope

Microphthalmia: small eye

Micturition: the act of passing urine

Milk teeth: the temporary teeth of young animals

Minerals: chemical elements of which small amounts are present in food

Miosis: excessive contraction of the pupil

Miotic: drug which makes pupil small, used to treat glaucoma

Mitosis: the process of cell reproduction

Mitral valve defect: defect in valves in the heart called mitral valves

Moniliasis: infection with monilia, a yeast

Monorchid: a male animal which has only one descended testicle

Morphine: a painkiller

Muco-purulent: consisting of pus and mucus

Mucous membrane: the tissue lining hollow organs and also covering the inside of the mouth

Mucus: the slimy secretion produced by mucous membranes

Murmur: a heart sound caused by abnormal flow of blood through the heart

Muscular dystrophy: a disease causing muscle weakness and wasting

Mutation: a permanent change in the characteristics of an animal caused by a change to the genetic information

Muzzle: the part of the head in front of the eyes

Mydriatic: a drug that dilates the pupil, e.g., atropine

Myelin: the insulation surrounding many nerves

Myocardial infarction: death of a portion of heart muscle, i.e., heart attack

Myocardium: heart muscle

Myopia: near-sighted, i.e., can only see clearly things which are close

Narcotics: drugs which induce a sleep-like state

Nasal solar dermatitis: skin of the nose is inflamed and made worse by the sun

Nasopharynx: the upper part of the throat which lies behind the nasal cavity

Nausea: the desire to vomit

Near-sighted: can only see things clearly which are close

Necrosis: death of cells or tissue while it is still within the living body

Neonatal: the period just after birth

Neoplasia: the formation of new tissue, the growth of which is not coordinated with the rest of the tissues of the body. This term is synonymous with tumor

Neoplasm: a new abnormal growth

Nephritis: inflammation of the kidney

Nerve block: a local anaesthetic applied near a nerve to block conduction along that nerve

Nervous system: the communication system of the body

Neuritis: inflammation in a nerve

Neuronal abiotrophy: hereditary nerve disease of the legs seen in the Swedish Lapland

Neuronal (canine) ceroidlipofuscinosis (CCL): storage disease due to enzyme deficiency causing blindness and death

Neutrophil: a common white blood cell which can move into tissues and eat foreign or damaged tissue or cells

Nictitans gland: gland of the third eyelid (in the dog this gland was formerly called the Harderian gland)

Nictitating membrane: the third eyelid which the animal may pull across its eye

Nodule: a small, firm swelling

Nyctalopia: night blindness

Nystagmus: a condition in which the eyeballs show constant fine jerky involuntary movements

Obese: overweight

Obstetrics: the branch of medicine dealing with pregnancy, labor, delivery and care of the newborn

Obstruction: blockage

Occiput: the part of the head which meets the neck

Ocular: pertaining to the eye

Oculist: eye doctor

Oedema: see Edema

Oesophageal achalasia: a malfunction of the gullet seen in Wire-haired Terriers

Oesophagus: it is the tube which conveys food and drink down into the stomach; the gullet

Oestrogens: female sex hormones

Oestrus: season or heat in the bitch

Olfactory nerve: the nerve concerned with smell

Oliguria: a decrease in the amount of urine produced

Oncology: the study of tumors

Opacity: cloudy area

Ophthalmia: severe inflammation of the whole eye

Ophthalmia neonatorum: purulent conjunctivitis in the newborn

Ophthalmic: pertaining to the eye

Ophthalmologist: eye specialist

Ophthalmology: study of the eye

Ophthalmoscopy: examination of the interior of the eye with an ophthalmoscope

Optic disc: the part of the optic nerve which can be seen in the eyeball

Optic nerve: the nerve which sends signals from the eye to the brain

Oral: pertaining to the mouth

Orbit: the bony socket which contains the eye

Orchitis: inflammation of the testicle

Organ: any discrete part of the body which has a specialized function

Organism: anything that can survive on its own

Orifice: an opening

Orthopedics: the branch of medicine dealing with bones and joints

Ossification: formation of bone tissue. This occurs normally in bone formation but may occur abnormally in other organs

Osteitis: inflammation of bone

Osteo: pertaining to bone

Osteochondritis: inflammation of bone and cartilage

Osteochondritis dissecans: inflammation of bone and cartilage resulting in the splitting of pieces of cartilage into the joint

Osteochondrosis: disease of bony growth centres seen in the spine of Foxhounds

Osteogenic sarcoma: bone cancer

Osteomyelitis: inflammation of bone and its marrow

Osteoporosis: brittle bones

Otitis externa: inflammation of the part of the ear outside the eardrum

Otitis media: middle ear infection

Outcrossing: the mating of unrelated individuals of the same breed

Ovaries: the organs in the female which produce the eggs

Ovariohysterectomy: surgical removal of the uterus and ovaries. This is also called spaying

Overshot jaw: lower jaw protrudes abnormally

Ovulation: release of eggs from the ovary

Ovum: an egg

Oxytocin: a hormone causing the uterus to contract during birth. It also stimulates milk letdown

Pad: sole of the foot

Palate: the structure which forms the roof of the mouth

Palpebral fissure: eyelid opening

Palsy: a nervous dysfunction

Pan-: a prefix meaning all or completely

Pancreas: an organ within the abdomen which produces substances which aid in digestion

Pancreatitis: inflammation of the pancreas

Pannus: newly inflamed tissue rich in blood vessels found on the cornea, also called CSK

Pannus, degenerative: inflamed cornea, third eyelid occurring in German Shepherds and their crosses

Papilloma: a wart

Paracentesis: the removal of fluid from the chest or abdomen

Paraffin: a lubricant often used to aid in defecation

Paralysis: the loss or impairment of the function of a part

Paraplegia: paralysis of the hind limbs

Parasite: an organism living totally off another

Parasympathetic nervous system: the portion of the nervous system which controls the minute-to-minute functioning of the body

Parathyroid glands: four small glands which secrete hormones involved in bone metabolism

Parenteral: the administration of a substance by a route other than the digestive tract, e.g., injection

Paresis: slight or incomplete paralysis

Parotid gland: one of the saliva-producing glands

Paroxysm: a violent attack

Parturition: birth

Patella: kneecap

Patella luxation: slipping kneecap

Patent ductus arteriosus: a small blood vessel in the chest between pulmonary artery and aorta which should close over at birth but remains open

Pathogen: an organism capable of causing disease

Pathology: the study of disease

Pelvis: the large bony structure supporting the hind limbs

Penetrance: the frequency with which an inherited trait is shown in animals carrying the gene which causes it

Penicillin: a commonly used antibiotic

Pepsin: a stomach enzyme which breaks down proteins

Perforation: a hole punched through a tubular organ

Pericarditis: inflammation of the covering membrane of the heart

Perineum: the region between the genetalia and the anus

Peripheral: away from the center

Peripheral nervous system: the part of the nervous system outside the brain and spinal cord

Peristalsis: the characteristic movement that takes place in muscular tubular organs. It causes the contents of the tube to be propelled in one direction

Peritoneum: the membrane lining the abdominal cavity

Peritonitis: inflammation of the peritoneum

Persistent hyperplastic primary vitreous (PHPV): tissue persists in the eyeball causing cloudy vitreous

Persistent pupillary membrane (PPM): strands which persist in the front of the eye which may cause opacity of the cornea or lens

Persistent right aortic arch: congenital defect in which the aorta in the chest is displaced forming a ring that can compress the windpipe and gullet

Pessary: a medication placed in the vagina

Pethidine: a strong pain killer

Pharmacology: the study of action of drugs

Pharynx: irregular funnel-shaped passage at the back of the mouth

Phenotype: the outward visible expression of the hereditary make-up

Phlebitis: inflammation of a vein

Photophobia: abnormal sensitivity to and discomfort from light

Photopic: pertaining to vision in the light, an eye which has become light adapted

Photoreceptor: a nerve end organ sensitive to light—rod or cone

PHPV: see Persistent hyperplastic primary vitreous

Pigmentary keratitis: deposition of brown pigment into the cornea

Pinkeye: conjunctivitis

Pinna: the major part of the external ear

Pituitary gland: a small gland found at the base of the brain which produces various hormones

Placenta: the organ which allows exchange of food, oxygen and wastes between mother and fetus

Plasma: the fluid portion of blood

Platelets: small structures found in the blood which help arrest bleeding

Pleura: the thin membrane which covers the lungs

Pleurisy: inflammation of the pleura

Pneumonia: inflammation of the lung

Pneumothorax: a collection of air in the pleural cavity. It occurs after a puncture wound to the chest

Polydipsia: excessive thirst

Polygenic: influenced by more than one gene

Polymorph: type of white blood cell

Polyuria: excessive urination

Popliteal: back of the knee

Post-: a prefix meaning after or behind

PPM: persistent pupillary membrane

Pre-: prefix meaning before

Prenatal: before birth

Prepuce: the sheath of the penis

Primary glaucoma: increased pressure in the eye due to an inherited deformed drainage angle

Progesterone: the hormone involved with the maintenance of pregnancy

Prognosis: a forecast of the probable outcome of an attack of disease

Progressive retinal atrophy (PRA): an inherited disease of the retina causing blindness

Prolapse: the slipping down of an organ or structure

Proliferative keratoconjunctivitis: inflamed growths on the cornea and conjunctiva tissue

Prophylaxis: measures undertaken to prevent disease

Prosthesis: artificial replacement of a body part

Proximal: closer to a given point

Pruritis: intense and persistent itching

Psoriasis: a type of skin disorder

Puberty: maturation of sexual function

Pulmonary: pertaining to the lungs

Pulmonic stenosis: narrowing of the opening between the heart and the artery to the lungs

Pulse: the result of the heart rapidly forcing blood into the major arteries

Pupil: the round hole in the center of the iris which corresponds to the lens aperture in the camera

Purgative: a substance which causes emptying of the gastro-intestinal tract. It may cause vomiting or have a laxative effect

Pus: a thick yellowish fluid resulting from certain types of inflammation. It contains dead and dying white blood cells plus dead and dying tissue and tissue fluid

Pyelonephritis: inflammation of the kidney and first portion of the urinary collecting system

Pyloric stenosis: narrowing of the opening between the stomach and duodenum

Pyogenic: producing pus or purulence

Quadriplegia: paralysis to all four limbs

Quiet eye: a non-inflamed eye

Radius: the inner of the two bones of the forearm. It is the weight-bearing bone of the forearm

Rales: moist sounds heard in the chest during various diseases

Ranula: a swelling under the tongue caused by collection of large amounts of saliva

Receptor: the end of a nerve which is sensitive to a particular stimulus

Recessive: a gene which is not expressed unless both members of a pair of chromosomes carry this gene

Rectum: the last few centimeters of the digestive tract

Red eye: inflamed eye

Reduction: refers to the realignment of the ends of a broken bone

Reflux: the backflow of stomach contents into the esophagus

Refraction:

  1. deviation in the course of rays of light passing from one transparent medium into another of different density

  2. determination of refractive errors of the eye and correction by glasses

Renal: relating to the kidney

Renal cortical hypoplasia: undeveloped part of the kidney called the cortex

Renal tubular dysfunction: faulty function of part of the kidneys called the tubules

Resection: the removal of part of an organ

Respiration: the processes associated with intake of oxygen into the blood stream and removal of carbon dioxide, i.e., breathing

Retina: the innermost coat of the back of the eye, formed of light-sensitive nerve elements

Retinal atrophy: thin retina

Retinal degeneration: a degeneration (thinning) of the retina, some are inherited

Retinal detachment: the separation of the retina from tissue behind it

Retinal dysplasia: abnormal development of retinal layers

Retro-: a prefix signifying behind

Rheumatism: a general term indicating pain and disability of muscles, joints, bones

Rhinitis: inflammation of the lining of the nose

Rickets: a disease of bone found in young animals due to a deficiency of calcium, phosphorus or Vitamin D

Rickettsia: a group of micro-organisms

Rigor mortis: temporary stiffening of the muscles several hours after death

Rigors: shivering fits

Ringworm: a contagious skin disease caused by a type of fungus

Rods: the part of the outer retina responsible for vision in dim light

-rrhaphy: a suffix meaning that an opening is being closed with sutures

Rupture: the bursting open of a body part

Sac: bag-like

Sacrum: the portion of the back just before the tail

Salicylic acid: an anti-bacterial and anti-fungal agent used on the skin

Saline: a salt solution used to replace body fluids

Saliva: fluid secreted in the mouth

Salmonella: a type of bacteria that can cause food poisoning

Sarcoma: a malignant tumor of tissues such as muscle, bone, cartilage

Sarcoptes: a genus of mite which causes mange in animals and man

Scapula: shoulder blade

Scar: fibrous tissue which has grown to repair injured tissue

Schirmer tear test: a method of measuring tear production

Scirrhus: the term applied to a hard growth

Sclera: the white part of the eyeball

Scleral ectasia: malformed eye tunic

Sclerosis: hardening

Scrotum: the pouch in which the testes are found

Seborrhea: a condition of the skin characterized by an accumulation of dry scurf, or excessive oily deposit on the skin

Sebum: the oil produced by skin glands

Secretion: a substance produced in a cell and then pushed out

-sectomy: a suffix meaning removal of

Sedative: a drug used to calm an animal

Semen: the fluid produced by the male which contains sperm

Semicircular canals: the portion of the ear responsible for balance

Sensitization: the process of developing immunity by giving a small amount of a substance; for example, an allergen, bacteria or virus

Sepsis: infection

Septicemia: carriage of bacteria or toxins through the blood stream, i.e., blood poisoning

Septum: a partition

Sequelae: effects which may follow a disease or injury

Sequestrum: a splinter of bone which has broken off bone. It dies and causes the formation of pus

Serous membrane: smooth glistening membranes lining certain organs

Serum: the fluid portion of blood with clotting factors removed

Shock: the condition of collapse following such things as injury or bleeding

Short-sightedness: the inability to focus on objects close to the eye

Sicca: dry eye

Side-effects: effects of a drug other than those desired

Sinus: a narrow, hollow cavity

Slipped stifle: dislocation of the kneecap

Slit lamp: provides a narrow beam of light used to aid in examination of the eye

Slough: the separation of a dead part from the healthy tissue

Smooth muscle: muscle not under voluntary control

Solar: pertaining to the sun

Spasm: involuntary muscle contraction

Spaying: the removal of the ovaries (and usually the uterus) of the female

Sphincter: a ring of muscle surrounding the opening of an organ

Sphygmomanometer: a device which measures blood pressure

Spinal cord: the collection of nerves running within the backbone

Spleen: an organ found on the left side of the abdomen which functions partly as a blood filter

Spondylitis: inflammation of the vertebrae

Sprains: the tearing of a ligament usually caused by the wrenching of a joint

Squamous cell carcinoma: a form of skin or eye cancer

Squint:
1. screwed up eyes—lids half closed
2. deviated eyeball

Staphylococcus: a type of bacteria

Staring coat: a dry, non-shiny coat

Steatorrhea: fat in the feces

Stenosis: unnatural narrowing of a body passage or opening, usually used in connection with blood vessels

Sternum: breastbone

Steroids: drugs closely related to certain chemicals produced by the body, such as the sex hormones, or some of the hormones produced by the adrenal glands

Stomach tube: a rubber tube inserted down the esophagus and into the stomach

Stomatitis: inflammation of the mouth

Stool: solid material passed from the anus

Storage diseases: products accumulate in the body due to enzyme deficiency

Strabismus: turned eyeball

Streptococcus: a type of bacteria

Streptomycin: a type of antibiotic

Stricture: narrowing of a body passage such as the bowel

Stroke: sudden rupture or occlusion of a blood vessel in the brain

Stud: an animal used for breeding

Stye: infection of the glands of the eyelid edge

Subaortic stenosis: obstruction in the heart below the aortic valve

Subluxation: (e.g., of lens or a joint) incompletely removed from its correct position

Sulphonamides: a group of antibacterial drugs

Superinfection: an infection which occurs even though the animal is already receiving antibiotics

Suppository: a mass which contains drugs which is inserted in the rectum

Suppuration: the formation of pus

Suspension: a pharmaceutical preparation in which ingredients are dispersed as visible particles and which is consequently turbid

Sutures: stitches

Sympathetic nervous system: the part of the nervous system which prepares the body for a reaction to fright, flight or fear

Syndrome: a group of symptoms occurring together

Synergists: drugs whose action together is more than the sum of their individual actions

Synovial membranes: the lining membrane of joints

Synovitis: inflammation of the lining of the joint

Systole: the contraction phase of a heartbeat

Tachycardia: speeding up of the heart rate

Tachypnea: speeding up of breathing

Tapetum: a layer at the back of the eye which helps night vision

Tear spill: overflow of tears down the face

Tear stain: white or lightly pigmented animals show facial staining from tear overflow

Tears: watery secretion of the tear glands

Tearing: excessive tear production

Tendon: the attachment of muscle to bone

Teratogen: an agent which can cause fetus malformation

Testes: the male gonads which produce spermatozoa and male hormones

Tetany: localized spasmodic muscle contractions

Tetralogy of Fallot: a combination of four congenital heart defects, including a hole in the heart

Thorax: chest

Thrombocytes: platelets

Thrombosis: the formation of a blood clot within the heart or blood vessel of a living animal

Thrombus: a blood clot within a vessel

Thymus gland: a gland found in the chest which helps in immunity

Thyroid gland: a gland found in the neck which produces certain hormones which control metabolism

Tibia: one of the bones of the hind leg. It is equivalent to the human shin bone

Tincture: a diluted alcoholic solution of certain medications

Tissue: the substance of an organ, e.g., liver, skin, bone formed by cells

-tomy: a suffix indicating an operation by cutting

Tonometry, eye: measurement of pressure within the eye

Tonsillectomy: the removal of the tonsils

Topical: a drug applied to the outside of the body

Torsion: twisting, usually of the intestine

Toxemia: the presence of a toxin in the bloodstream

Toxin: a bacterial poison

Toxoid: a toxin made harmless by physical or chemical means (used in the treatment of some conditions)

Trachea: air passage from the throat to the lungs

Tract: a collection of nerves having the same origin, function and termination

Traction: pull

Trauma: a disorder which is the result of direct injury

Tremors: very fine, jerky muscle contractions

Trichiasis: a condition where the eyelashes turn inwards and rub on the eyeball

Trypsin: one of the digestive enzymes

Tumor: a solid swelling resulting from abnormal growth, or a hollow swelling containing fluid

Tympanic membrane: ear drum

Tympany: the expansion of a hollow organ with gas

Uberreiter's syndrome: red mass, e.g., on the cornea, CSK, pannus

Ulcer: a breach in a surface which tends not to heal

Ulcer, corneal: a break in continuity of the cornea. It is often slow to heal and may suddenly deepen to cause perforation of the eye

Ulna: the longer of the two bones of the forearm

Umbilical cord: the connection between fetus and placenta

Umbilical hernia: a hernia of fat and sometimes intestines in region of the navel, where the umbilical (birth) cord exited

Umbilicus: navel

Undershot jaw: upper jaw protrudes abnormally

Urea: the substance which mammals use to excrete nitrogen-containing wastes. The level of urea in the bloodstream is a useful measure of kidney function

Uremia: build-up of waste products in the blood due to kidney disease

Ureter: the tube from the bladder to the external surface of the body

Urinalysis: testing of the chemical and cellular elements of urine

Urination: the act of voiding urine

Urinary: purtaining to urine

Urine: the excretion produced by the kidneys

Urolithiasis: formation of kidney or bladder stones

Urticaria: a skin rash characterized by small raised red lumps

Uterus: womb

Uvea: the bloody coat within the outer wall of the eyeball. Includes the iris
Uveitis: inflammation within the eye of the iris, ciliary body, choroid

Vagina: the muscular canal extending from the uterus to the outside of the body
Vagus nerve: an important nerve which sends branches to the heart, lungs, liver, stomach and bowels
Vascular: pertaining to blood vessels
Vasoconstriction: a drug which decreases the diameter of blood vessels
Vasodilator: a drug which increases the diameter of blood vessels
Vasopressor: a drug which raises blood pressure
Vertebrae: the bones of the back
Viscera: the internal organs of the body
Voluntary muscles: muscles under conscious control
Vulva: female external genitals

Wall eye: lack of color in the iris so the eye appears wholly or partly bluish or greyish white
Wart: small, solid growth arising upon the skin or mucous membrane
Watch eye: an eye partly colored blue with the rest colored yellow or brown
Weal: raised white area of skin with a reddened edge
Weaning: the separation of young animals from the mother
Whelping: giving birth in the dog
Winking: quick closing and opening of the eyelids

X-rays: rays of electromagnetic energy used to display internal structures within the body

Y-Chromosome: the chromosome which causes the development of male characteristics

Zonules: the numerous fine tissue strands (ligaments) which hold the lens in place in the eye; inherited weakness occurs in some breeds
Zoonosis: a disease of animals which may be communicated to man—the common eye diseases are not communicated to man

Index